THE A TO Z OF

ADDICTIONS AND
ADDICTIVE BEHAVIORS

THE A TO Z OF

ADDICTIONS AND ADDICTIVE BEHAVIORS

Esther Gwinnell, M.D.
Christine Adamec

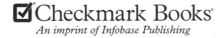
Checkmark Books®
An imprint of Infobase Publishing

The A to Z of Addictions and Addictive Behaviors

Checkmark Books
An imprint of Infobase Publishing
132 West 31st Street
New York NY 10001

Library of Congress Cataloging-in-Publication Data

Gwinnell, Esther.
The encyclopedia of addictions and addictive behaviors / Esther Gwinnell, Christine Adamec.
p. ; cm.
Includes bibliographical references and index.
ISBN 0-8160-5707-9 (hc: alk. paper)—ISBN 0-8160-6932-8 (pbk : alk. paper)
1. Substance abuse—Encyclopedias. 2. Drug abuse—Encyclopedias. 3. Compulsive behavior—Encyclopedias.
[DNLM: 1. Behavior, Addictive—Encyclopedias—English. 2. Substance-Related Disorders—Encyclopedias—English. WM 176 G994e 2006] I. Adamec, Christine A., 1949–   II. Title.
RC564.G95 2006
362.29′03—dc22   2004023866

Checkmark Books are available at special discounts when purchased in bulk quantities for businesses, associations, institutions, or sales promotions. Please call our Special Sales Department in New York at (212) 967-8800 or (800) 322-8755.

You can find Facts On File on the World Wide Web at http://www.factsonfile.com

Text design by Cathy Rincon

Graphs by Sholto Ainslie

Printed in the United States of America

VB Hermitage 10 9 8 7 6 5 4 3 2 1

This book is printed on acid-free paper.

Esther Gwinnell would like to dedicate this book to
her patients and to her students, who have always taught
as much as they learned—and more.

Christine Adamec would like to dedicate this book
to her husband, John Adamec,
for his continued patience and support throughout this project
as well as for his assistance with the creation
of some of the more graphically challenging charts.

CONTENTS

FOREWORD

Psychiatrists often treat both the causes and the consequences of addictive behaviors. As a psychiatrist, I have treated many people with serious addictive behaviors ranging from cocaine addiction to kleptomania. I have also treated patients who have come to me with a broad range of other psychiatric problems. In addition, some of my patients have had problems with both addictive behaviors and psychiatric problems. In fact, studies indicate that many people with addictive behaviors also suffer from underlying psychiatric problems that must be identified and treated.

Whether the psychiatric problem came before or after the addiction is not always clear. Did the alcoholic begin abusing alcohol because of an underlying depression? Did years of alcohol abuse instead cause the individual to develop a depressive disorder? Knowing the answer may be hard or impossible. What most psychiatrists do know is that *both* disorders need to be treated.

In such cases, treating the addiction alone (and ignoring the depression or other underlying psychiatric problem) might temporarily resolve one particular addiction, but the patient will often develop problems in another area. For example, a person who is obsessed with spending time on the Internet, while ignoring her children and her spouse, may eventually learn to stay away from the Internet. However, if the underlying problem that caused this addiction is not identified and dealt with, she may then develop another compulsive problem such as gambling or compulsive overeating. For this reason, both the addiction and any accompanying emotional disorders need to be addressed.

People generally come to psychiatrists complaining of depression, anxiety, obsession, or other disorders. What they may not realize, however, is that these often previously undiagnosed illnesses may be the underpinnings for addictive behaviors that are causing havoc in their lives. In many cases, they do not recognize or acknowledge that they have these problems. It can actually be liberating for these patients to discover that there were reasons for such behaviors and there are also ways to overcome them.

Of course, it is not easy for psychiatrists, other physicians, or anyone else to determine readily the cause of addictive behaviors in general or of one person's addiction in particular. People are complex. Emotions, experience, genetic factors, educational levels, intelligence levels—and a myriad of other factors—affect how people view situations and react to them. Thus, there are no overnight cures for addictions. It may take months or even years to recover from addictive behaviors and/or psychiatric illness.

It is also true that some people can recover from some addictions without therapy; for example, most people can quit smoking without seeing a mental health professional. Nicotine replacement therapy is available over-the-counter, and many primary care physicians prescribe bupropion (Zyban or Wellbutrin).

With other addictive behaviors, such as alcoholism or drug addiction, more aggressive help is often needed. Groups such as Alcoholics Anonymous or Narcotics Anonymous have been of enormous benefit for many people with these addictions.

In addition to treating people with addictions, psychiatrists often treat those who are affected by the behaviors of addicted individuals. People in the grips of an addiction may become extremely violent and even homicidal with their family members. Conversely, addicts may be completely neglectful of them. The physical pain of frequent beatings, as well as the emotional scarring of emotional (and sometimes actual) abandonment, can be extremely difficult for children or spouses to cope with. Children of addicted parents may themselves act out in similar addictive ways or in other destructive and addictive ways throughout their childhood and into adulthood. Only by breaking the addictive pattern can this damaging chain be broken.

As far as the addict is concerned, as long as the patient's body is still reasonably healthy, there is nearly always hope for dramatic physical and psychological recovery. For example, once drinking ends, if cirrhosis has not developed, the liver will recover. Once drug abuse ends, the body and the psyche can usually begin to heal. In some cases, the healing can be remarkable.

It is important to understand, however, that there are some cases in which there are no second chances. Those cases cannot usually be predicted. Sometimes the first use of a drug may result in death. We have seen this occur with abuse of inhalants or with hallucinogenic drugs such as Ecstasy. It is also true that sometimes harm comes from the indirect results of addictive behaviors. Driving while intoxicated with any substance can lead to car crashes that kill and maim people, destroying lives and entire families.

Although addictive behaviors can be devastating, those who suffer from them need not lose heart. Relief may be found with medications, therapy, or even sometimes with incarceration. Sometimes a person has to experience a painful lesson to realize that he or she has a serious problem, regardless of the specific addiction. Denial is common in individuals exhibiting all addictive behaviors.

Yet transformation is possible. The right insights can help people avoid making the same mistakes over and over. These insights can lead to learning new patterns and eventually to a better life—for addicts, for families, and in the end, for all of us.

I hope that this volume will enrich readers and provide them with the information and the knowledge that they seek.

—Esther Gwinnell, M.D.

INTRODUCTION

Millions of Americans are ruled by addictive behaviors. These behaviors sometimes destroy their lives as well as the lives of their families, their friends, and even complete strangers. The drunken driver did not really mean to crash into and kill the pregnant woman whose car was stopped at a red light. He was just in a rush to get to the liquor store before it closed because he felt like he needed some bourbon to calm his jangled nerves. The drug addict did not really mean to wipe out her parent's life savings with the payments for her bail and the legal and court fees that she has incurred so far. She has explained to herself, her family, and others that she has needed cocaine to get by sometimes. The father who gambled away all the money that he and his wife saved for their children to go to college was no monster who hated his family. In fact, he loved his children. It is just that he *knew* that his luck was going to change and that *this time*, he was going to win really big, because things were going to be different.

All of these individuals were exhibiting addictive behaviors. Addictive behaviors are repeated actions that form a negative pattern and that cause harm to the individual and often to their family members, friends, and society at large. The costs may come in terms of the health of the addicted person or family members as well as emotional, psychological, and financial costs.

Addicts may realize that they are addicted. More frequently they deny their addiction, insisting that they can "give up" the behavior anytime that they feel like it. (They often rationalize that they just never actually feel like giving it up.) For example,

according to *A National Drug Control Strategy*, a White House report released in 2004, about 6 million of the 7.7 million people in the United States who need drug treatment do not receive it because they do not believe that they have a problem.

Of course, denying that a problem exists does not make it vanish. Only by first acknowledging it and then by beginning to deal with it can a person begin to manage or cope with an addictive behavior if not eliminate it altogether.

Who Has Addictions

All sorts of people develop addictive behaviors. Some people think that it is primarily glamorous rock stars or television or movie personalities who become addicted to drugs, alcohol, and other substances. Sometimes people in the public eye do develop serious addictions. However, the average nonwealthy person may also become addicted to substances as well as to gambling, compulsive sexual behaviors, and other behaviors. The working-class addict may not be addicted to drinking expensive Cristal champagne, but low-cost red wine can feed the same type of underlying addiction.

Professionals, such as doctors, lawyers, airline pilots, and others who work in trusted professions, sometimes become addicted to illegal or prescribed drugs or to alcohol. Individuals in such professions sometimes feel that they are immune to becoming addicted because they are very intelligent and thus can "handle" the problem. However, their body chemistry is basically the same as everyone else's. If they repeatedly use addictive substances, they too may develop addictions. Fortunately, studies have shown that when treated, some professionals, such as physicians, have a high recovery rate.

Adolescents and even children may develop addictions to alcohol, and drugs, as well as other behaviors that can cause severe harm to the body and mind. In general, however, most addicted people are young adults in the 18–25 age range, and they are often male.

People of all races and ethnicities can develop addictions. In many cases, however, Native Americans, whites and Hispanics have the highest percentages of addictions to drugs and alcohol, while Asians have the lowest levels. African Americans have a greater risk of addictive behaviors than Asians.

People of all educational levels can develop addictions, although generally, the lower the education, the higher the risk of addiction. For example, a college graduate has a much lower risk of becoming a smoker (about 9 percent) than someone with a high school diploma (24 percent).

Myths About Addictions

There are many fears and myths about addictions and addicted people. Some of them have some underlying truth, while others have none. The following are three common myths about addiction.

Myth #1: Taking Narcotics Always Turns People Into Drug Addicts

Doctors sometimes prescribe narcotic painkillers for very ill patients with pain from cancer or for patients with severe pain stemming from chronic conditions, such as severe back pain. Yet many people, including some physicians, fear the use of narcotic analgesics because they are worried that opiates will transform patients into drug addicts. Physicians may also fear being prosecuted by overly zealous law enforcement officials for prescribing opiates. So they may hold back when patients need pain medication. These fears can thus lead to undertreatment of patients with chronic pain. In fact, a study of nursing home patients with cancer, reported in a 1998 issue of the *Journal of the American Medical Association*, revealed that elderly patients with cancer often received no pain med-

ication at all, especially if they were over age 85, female, and nonwhite.

In another study reported in a 2000 issue of the *New England Journal of Medicine*, researchers found that pharmacies in nonwhite neighborhoods of New York City refused to carry sufficient stocks of opioid pain medications. Only 25 percent of the pharmacies carried a sufficient stock of opioid pain medications, while 72 percent of the pharmacies in predominantly white neighborhoods carried sufficient stocks. Said the researchers, "These results suggest that nonwhite patients may be at even greater risk for the undertreatment of pain than previously reported."

What is the reality? Can patients who use narcotics for pain become addicted? Yes, they can, although most do not. Addiction to narcotics is most likely to occur if the patient has a prior history of drug addiction. However, various studies have indicated that most patients who take narcotics for pain do not become addicted to the drug. It simply relieves their pain.

As stated by H. Westley Clark, M.D., director of the Center for Substance Abuse Treatment, Substance Abuse and Mental Health Services Administration in his testimony before the Senate in 2002 on the narcotic drug OxyContin, "Most people who take OxyContin and other prescription opioids, as prescribed, do not become addicted. With prolonged use of opioids, however, pain patients often do become tolerant, that is, require larger doses, although this does typically reach a plateau, which can vary markedly between different patients and different pain conditions. Chronic pain patients can also become physically dependent on their medications. However, most patients who receive opioids for pain, even those undergoing long-term therapy, do not become addicted to these drugs."

He further stated, "In short, most individuals who take their prescribed OxyContin, or any other opioid such as hydrocodone or morphine, under medical treatment for pain, will not become addicted, although some may become physically dependent on the drug and may need to be carefully withdrawn after their pain problem is otherwise resolved. Patients who are taking these drugs as prescribed should continue to do so, as long as they and their physician agree that taking the drug is a medically appropriate way for them to manage pain."

Some patients apparently do become addicted to their narcotic painkillers, including some very high-profile people. In 2004, radio personality Rush Limbaugh publicly acknowledged that he had become addicted to drugs and was undergoing treatment for his addiction. According to Limbaugh, he took drugs for medical problems and subsequently developed an addiction. However, Limbaugh does not represent the average pain patient in the United States, and thus it should not be concluded that taking pain drugs inevitably leads to addiction.

Nonetheless, precautions do need to be taken with narcotics, and responsible doctors take those precautions. Doctors who treat patients with chronic pain take careful medical histories and perform complete medical examinations. They urge patients to contact them about changes or about increased or decreased pain. Many doctors ask patients to sign a treatment agreement, which is an agreement between the physician and the patient that the doctor will be in charge of pain medication for the patient. This will reduce the risk of doctor shopping, in which the patient goes from doctor to doctor, obtaining many different medications, risking an accidental overdose if he or she has an adverse reaction to mixing drugs.

Myth #2: Most Addicts Are Minority Members

Whether because of television shows, racial bias, or other reasons, some people believe that large numbers of addicts are nonwhite. In fact, white people either lead or come in second when it comes to many addictions, such as alcoholism, drug addiction, and smoking. Some racial groups, however, such as Native Americans and Hispanics, do have high rates of alcohol abuse. For example, according to the National Institute for Alcohol Abuse and Alcoholism, nearly 16 percent of Native Americans between the ages of 18–29 years were alcoholics in 2002, as were 15 percent of white males in this age group.

When considering binge drinking, according to the findings from *Results from the 2002 National Survey on Drug Use and Health: National Findings*, the largest percentage of binge drinkers was found among Native Americans/Alaska Natives (27.9 per-

cent), followed by Native Hawaiians and other Pacific Islanders (25.2 percent), Hispanics (24.8 percent), whites (23.4 percent), and African Americans (21.0 percent).

When considering drug abuse, whites are often heavy drug abusers. For example, in 2002, 2.8 percent of white high school seniors used a drug within the month before the survey compared with less than 1 percent (0.2 percent) of African-American seniors.

Myth #3: Most People Grow Out of Addictive Behaviors

Many people think it is acceptable for young people to sow some wild oats when they are still teenagers or young adults and that these young ones can become more serious and sober adults later on. They believe that if younger people smoke and abuse alcohol or some drugs, or if younger people engage in other activities that may be addictive, such as gambling, that these individuals have plenty of time to "grow up" and act in a more responsible manner at a later time. (The one exception to this attitude is if the addictive behaviors of younger people cause harm to others, in which case many people believe that punishments should be meted out.)

Yet studies have shown that behavior that occurs in early and midadolescence has long-reaching effects into adulthood. The most obvious example is with smoking. Most smokers began their habit when they were in their early teens. They continue smoking well into adulthood, often experiencing great difficulty in wresting themselves free from this addiction. In addition, problems with alcohol abuse and drug abuse that begin in adolescence do not usually go away in adulthood.

Elements of Addictions

An addiction—whether to illegal or prescription drugs, alcohol or gambling, or to a broad array of other behaviors—involves certain common features. These include a craving for the substance or behavior, centering the life around the behavior, and changing one's life in negative ways as a result of the behavior.

In some cases of addiction, the individual develops a physical tolerance so that greater amounts of the substance are needed to achieve the same effect. If the substance or behavior cannot be used or performed, the individual feels physical and psychological side effects. In the worst cases, these withdrawal effects are extreme, as with the delirium tremens of the alcoholic or the extreme nausea and vomiting of the drug addict withdrawing from drugs without medical assistance.

Craving and Subsequent Rush/Euphoria

Addicts experience a compulsive craving. They may also experience a pleasurable feeling when the addictive behavior is performed. Some people call this feeling a "rush" or "euphoria." If they do not actually feel pleasure when performing the addictive behavior any longer, they may instead avoid the pain that they would experience if the behavior were not performed. For example, withdrawal from alcohol or drugs can be extremely painful to the addicted person, both physically and psychologically. As a result, addicts are in a sort of push-pull situation. They are drawn (pulled) to perform the behavior and also feel pushed to perform it, because avoiding the behavior feels much harder than performing it.

Life Centered Around Addictive Behavior

When an individual is addicted, the addiction becomes the center of his or her world, whether the person is addicted to exercising 60 hours per week or addicted to heroin. For the addict, "normal life" can seem like an intrusion. Employers or family members may make demands that can interfere with the ability to obtain what is needed to perform the addictive behavior.

Problems that Result from Addictive Behavior

The addicted person often suffers from health and/or emotional problems. The addict may ignore his or her own bodily needs as well as those of children and other family members. Severe financial problems often result from an addiction; many addictive behaviors are exceedingly expensive.

Physical Tolerance and Withdrawal

After individuals become addicted to nicotine, alcohol, or drugs, their bodies have become accustomed to these substances. They need them to feel "normal." It may seem odd to many people to compare the need that the heroin addict has for an injection of heroin to the need the smoker has for a cigarette or the need the alcoholic has for a shot of whiskey. For an addict, though, the needs are similar. When the addicted person is unable to obtain the substance or tries to stay off the substance on his or her own, the body fights back.

For this reason, doctors offer medications to patients withdrawing from alcohol and drugs. Medications are also available for patients who decide to quit smoking, such as nicotine replacement therapy or bupropion (Zyban or Wellbutrin). Nicotine replacement therapy in its different forms (gum, skin patch, nasal spray, and so on) enables the user to taper off from the use of nicotine. Bupropion is an antidepressant that also works to decrease the individual's craving for nicotine. Some studies have demonstrated that the most effective smoking cessation technique has combined nicotine replacement therapy with bupropion.

If the patient has been dependent on alcohol or drugs for a long time or is elderly, pregnant, or has medical problems making outpatient treatment unfeasible, he or she should receive inpatient detoxification in a facility that is staffed by experienced and trained individuals. Withdrawal can be difficult, but most people can complete the process. For many individuals, however, the craving to perform the addicted behavior persists even after detoxification occurs. For this reason, membership in a self-help group, such as Alcoholics Anonymous or Sex Addicts Anonymous, may provide the support that individuals need to fight against the cravings.

Types of Addictive Behaviors

The most commonly noted addictions are to alcohol and to illegal drugs such as heroin or cocaine; however, there are many other addictions. For example, millions of people are addicted to prescription drugs, particularly to benzodiazepine medications (antianxiety medications) and to narcotic painkillers. Other people are so addicted to gambling that they would spend their last dollar to buy a scratch-off lottery ticket.

Others are sex addicts, engaging in risky and compulsive sexual behaviors. Some people are specifically addicted to Internet sex, spending thousands of dollars on their credit cards charged to businesses that are eager to supply whatever form of pornographic materials is requested.

Compulsive shopping is a problem for many people, who will overspend on their credit cards for items that they do not need. Compulsive shoppers may find themselves facing financial ruin.

Some people are addicted to food, which has caused them to become obese or even morbidly obese (weighing 100 pounds or more than normal for one's height). Some people engage in binge eating, often seeming to be in a trance as they eat. As with smoking, succumbing to a food addiction is a perfectly legal activity, yet it is also a highly destructive one. It can lead to the development of diabetes, heart disease, arthritis, stroke, and many other medical problems.

Smoking

Tens of millions of people in the United States and other countries are addicted to tobacco. The Surgeon General's office and other sources have estimated that smoking cigarettes kills an estimated 440,00 people per year from heart disease, lung cancer, and other health problems in the United States. Smoking is the number one preventable form of death in the United States. It is also an addictive behavior that many people begin in their youth or early adulthood.

In 2004, the Surgeon General's office released a new report on smoking and health that revealed that in addition to the already-known health effects of smoking cigarettes are additional risks. For example, the Surgeon General further expanded the list of cancers that were caused by cigarette smoking to include cervical cancer, kidney cancer, pancreatic cancer, and stomach cancer as well as acute myeloid leukemia.

In 2000, the Centers for Disease Control and Prevention (CDC) in its *Healthy People 2010* set goals for the year 2010. The smoking goal was to reduce smoking from 24 percent of the population in 1998 to 12 percent by 2010.

Alcohol Abuse and Alcoholism

Alcohol abuse and alcoholism are major problems in the United States and other countries. In the United States, the NIAAA reported that 4.7 percent of the population of the United States, or 9.7 million people, were alcohol abusers in 2002. In addition, it is important to note that the NIAAA also said an estimated 3.8 percent of the population was estimated to have a problem with alcoholism (also known as "alcohol dependence") or about 7.9 million people in the United States were alcoholics. (Some estimates are slightly lower, such as the *2002 National Survey on Drug Use and Health*, which set the estimated national level of alcoholism at 3.50 percent.)

Alcoholism causes numerous health problems, including cirrhosis of the liver, liver cancer, gastrointestinal diseases, alcoholic hepatitis, and other diseases. In 2000 in *Healthy People 2010*, the CDC set goals to reduce the deaths from cirrhosis of the liver from 9.5 per 100,000 people in 1998 to a goal of no more than 3.0 deaths per 100,000 people by 2010.

In addition, a further goal was to reduce alcohol-related deaths from 5.9 per 100,000 people to no more than 4 per 100,000 people. Of course, no deaths at all would be preferable, but that would be an unrealistic goal. Another goal was to reduce the rate of alcohol-related injuries from 113 per 100,000 to no more than 65 per 100,000.

Drug Abuse and Drug Addiction

Drug abuse and addiction is another serious problem for many people in the United States and the world. Although the use of some drugs, such as heroin, has decreased, other drugs, such as cocaine, continue to be abused by many people of all ages. According to the *2002 National Survey on Drug Use and Health*, there were about 166,000 heroin users in the United States in 2002. Most were male and older than age 18.

According to the *2002 National Survey on Drug Use and Health*, an estimated 2 million people in the United States were current cocaine users in 2002 and of these, 567,000 were crack cocaine users. Most cocaine users are male and older than age 18. However, significant numbers of youths use cocaine and become addicted to the drug.

According to *Healthy People 2010*, in 1998, 55 percent of the drug-related episodes in hospital emergency departments occurred to people between the ages of 16–34 years old. A total of

542,544 drug-related emergency department episodes occurred in 1998. The goal for 2010 is a reduction to 350,000 patients, which would be a 35 percent decrease.

Another major goal is to decrease the number of drug-induced deaths. In 1998, there were about 6.3 deaths for 100,000 people, according to the CDC. The goal for 2010, according to *Healthy People 2010,* is to decrease this drug-induced death rate dramatically to 1.0 per 100,000.

Gambling

People who become addicted to gambling may lose all their money in pathological gambling behavior. Such individuals usually are also engaged in other addictive behaviors such as smoking and heavy drinking. Organizations such as Gamblers Anonymous, modeled on Alcoholics Anonymous, strive to help them overcome their addictive behavior.

Other Addictive Behaviors

Some people cannot seem to stay off the Internet. Some mental health professionals say that such individuals have an addiction, although it is not one that is recognized by the American Psychiatric Association. Such individuals may be fascinated by computer games, or they may be mesmerized by pornographic images. Still others engage in illicit "affairs" online, sometimes destroying their own long-term marriages. The euphoria of the attention that they receive, whether it is from a game or another person, pulls them in and holds them, and they do not want to let go. The Internet can provide a seeming escape from the problems and the difficult life that many people face. However, when Internet use becomes an addictive behavior and controls the individual's life, this behavior creates more problems.

Not Everyone is Addicted

Some people might wonder to themselves if everyone could be regarded as addicted to something, whether their morning coffee, having sex at certain times, playing golf on Sundays, or other personal habits that people may often display. Most people are creatures of habit. Yet there is a difference between habitual behavior and addiction.

Consider this hypothetical example: Joe X owns several boats and looks forward all week long to his weekend boating excursions. All Joe X talks about is boats, boats, and more boats. Is Joe addicted to boating? If Joe simply likes boating a lot, that affinity alone does not signify an addiction. However, if Joe spends all his money on boats, has missed numerous mortgage payments, and is in danger of losing his home, his financial problem is one indicator of addiction. If Joe's daughter is in a car crash but Joe just cannot seem to get to the hospital right away because he has to go pick up that very special engine, Joe is putting boats far too high on his priority list. He is probably essentially addicted to boating, a hobby that is harmless or positive for most people.

Causes of Addictions

People develop addictive behaviors for many different reasons. Often knowing what the causes are in any individual is hard. However, researchers continue to study this issue, searching for answers.

Genetic Links

Many studies indicate a possible genetic link in addictions. Some adoption studies of children raised apart from their biological parents have shown that the biological children of alcoholics and drug addicts have an above-average risk of becoming addicts themselves. This does not mean that adopted children born to alcoholics or drug addicts are doomed to develop addictions. Instead, it means the risk for addictive behavior is increased. Some studies have shown that adopted children have a lower risk for alcoholism than among biological siblings reared by birthparents, indicating the importance of environment.

Parental Influences

Normal parents do not want their children to become alcoholics or drug addicts. Yet parents have a profound influence on their children. If parents are alcohol and/or drug abusers or addicts, their children are more likely to abuse or become addicted to alcohol or drugs as well.

Some studies have shown that alcohol and drug use in youths can be predicted based on parental alcohol and drug use. Such a study was performed by Dr. Joseph Biederman and colleagues and reported in a 2000 issue of *Pediatrics*. The researchers evaluated the subjects at the average age of 12 years and performed a follow-up four years later. The researchers found that 9 percent of the parents were alcoholics, as were 6 percent of the teenagers.

Peer Influences

Individuals are affected by the behaviors of their peers. Teenagers wish to dress and act like their friends. If all or most of their friends are drinking and smoking, then they will often wish to drink and smoke too. Adults are also affected by the behaviors of their peers. In many cases, they must stop interacting with their friends and sometimes even family members who share their addictions and who may actively undermine their recovery from addiction.

The Ramifications of Addictive Behaviors

As addiction becomes the center of an addict's world, the addict becomes increasingly disinterested in caring for and interacting with the people who care the most about the person.

Work may become impossible for the addict because of his or her overwhelming preoccupation with the addictive activity and/or because of the impact that the addiction (drunkenness, euphoria, depression, lack of sleep, or other psychological effects) has on the individual's work performance. Some addicted individuals may be able to maintain their jobs and fool their family, friends, and colleagues about the severity of their addiction. However, most are unable to maintain the illusion of normalcy for a significant length of time.

Violence and other criminal behavior often emanate from addictions, particularly from drinking and drug abuse. Study after study have shown that addicts are more likely than others are to commit violent crimes against their family members and others.

Law enforcement is another area affected by addictive behaviors. In the United States, billions of dollars are spent each year to identify, arrest, prosecute, and lock up people who violate drug and alcohol laws. In addition, sex addicts violate existing laws against public sex, indecent exposure, and other federal, state, and city laws and ordinances. There are also laws against illegal gambling. Identifying and prosecuting the offenders against these laws costs money. (Ironically, most states actively promote compulsive gambling by selling lottery tickets to supplement tax revenue to support law enforcement expenses.)

Psychiatric Issues and Addictions

Researchers and psychiatrists disagree as to the cause and effect relationship of psychiatric illness and addiction. It is not clear whether people who are depressed or anxious are more likely to engage in addictive behaviors or whether addictive behaviors themselves somehow trigger psychiatric problems. However, many psychiatric illnesses, such as major depressive disorder, anxiety disorders, and bipolar disorder, are associated with addictions. Clinical researchers have studied this issue for years, and they will continue to study it. The only conclusions that most researchers can agree on is that a link indeed exists between many addictive behaviors and psychiatric disorders and that people who exhibit addictive behaviors have a significantly higher rate of psychiatric problems than people who do not have addictions.

Youth and Addictions

Youths ages 12–17 or 18 years old are more likely than adults to exhibit risky behavior with addictive substances that can cause them to suffer from lifelong consequences. For example, most adult smokers started their habit when they were about 14 years old, primarily to impress others, to feel adult, or because of pressure from their peers. They became addicted to tobacco and later, when smoking no longer seemed glamorous or fun, found quitting to be very difficult.

When they are under the influence of alcohol or drugs, youths are more likely to commit crimes, assault others, and engage in risky sexual behavior. Binge drinking (having five or more drinks on at least one occasion during a two-week time period) is another common problem among youths. According to the May 9, 2003 *NHSDA Report* (National Household Survey on Drug Abuse), published by the Substance Abuse and Mental Health

Services Administration, nearly one in five individuals ages 12–20 years old has engaged in binge alcohol drinking. Adolescents and young adults also engage in risky behaviors that may be addictive, such as taking illegal drugs, smoking, gambling, and so forth.

Youths and Drinking

Many teenagers in the United States have had some experience with alcohol, based on such surveys as the annual "Monitoring the Future" survey. According to this data, most high school seniors (78.4 percent), 10th graders (66.9 percent), and nearly half of all eighth graders (47 percent) used alcohol as of 2002. Of even more concern for most parents, teachers, physicians, policy makers, and others is that some students abuse alcohol on a daily basis: 3.5 percent of 12th graders, 1.8 percent of 10th graders, and less than 1 percent (0.7 percent) of eighth graders drank alcohol every day in 2002.

Binge drinking is another serious problem for many adolescents in the United States (as well as other countries). Binge drinking is behavior that is associated with car crashes and other risky behavior, such as having sex without condoms or driving in cars with people who are intoxicated or without wearing seat belts. In 2002, 28.6 percent of high school seniors were binge drinkers, as were 22.4 percent of 10th graders and 12.4 percent of eighth graders.

Alcohol abuse or alcoholism that starts at an early age often sets a pattern. Studies have shown that people who start drinking as teenagers are more likely to develop a problem with alcohol, or even become alcoholics, than others.

Youths and Smoking

Smoking is linked to poor grades, many school absences, and even dropping out of high school. It also affects future adult life. A study in a 2004 issue of the *American Journal of Public Health* looked at the behavior of adolescents when they were high school seniors compared with when they were 35 years old. The study found that when 12th graders smoked, they were 12 times more likely to be smokers when they were age 35. If they were daily smokers as seniors in high school, they were 42 times more likely than high school nonsmokers to be smokers at the age of 35. Clearly, high school

behavior can and does affect the behavior of many adults.

Youths and Drug Use

Illegal drug use may begin in early adolescence as experimentation, especially with marijuana or with household products used illegally as inhalants. More than half (53 percent) of all high school seniors have used illicit drugs as of 2002. Nearly half (44.6 percent) of all 10th graders have used drugs. The most popular drug for most adolescents is marijuana, and nearly half of all 12th graders (47.8 percent) have used this drug. Inhalants are most popular among eighth graders. About 15 percent have used the drug as of 2002, compared with about 8 percent of 10th graders and about 12 percent of 12th graders.

Youths and Other Addictive Behaviors

Because of an excessive and unrealistic concern over appearance, some adolescents and young adults develop an unhealthy body image and become anorexic or bulimic. The anorexic person avoids eating, while the bulimic person will overeat in a binging fashion and then force himself or herself to vomit the food. Both behaviors are dangerous to the health.

People who are anorexic or bulimic may become attracted to drugs, such as diet drugs or stimulants, particularly if they believe the drugs will cause them to lose weight, bulk up their muscles (if they are males), or somehow enhance their appearance. They may become addicted to steroids, stimulants, or cocaine. Some people start smoking because they think it will help them lose weight. Once they start smoking, they fear quitting, thinking that if they do so, they will become obese.

College Students and Addictions

For many young adults, college is an opportunity to leave the nest and spread their wings. Unfortunately, for many students, it is also a time when they begin (or continue) a cycle of addictive behaviors. The most common addictive behavior among college students is alcohol abuse, including binge drinking. Many college students also smoke, using all forms of tobacco (with the exception of pipe tobacco, which is not popular among most college students today).

Many college students abuse drugs as well, and marijuana is the most commonly abused drug. Nearly half (49.5 percent) of all full-time college students have used marijuana, and about 4 percent use the drug every day.

Some students are compulsive gamblers. In a study reported in a 2004 issue of the *Journal of American College Health,* the researchers found that 4 percent of the females and 18 percent of the males had gambling behaviors that were problematic. The students who were reported as problem gamblers also had a greater risk for heavy drinking and regular tobacco and marijuana use.

Conflicts About Addictions

There are many different views about addictive behaviors. Sometimes these views clash, often depending on whether it is the view of the physician, the police officer, or the politician trying to get reelected. The patient suffering from chronic pain that is relieved by narcotic painkillers prescribed by a physician may also have a different view from the opiate addict who does not take the drug for pain relief and buys the drug illegally, but the rules and regulations that are created to control opiates may be determined by fears centered around addiction.

Addictions: Punishable Behaviors or Treatable?

When should a person who is addicted to drugs, alcohol, or another substance be considered a patient with an illness rather than a person whose bad behavior is out of control? This is a question that will probably continue to be debated for years to come and that cannot be resolved in this volume. However, it is a question worthy of consideration. Most people seem to accept that alcoholism is a disease and that alcoholics are people who need treatment. They acknowledge that the alcoholic may not be willing or able to see that he or she has a problem or to get treatment. They understand it is the disease that is blinding him or her, not a weak moral character.

With other addictions, however, the picture becomes less clear. For example, the sex addict or the drug addict may also need therapy, but many people may be less willing to view these addictions as diseases. Many people feel that individuals should know intuitively that they should not engage in promiscuous sexual behavior or that

they should not gamble and should simply decide to forgo these activities. However, these individuals are acting out compulsively, which is a key aspect of many addictive behaviors. The reality is that behavioral addictions can be just as powerful and difficult to overcome as chemical addictions, such as those to alcohol and drugs.

Pressured Into Treatment or Under Their Own Terms?

Another issue under debate is whether people exhibiting addictive behaviors should be allowed to choose to enter treatment or whether they should be compelled to have treatment for their own good or the good of society. Strong arguments can be made for both positions. Unless the individual is committing crimes, most people, including adolescents, cannot be forced into treatment for alcohol or drug abuse or for most other addictive behaviors. When the addicted person exhibits behavior that harms other people, such as sexually harassing others at work or stealing money for the purposes of gambling, it is more likely that treatment will be legally mandated.

Smoking rarely falls into this area. In recent years, though, many states have passed laws prohibiting people from smoking in restaurants and public areas. As a result, smokers can be arrested for violating the law, although currently, mandated treatment is not a common sentence.

Recovering From Addictions: Individual Acknowledgment is Crucial

One key to recovering from any addiction is that the individual must acknowledge that he or she has a serious problem. Without self-awareness of the destructiveness of the addictive behavior, the behavior will continue.

To many people, the risks that addicted people take in continuing their addiction are obvious, and it is painstakingly clear that the addiction should end as soon as possible. However, the boss who starts drinking on the job at 4:30 P.M. and is drunk and verbally threatening to fire workers an hour later does not allow himself to be aware that he is not only hurting himself but is also hurting others. The pregnant woman who smokes cigarette after cigarette does not admit to herself that she is not only risking developing medical problems herself but is also causing problems in the child she plans to bear. Without this awareness, addicts can be restrained sometimes by others from their particular addictive behavior, but they do not recover from it.

Other Steps to Healing: A Desire and Willingness to Change

Other key elements in recovery from addictions are both the desire to change and the willingness to take the actions needed to effect that change. Many people may have a vague desire to change. Others may have an intense desire to change, for example, wishing that they were not alcoholic or obese but are unwilling to take the steps needed to resolve their addictions. To combat alcoholism or obesity, one must not only give up drinking or overeating but must also attack the underlying problems associated with these addictions. This is usually done through a combination of recovery programs, exercise, and therapy.

Treatment is Available

Many people who suffer from addictions do recover. Some of them recover through self-help programs, such as those run by Alcoholics Anonymous or Narcotics Anonymous. Others recover thanks to inpatient rehabilitation hospital treatment or intensive institutional programs, such as Betty Ford-type clinics. For some addictive behaviors, few or no special programs are available. However, addicts with such problems may successfully struggle through their personal conflicts with the help of psychiatrists and psychologists and benefit from 12-step programs directed toward other kinds of addiction.

A wide variety of treatment programs are available for individuals who wish to recover. These range from a punitive model that generally favors strict rules with incarceration for repeated minor offenses to a more supportive model that favors therapy and discovering the underlying causes of addiction.

There are primarily medical models, which rely on medications such as preventive drugs for alcoholism and drug abuse (such as Antabuse and Naltrexone) and other drugs for maintenance and

tapering (such as methadone). As mentioned, the underlying cause of many addictions may be a psychiatric disorder (such as depression, bipolar disorder, or impulse control disorders). Thus existing psychiatric disorders may need to be treated before an individual can overcome addictive behaviors.

The law enforcement community and the medical community sometimes clash over the best way to cope with an addicted person who has committed a crime. Did he or she commit the crime because of the addiction, for example, in order to obtain an illicit substance? If so, does it matter? The debate between proponents of punishment and incarceration versus the advocates of mandated treatment continues.

Self-Help Programs

The most commonly known self-help program for combating addictions is Alcoholics Anonymous, formed in 1935 by a man known as Bill H., who realized that his alcoholism was a disease but one that could be controlled through hard work and sharing his message with others. Many recovery programs are modeled on Alcoholics Anonymous, such as Gamblers Anonymous, Narcotics Anonymous, and Sex Addicts Anonymous. The underlying premise of each of these groups is that the member will completely give up the addictive behavior through group support and a shared experience.

What Society Thinks Does Matter

Another key factor in facilitating healing from addiction is the attitude of others, including the addicted individual's family, friends, and society in general. Our culture has trouble deciding whether people with addictive behaviors should be punished or need to have their illness treated. Complicating the issue further is that people with addictive behaviors are often more likely to commit violent crimes and to end up in the criminal justice system, regardless of which model of addiction is accepted.

Social acceptance of addiction can also hamper recovery. When smoking was an accepted and ordinary behavior, allowed in any setting, the percentage of Americans who smoked was substantially higher than it is now. As smoking became less and less acceptable, the percentage of smokers slowly dropped. Peer acceptance for drug abuse, alcohol abuse, and even binge eating with purging all increase the likelihood of continued addiction, while peer rejection increases the chance of recovery.

Strong condemnation of addiction can also create problems for recovery. If one's physician evinces contempt for addicts, a patient is unlikely to admit concerns about alcohol use or drug use. In addition, if the addicted person believes (or knows) that revealing his or her drug addiction could mean loss of his or her job, money, power, and prestige as well as the respect of the people who matter to the individual, then the person will actively work to hide his or her addiction as much as possible.

Another issue affecting how addiction is regarded is a view of individual rights. Some individuals, spanning the political spectrum from liberal to conservative, believe that federal and state governments should stop punishing individuals for using or possessing illegal drugs. Their argument is that treatment is far less expensive than a war on drugs, including the attempts to prevent drug sales, possession, and use as well as the arrest, trials, and incarceration of individuals who use or sell drugs.

The attitudes of adolescents toward substance abuse are significant because their attitudes affect whether they decide to use drugs and alcohol as well as which substances they choose to abuse, if any. Large annual surveys measure such attitudes. Researchers, policy makers, and educators use the data from these surveys to try to improve the situation so that fewer adolescents will become drug and alcohol abusers.

Looking Ahead

As researchers and physicians learn more about the human brain and how and why individuals develop addictive behaviors, it is increasingly likely that they will also develop more effective means to enable individuals to combat their addictions. Despite a hopeful future, however, there will always be some individuals who become addicted to substances or behaviors and who will find refraining from using these substances or refraining from these behaviors to be extremely difficult. The conundrum of a free society is that often individuals are still free to make choices—even bad choices.

Biederman, Joseph, M.D., et al. "Patterns of Alcohol and Drug Use in Adolescents Can Be Predicted by Parental Substance Use Disorders." *Pediatrics* 106, no. 4 (October 2000): 792–797.

Clark, H. Westley, J.D., M.D. "The Treatment of OxyContin Addiction and the Prevention of Further Drug Abuse." Statement before the Senate Committee on Health, Education, Labor, and Pensions, February 12, 2002. Available online. URL: http://www.hhs.gov/asl/testify/t020212.html. Accessed on July 10, 2004.

Engwall, Douglas, Robert Hunter, and Marvin Steinberg. "Gambling and Other Risk Behaviors on University Campuses," *Journal of American College of Health* 52, no. 6 (May/June 2004): 245–255.

Merline, Alicia, et al. "Substance Use Among Adults 35 Years of Age: Prevalence, Adulthood Predictors, and Impact of Adolescent Substance," *American Journal of Public Health* 94, no. 1 (January 2004): 96–102.

Morrison, R. Sean, M.D., et al. " 'We Don't Carry That'—Failure of Pharmacies in Predominantly Nonwhite Neighborhoods to Stock Opioid Analgesics." *New England Journal of Medicine* 342, no. 14 (April 6, 2000): 1,023–1,026.

National Center on Addiction and Substance Abuse at Columbia University. *Report on Teen Cigarette Smoking and Marijuana Use.* New York: National Center on Addiction and Substance Abuse, September 2003.

Sorensen, James L., et al., ed. *Drug Abuse Treatment Through Collaboration: Practice and Research Partnerships That Work.* Washington, D.C.: American Psychological Association, 2003.

Substance Abuse and Mental Health Services Administration (SAMHSA). *Results From the 2003 National Survey on Drug Use and Health: National Findings.* Office of Applied Studies, NHSDA Series H-22, DHHS Publication Number SMA 03-3836. Rockville, Md.: SAMHSA, 2003.

United States Department of Health and Human Services. *The Health Consequences of Smoking: A Report of the Surgeon General.* Washington, D.C.: U.S. Department of Health and Human Services, Centers for Disease Control and Prevention, National Center for Chronic Disease Prevention and Health Promotion, Office on Smoking and Health, 2004.

United States Department of Health and Human Services. *Healthy People 2010: Understanding and Improving Health and Objectives for Improving Health,* 2nd ed. Washington, D.C.: U.S. Department of Health and Human Services, November 2000.

Vastag, Brian. "Addiction Poorly Understood by Clinicians." *Journal of the American Medical Association* 290, no. 10 (September 10, 2003): 1,299–1,303.

The White House. *National Drug Control Strategy: Update.* Washington, D.C.: The White House, March 2004.

Wright, D. *State Estimates of Substance Use from the 2002 National Survey on Drug Use and Health.* Department of Health and Human Services Publication No. SMA 04-3907, NSDUH Series H-23. Rockville, Md.: Substance Abuse and Mental Health Services Administration, Office of Applied Studies, July 2004.

ENTRIES A–Z

abstinence Refraining altogether from a specific activity, such as drinking alcohol, smoking cigarettes, eating in binges, or using the Internet to excess. Some behaviors do not lend themselves to abstinence. For example, sex addicts are probably not willing to give up all sexual acts forever, and binge eaters obviously cannot give up eating.

The importance of abstinence is a core belief of many recovery organizations, such as ALCOHOLICS ANONYMOUS and NARCOTICS ANONYMOUS. Yet some individuals and organizations believe that it is possible for some people to limit their addictive behavior to a mild level that stops short of abstinence. Supporters of abstinence in the treatment of addiction believe that an addict cannot take just one drink or smoke just one cigarette, and so forth. They are convinced that consuming even a very small amount of the addictive substance will ultimately and inevitably lead to a complete lack of impulse control and back to a full-blown addiction. This debate will likely continue for years.

See also ANTABUSE; CRAVING.

abuse Excessive use of a substance, whether it is alcohol, tobacco, prescribed medications, or other items. Individuals who exhibit an abusive behavior may escalate their behavior into an addiction, which includes both a physical and psychological need to perform the harmful behavior repeatedly.

Some individuals can abuse drugs, alcohol, and other substances on one or more occasions without the behaviors developing into addictions. This does not mean that substance abuse is harmless. For example, an individual could drink to excess and subsequently cause a severe car crash leading to loss of lives. Alternatively, a person could have unprotected sex with many individuals over a short period and contract a sexually transmitted disease that he or she may subsequently spread to others.

See also ADDICTION; ADDICTIVE BEHAVIORS; ALCOHOL ABUSE; ALCOHOLISM; ALCOHOL POISONING; DRUG ABUSE; DRUG ADDICTION.

accidental overdose Excessive use of a substance, such as alcohol, legal or illegal drugs, or a combination of alcohol and drugs, but without the intent of committing suicide or homicide. An accidental overdose can cause severe medical problems, such as coma, permanent brain and organ damage, or even death. People who use HEROIN are particularly susceptible to an accidental overdose that may be fatal. According to the National Center for Health Statistics, 2,718 people in the United States died of accidental overdoses from the use of opiates and related narcotics in 1998.

In some cases, such as when a person has died from an overdose of drugs or a combination of drugs and alcohol, knowing whether the overdose was accidental or if the individual was completing a SUICIDE is difficult or impossible.

See also OVERDOSE.

Executive Office of the President, *The Economic Costs of Drug Abuse in the United States, 1992–1998.* Office of National Drug Control Policy, Washington, D.C.: September 2001. Available online. URL: http://www.whitehousedrugpolicy. gov/publications/pdf/economic_costs98.pdf. Accessed on May 15, 2004.

accidents Unplanned events, such as falls, car crashes, injuries, and other occurrences. Accidents are more likely to occur in the face of addictions that impair the individual's thinking and physical abilities. For example, a person who is intoxicated on drugs or alcohol is more likely than a sober person to cause a car crash. Some accidents occur as a result of carelessness that is not related to addictive behavior. Sometimes it is difficult to determine whether the accident was caused because of an individual's impairment or if it could not have been prevented even if he or she were not impaired by an addictive substance.

See also ACCIDENTAL OVERDOSE; ALCOHOL POISONING; DRIVING, IMPAIRED; DRIVING WHILE INTOXICATED/DRIVING UNDER THE INFLUENCE.

acknowledgment of addiction   An individual's acceptance that he or she has an addictive problem, which is an essential part of recovery. Of course, awareness alone is not sufficient, but it is one necessary element of overcoming an addiction.

Many addicts initially deny that they have a problem at all, insisting that they can stop the addictive behavior anytime that they feel like it (and they just have not felt like stopping it to date). They are also often in denial. Many addicts have actually tried to stop the behavior in the past and failed. They then bury this memory and convince themselves that if they *really* wanted to stop the behavior, they could do so.

Even in the face of clear evidence of a major problem, such as losing one's job, becoming divorced, or causing the death of another person in a car crash due to alcohol- or drug-impaired driving, some people will continue to deny their addiction. Until such an acknowledgment occurs, no treatment program is effective—other than incarceration. That is effective only until the person is released into society again. (Illegal substances are often available in jails and prisons.)

Compelling a person who does not acknowledge an addiction to go to a treatment program often means that he or she will attend the sessions in order to avoid consequences for not attending (such as losing a driver's license, losing custody of a child, or going to jail). However, without acknowledgment, the person is still likely to resume the addictive behaviors that led to his or her problems.

Compulsory treatment programs can lead people to an awareness and acknowledgment of their addiction and therefore can be effective, regardless of how an individual came to treatment.

Sometimes even when individuals accept that they are addicted, compulsory programs may be the only way they will finally enter treatment. For some individuals, including those who acknowledge their addiction, the threat of serious legal consequences may be necessary to keep them in treatment.

Fortunately, many people do finally realize and accept that they have an addiction. Such individuals can benefit from rehabilitation programs and self-help groups such as ALCOHOLICS ANONYMOUS, GAMBLERS ANONYMOUS, and similar support groups for addicted individuals.

Some experts recommend that family and friends stage an INTERVENTION, a confrontational session with the addicted person, in which they tell him or her how they feel about the addictive behavior and how it causes the individual financial and emotional pain. This intervention is designed to break through the denial and bring home the many ways in which the family and friends have been harmed by the addiction. Generally the plan is for the addicted individual to go directly from the session into a rehabilitative facility.

Interventions should always involve a professional counselor. Most family members are not trained in addiction medicine or psychiatry and may inadvertently cause the flight (or even the suicide) of the addicted person rather than the desired acknowledgment of the addictive behavior and the agreement to enter treatment.

See also ADDICTION; CODEPENDENCY; ENABLERS.

addiction   The emotional and often physical need to perform a certain behavior, whether it is consuming large quantities of alcohol, taking illegal drugs, or acting on other compulsions. Some experts use the word "dependence" as a substitute for "addiction." Most addictive behaviors have both a physical and a psychological dimension.

People who take narcotics for severe pain over the short term rarely develop a problem with addiction unless they have a tendency toward addictive behaviors. They will, however, develop a need for greater amounts of narcotic medications over time to achieve the same level of pain control.

Addiction implies not only a physical need for a substance or a psychological need to perform a behavior but also a series of behaviors associated with the physical or psychological need. These behaviors have the potential to cause serious negative consequences, not only to the individual, but also to others that surround the individual, such as his or her family, friends, and coworkers.

Adults can become addicted to legal substances, such as alcohol, cigarettes, or prescribed painkilling medications as well as to a variety of illegal substances, such as heroin. They can also become addicted to legal behaviors, such as gambling, consensual adult sex, and shopping.

Elements of Addictive Behaviors

Several key elements are present in an addiction, whether the addiction is to drugs, shopping, sex, or other forms of behavior. First, individuals feel irresistibly drawn to perform the behavior, and they generally feel that they cannot resist this impulse.

Next, the behavior has negative consequences. In many cases, the person's health is compromised, such as when he or she smokes or drinks at addictive levels. In most cases, the individual's financial status is affected. As a result, the person may resort to performing criminal acts in order to obtain the money needed to perform the addictive behavior, to view for-pay Web sites of pornography on the Internet, to buy illegal drugs, or to gamble at the track.

Another element of addiction is that the individual cannot perform this act only once or twice but continues to wish to repeat the act. Excessive drinking on a Saturday night and the subsequent severe headache on Sunday morning is not sufficient to deter the person addicted to alcohol from wishing to drink again and usually to drink again as soon as possible. Thus, painful consequences from the addictive behavior do not deter the individual from the addiction.

Many people with addictions appear to be cued by certain stimuli. One of the most classic examples is the desire to smoke a cigarette after having sex or after eating dinner. Often these cues are subtle and are not understood by the individuals affected by them. Individuals can learn to identify and to reprogram their own behaviors, although doing so can be difficult but not impossible. Many treatment programs focus on teaching addicted individuals to recognize and overcome these powerful signals to use a substance or to perform a behavior.

Support groups composed of other individuals who are facing the same problems can help. Sometimes medications can help, depending on the nature of the problem. Therapy of various forms may also be helpful. Some people with addictive behaviors require inpatient rehabilitation to remove them, as much as possible, from access to a drug or behavior while they learn new coping mechanisms and behaviors.

See also ACKNOWLEDGMENT OF ADDICTION; ALCOHOLISM; BEHAVIOR MODIFICATION; DRUG ADDICTION; PHYSICIANS AND HEALTH CARE PROFESSIONALS AND ADDICTION.

addiction medicine Refers to a branch of medicine that specializes in the care of individuals with substance abuse problems with the goal of helping them overcome their addictions. Physicians who specialize in addiction medicine concentrate largely on the abuse of alcohol, illegal drugs, and/or prescribed drugs with addictive potential, such as narcotic painkillers.

Doctors who specialize in addiction medicine may also wish to obtain certification from the American Society of Addiction Medicine so they may obtain permission to treat patients with BUPRENORPHINE, an alternate drug to METHADONE for the treatment of opiate addiction.

See also ALCOHOLISM; DETOXIFICATION; DRUG ADDICTION; OPIATES.

For further information, contact:

American Society of Addiction Medicine
4601 North Park Avenue
Arcade Suite 101
Chevy Chase, MD 20815
(301) 656-3920
http://www.asam.org

addictive behaviors A pattern of actions that an individual has great difficulty changing or cannot change without assistance and that causes emotional, financial, health, and other consequences to him or her and to others. For example, ALCOHOLISM causes many health problems and may also cause the individual to lose his or her job, marriage, and any savings or wealth. The same can be said for the person who is addicted to illegal drugs or who has developed a problem with pathological gambling.

When people are addicted, they are nearly always thinking about the item they are addicted to. They are either using the item or are thinking about how they are going to acquire the item, whether it is BEER, COCAINE, pornography (in the case of a sex addiction), or cigarettes. Of course, not everyone who uses beer (or pornography or even cocaine) is an addict. The compulsiveness of use, despite the consequences, is one of the key features of addiction. Another key feature is tolerance, or the desire for greater amounts of the substance. The amount that was once satisfying is no longer enough.

Some addictive behaviors are common, such as alcoholism. Others are rare, such as an apparent addiction to exercise or extreme sports. No one really knows how extensive some addictions are, such as an addiction to the use of the Internet. However, many people clearly seem to be mesmerized by this new force and have an extreme difficulty in breaking away, whether they use it for sexual gratification, friendships, games, or other reasons.

See also ADDICTION; EXERCISE ADDICTION/DEPENDENCE; GAMBLING, PATHOLOGICAL; INTERNET ADDICTION DISORDER; TOLERANCE.

addictive personality   A personality type in an individual who is significantly more likely to develop addictive behaviors than other people. Whether such a personality exists is highly debated among physicians and other experts in the field of addiction. Whether this concept is a useful one is also not clear.

In their April 2002 report, the Task Force of the National Advisory Council on Alcohol Abuse and Alcoholism stated, "Decades of research have failed to identify an 'addictive personality.' However, certain personality traits have been related to drinking habits. For example, sensation-seeking has been related to higher rates of consumption, while religiosity has been related to lower rates. Personality traits are typically seen as mediating or moderating the relationship between biological, psychological, social, and environmental factors and subsequent alcohol use and misuse."

Other factors may play a role in an "addictive personality." For example, individuals with undiagnosed and/or untreated ATTENTION DEFICIT HYPERACTIVITY DISORDER may have problems with impulsivity and distractibility. These individuals may be drawn to addictive behavioral choices.

Many experts believe that genetic factors are at work that cause a predisposition to addictive behaviors. Others say that addictive behaviors are not inherited but psychiatric problems are, such as BIPOLAR DISORDER, DEPRESSION, ANXIETY DISORDERS, attention deficit hyperactivity disorder, OBSESSIVE-COMPULSIVE DISORDER, and other conditions that increase an individual's likelihood of exhibiting addictive behaviors, as a form of distraction, as the result of compulsive or obsessive behaviors, or for self-medication.

Environmental factors cannot be ignored. Children who are reared in families where parents are heavy abusers of drugs or alcohol may be affected by both genetic and environmental impacts. Separating the two issues is difficult.

Physicians and other experts who believe that such a phenomenon as an addictive personality exists also believe that individuals are prone to developing a variety of addictions. For example, if individuals drink alcohol, they are more likely to drink to excess and become alcoholics. If they gamble, they are more likely to be drawn toward compulsive gambling. They are drawn to the excitement and random reinforcement of gambling. In fact, individuals with this type of personality are likely to go from addiction to addiction, replacing one with another.

Another school of thought concerns development of changes in the brain in response to the use of addictive substances, or neuroadaptation. This change in brain chemistry can theoretically lead to a need for stimulation associated with many kinds of addictions. Once an individual has developed these brain changes, the risk of developing a new addiction is very high, as the brain is trained to respond in the specific addictive pattern.

Task Force of the National Advisory Council on Alcohol Abuse and Alcoholism. *High Risk Drinking in College: What We Know and What We Need to Learn: Final Report on Contexts and Consequences.* Washington, D.C.: National Institute on Alcohol Abuse and Alcoholism, April 2002.

Available online. URL: http://media.shs.net/collegedrinking/FINALPanel1.pdf. Accessed May 2004.

Al-Anon An international support group organization and a subset of ALCOHOLICS ANONYMOUS specifically designed for individuals who have family members or friends who are addicted to alcohol. An estimated 26,000 Al-Anon and ALATEEN groups (designed for adolescents with family members addicted to alcohol) meet in 115 countries worldwide. Al-Anon does not charge any membership fees. It operates under the 12-step principles of Alcoholics Anonymous.

Based on a 2003 study commissioned by the organization, most members of Al-Anon are female (88 percent), and most (57 percent) are married. About two-thirds have an education beyond high school up to and including a college degree or postgraduate studies. Most members (69 percent) are employed.

Among Al-Anon members, 86 percent said that they believed that someone else's drinking had affected their mental health, and 63 percent said that their overall health status was affected by someone else's drinking. About half the Al-Anon members (52 percent) named their current spouse as the alcoholic person while others named other relatives and family members. Interestingly, according to the survey, "More Al-Anon members now list a parent as an alcoholic in their lives when compared to 1999 findings (48% vs. 36%)." Perhaps this is due at least in part to greater media exposure of the effects of alcoholism on adult children of alcoholics.

Most Al-Anon members (78 percent) joined the organization as a result of a personal referral, such as family members and close friends.

See also ALCOHOLISM; TWELVE STEPS.

For further information, contact:

Al-Anon Group Headquarters
1600 Corporate Landing Parkway
Virginia Beach, VA 23454
(757) 563-1600
http://www.al-anon.org

Southeastern Institute of Research, Inc. *Research Report: 2003 Al-Anon/Alateen Membership and Alateen Sponsor Survey, January 13, 2004.* Richmond, Va.: Southeastern Institute of Research, Inc., 2004.

Alateen An organization that is a subset of ALCOHOLICS ANONYMOUS and is specifically designed for adolescents who are related to others who are alcoholics, such as parents or siblings and other individuals who are important in their lives. An estimated 2,300 Alateen groups exist throughout the United States and other countries. The organization does not charge dues and only requires that members have a relative or friend who is an alcoholic. The organization operates under the 12-step principles of Alcoholics Anonymous as a means to recovery.

In a survey performed in 2003 of Alateen members, the results showed that 94 percent were influenced to attend their first meeting by a recommendation of another person. More than 90 percent of Alateen members reported having parents or stepparents who were alcoholic.

See also AL-ANON; ALCOHOLISM; TWELVE STEPS.

Alateen shares their corporate headquarters with Al-Anon. For further information, contact:

Al-Anon Group Headquarters
1600 Corporate Landing Parkway
Virginia Beach, VA 23454
(757) 563-1600
http://www.al-anon.org

alcohol abuse The excessive use of alcohol. Alcohol abuse can develop into an addiction, although some individuals abuse alcohol on one or more occasions and never develop an addictive need for alcohol. According to the NATIONAL INSTITUTE ON ALCOHOL ABUSE AND ALCOHOLISM (NIAAA) in the United States, alcohol abusers fit at least one of the following criteria caused by their excessive drinking:

- They fail to fulfill their responsibilities at work, school, or home.
- They drive or operate dangerous equipment while under the influence of alcohol.
- They have been arrested for an alcohol-related problem, such as driving while intoxicated or assaulting another person when drunk.
- They drink despite family or personal relationship problems that are either created or worsened by the excessive drinking.

According to the NIAAA, 4.7 percent of the population of the United States, or 9.7 million people, were alcohol abusers in 2002. This is an increase from the levels in 1992, when an estimated 3 percent of the population and 5.6 million people were alcohol abusers. Abuse rates were up for all racial and ethnic groups except Native Americans and were significantly increased for whites, blacks, and Hispanics. Significant increases also occurred for both men and women. Further studies are needed to determine why these increases may have happened.

Of importance, however, is that over the same time frame, the estimated rate of alcoholism declined from 4.4 percent of the population in 1992 (and 8.2 million people) to 3.8 percent of the population in 2002 (and 7.9 million people). These prevalence statistics on both alcohol abuse and alcoholism were based on a study published in a 2004 issue of *Drug and Alcohol Dependence*.

See also ALCOHOL/ALCOHOL CONSUMPTION; ALCOHOLISM; ALCOHOL POISONING; BINGE DRINKING; COLLEGE STUDENTS; TEENAGE AND YOUTH DRINKING.

Grant, Bridget F., et al. "The 12-Month Prevalence and Trends in DSM-IV Alcohol Abuse and Dependence: United States, 1991–1992 and 2001–2002," *Drug and Alcohol Dependence* 74, (2004): 223–234.

alcohol addiction See ALCOHOLISM.

alcohol/alcohol consumption Alcohol is a fluid that is made from grains, fruits, and vegetables. It contains a substance known as ETHANOL and causes intoxication if consumed in sufficient quantities. "Consumption of alcohol" in this text refers to the aggregate amount of alcohol drunk by a population, whether it is men or women in the United States, individuals within a specific age group, or other specific populations, such as groups divided by age, race, or ethnicity.

Experts measure the actual consumption of alcohol, whether beer, wine, or distilled spirits (alcoholic beverages that are not beer or wine) in gallons, and they also measure the consumption of ethanol. Ethanol, which is an intoxicant, is one type of alcohol. It comprises only a small part of beer (about 3–6 percent or less). It comprises a greater portion of wine (about 13 percent) and a much larger portion of distilled spirits (about 40 percent, depending on the type of spirit that is consumed). Alcohol is also in some forms of liquid cold medicine, which is one of the key reasons why it causes consumers to fall asleep.

When considering the different major categories of alcohol and their alcohol contents, 12 ounces of beer is equal to 5 ounces of wine and to 1.5 ounces of 80-proof distilled spirits. Clearly, a smaller absolute quantity of distilled spirits would need to be consumed for a person to become intoxicated than if the individual were drinking only beer or wine.

Some forms of alcohol are measured by the "proof," which is an indication of its alcohol content. For example, an alcohol that is 80 proof is comprised of 40 percent alcohol. In general, beer and wine containers do not provide information on the proof of the alcohol, and this information is limited to spirits only (such as bourbon, whiskey, rum, and so forth). Some states specifically define the alcohol content that can be present in beer or wine.

All Forms of Alcohol Can Be Addicting

Because of the significantly lower alcohol content that is present in both wine and beer compared with other forms of alcoholic beverages, some people mistakenly believe that addiction is impossible or unlikely to occur as long as the individual continues to drink only beer and/or wine. The reality is that many people become addicted to beer or wine because they drink large quantities of them and thus ingest large quantities of ethanol.

Considering Gender, Age, and Ethnic Differences in Alcohol Consumption

In general, men are heavier drinkers than women. According to the National Center for Health Statistics, in 2001, 39.7 percent of all women age 18 and over in the United States were regular drinkers, compared with 56.6 percent of all men. (See table at top of page 7.) Note that not all regular or current drinkers have an alcohol abuse or alcoholism problem.

Women are more likely to be lifetime abstainers than men, or 29.2 percent of women compared with 15.2 percent of men.

More young people drink than older people. As people age, drinking declines for many individuals.

ALCOHOL CONSUMPTION BY PERSONS 18 YEARS OF AGE AND OLDER, ACCORDING TO DRINKING STATUS, UNITED STATES, 2001

Drinking Status	Both Sexes	Male	Female
All	100.0	100.0	100.0
Lifetime abstainer	22.6	15.2	29.2
Former drinker	14.9	16.0	14.0
Current drinker	62.5	68.8	56.8
Infrequent	12.8	9.2	16.2
Regular	48.7	56.6	39.7

Source: Fried, V. M., et al. *Chartbook on Trends in the Health of Americans. Health, United States, 2003.* Hyattsville, Md.: National Center for Health Statistics, 2003.

When isolating the factors of race and ethnicity, people of two or more races had the largest percent of current drinkers (68.5 percent), followed by whites (65.8 percent) and then American Indians and Alaskan Natives, at 51.5 percent. (See table below.) Asian individuals are the least likely to consume alcohol (44.7 percent) particularly Asian females (30.1 percent).

ALCOHOL CONSUMPTION BY PERSONS 18 YEARS OF AGE AND OLDER, ACCORDING TO PERCENT OF CURRENT DRINKERS, UNITED STATES, 2001

	Both Sexes	Male	Female
Age			
18–44 years	69.0	75.0	63.2
45–64 years	62.5	67.8	57.5
65 years and older	42.0	50.9	35.5
Race			
White only	65.8	71.0	61.0
Black only	46.6	56.9	38.6
American Indian and Alaska Native only	51.5	62.8	38.6
Asian only	44.7	59.7	30.1
Two or more races	68.5	69.9	67.1

Source: Fried, V. M., et al. *Chartbook on Trends in the Health of Americans. Health, United States, 2003.* Hyattsville, Md.: National Center for Health Statistics, 2003.

Alcohol Consumption Nationwide

States vary radically in their consumption of alcohol. According to the NATIONAL INSTITUTE ON ALCOHOL ABUSE AND ALCOHOLISM, in considering the ethanol content of alcohol alone, there is a high per capita consumption in New Hampshire (4.00) and Nevada (3.67) and a lower than average consumption in Utah (1.27), West Virginia (1.64), and Oklahoma (1.69).

Americans consumed about 493 million gallons of all forms of alcohol in 2000. In terms of ethanol content alone, the per capita (per person) ethanol consumption was 2.18 gallons. (See table on page 8 for comparative data on states, regions, and the United States as a whole.)

The per capita consumption of ethanol from all forms of alcoholic beverages increased from 2.16 gallons in 1999 to 2.18 gallons in 2000, the same level as in 1994. This increase was primarily due to an increase in the per capita consumption of spirits from 0.63 gallons in 1999 to 0.65 gallons in 2000.

See also ALCOHOL ABUSE; ALCOHOLISM; ALCOHOL POISONING; BINGE DRINKING; BLOOD ALCOHOL LEVELS.

Nephew, Thomas M., et al., *Apparent Per Capita Alcohol Consumption: National, State, and Regional Trends, 1977–2000.* Bethesda, Md.: National Institute on Alcohol Abuse and Alcoholism, National Institutes of Health, August 2003.

alcohol breath tests Studies that determine the amount of alcohol on a person's breath in order to determine if he or she has a BLOOD ALCOHOL LEVEL that constitutes the individual is DRIVING WHILE INTOXICATED.

The earliest test for alcohol on the breath was the Breathalyzer, a device that was invented in 1954 by Robert Borkenstein. Other, more sophisticated devices were subsequently created. In general, a person who appears to be driving erratically or who has been involved in a car crash and appears to be intoxicated is challenged by a police officer. Some police departments use portable alcohol breath devices, while others require the individual to go to the police station to take the breath test. Some individuals opt for a blood test of their alcohol levels, while others may take a urine test.

APPARENT ALCOHOL CONSUMPTION FOR STATES, CENSUS REGIONS, AND IN THE UNITED STATES, 2000 (VOLUME AND ETHANOL ARE IN THOUSANDS OF GALLONS, AND THE PER CAPITA [PC] ETHANOL CONSUMPTION IS IN GALLONS, BASED ON THE POPULATION AGES 14 AND OLDER.)

State or Region	Beer			Wine			Spirits			All Beverages	
	Volume	Ethanol	PC	Volume	Ethanol	PC	Volume	Ethanol	PC	Ethanol	PC
Alabama	94,530	4,254	1.19	4,934	636	0.18	4,485	1,843	0.51	6,734	1.88
Alaska	14,373	647	1.35	1,379	178	0.37	1,076	442	0.92	1,267	2.63
Arizona	134,336	6,045	1.48	9,869	1,273	0.31	7,055	2,900	0.71	10,218	2.50
Arkansas	52,053	2,342	1.09	1,993	257	0.12	2,796	1,149	0.53	3,749	1.74
California	637,080	28,669	1.07	99,930	12,891	0.48	41,327	16,985	0.64	58,545	2.19
Colorado	103,734	4,668	1.35	9,845	1,270	0.37	7,503	3,084	0.89	9,022	2.60
Connecticut	57,491	2,587	0.94	10,521	1,357	0.49	4,959	2,038	0.74	5,982	2.18
Delaware	19,156	862	1.36	2,382	307	0.48	1,622	667	1.05	1,836	2.89
District of Columbia	14,428	649	1.35	2,597	335	0.70	1,724	709	1.48	1,693	3.53
Florida	388,796	17,496	1.32	41,383	5,338	0.40	26,422	10,860	0.82	33,694	2.55
Georgia	177,061	7,968	1.22	12,902	1,664	0.26	10,999	4,520	0.69	14,153	2.17
Hawaii	29,065	1,308	1.33	3,002	387	0.39	1,434	589	0.60	2,285	2.33
Idaho	26,257	1,182	1.16	5,142	663	0.65	1,253	515	0.51	2,360	2.32
Illinois	282,189	12,698	1.28	24,663	3,182	0.32	15,281	6,281	0.63	22,161	2.24
Indiana	125,490	5,647	1.16	7,738	998	0.21	7,261	2,983	0.61	9,629	1.98
Iowa	71,323	3,210	1.35	2,353	304	0.13	2,863	1,177	0.50	4,690	1.98
Kansas	54,832	2,467	1.15	2,518	325	0.15	2,692	1,106	0.52	3,898	1.82
Kentucky	78,055	3,512	1.07	3,460	446	0.14	4,278	1,758	0.54	5,717	1.74
Louisiana	117,937	5,307	1.50	6,159	794	0.22	6,043	2,484	0.70	8,585	2.43
Maine	27,370	1,232	1.17	3,179	410	0.39	1,861	765	0.73	2,406	2.29
Maryland	97,754	4,399	1.04	10,009	1,291	0.30	7,735	3,179	0.75	8,869	2.09
Massachusetts	133,990	6,030	1.16	20,635	2,662	0.51	11,031	4,534	0.87	13,225	2.55
Michigan	209,608	9,432	1.19	14,757	1,904	0.24	13,360	5,491	0.69	16,827	2.12
Minnesota	108,478	4,882	1.24	7,918	1,021	0.26	8,359	3,435	0.87	9,338	2.37
Mississippi	71,823	3,232	1.44	1,657	214	0.09	3,273	1,345	0.60	4,791	2.13
Missouri	135,246	6,086	1.35	8,144	1,051	0.23	7,302	3,001	0.67	10,138	2.25
Montana	25,257	1,137	1.55	1,671	216	0.29	1,213	499	0.68	1,851	2.53
Nebraska	43,943	1,977	1.44	1,791	231	0.17	2,061	847	0.62	3,055	2.23
Nevada	64,055	2,882	1.79	7,745	999	0.62	4,913	2,019	1.26	5,901	3.67
New Hampshire	39,001	1,755	1.75	4,373	564	0.56	4,107	1,688	1.69	4,007	4.00
New Jersey	144,883	6,520	0.96	24,472	3,157	0.47	12,681	5,212	0.77	14,888	2.19
New Mexico	48,624	2,188	1.53	2,771	357	0.25	2,113	868	0.61	3,414	2.38
New York	313,158	14,092	0.92	44,840	5,784	0.38	21,657	8,901	0.58	28,777	1.88
North Carolina	173,293	7,798	1.19	11,486	1,482	0.23	8,204	3,372	0.52	12,651	1.94
North Dakota	17,018	766	1.47	591	76	0.15	1,003	412	0.79	1,254	2.40
Ohio	263,287	11,848	1.30	13,693	1,766	0.19	11,091	4,558	0.50	18,173	1.99
Oklahoma	69,346	3,121	1.13	2,672	345	0.12	2,998	1,232	0.44	4,698	1.69
Oregon	74,313	3,344	1.20	9,409	1,214	0.44	4,309	1,771	0.64	6,329	2.28
Pennsylvania	270,006	12,150	1.21	16,553	2,135	0.21	11,576	4,758	0.47	19,043	1.90
Rhode Island	21,988	989	1.15	3,033	391	0.46	1,461	600	0.70	1,981	2.31
South Carolina	104,116	4,685	1.45	5,611	724	0.22	5,545	2,279	0.70	7,688	2.37
South Dakota	19,349	871	1.44	680	88	0.15	996	409	0.68	1,368	2.27
Tennessee	124,041	5,582	1.21	5,290	682	0.15	5,644	2,320	0.50	8,584	1.86

State or Region	Beer			Wine			Spirits			All Beverages	
	Volume	Ethanol	PC	Volume	Ethanol	PC	Volume	Ethanol	PC	Ethanol	PC
Texas	556,051	25,022	1.53	27,653	3,567	0.22	19,897	8,178	0.50	36,767	2.25
Utah	28,797	1,296	0.77	1,416	183	0.11	1,629	669	0.40	2,148	1.27
Vermont	13,656	615	1.23	1,824	235	0.47	767	315	0.63	1,165	2.34
Virginia	148,362	6,676	1.16	14,010	1,807	0.31	6,925	2,846	0.50	11,330	1.97
Washington	115,148	5,182	1.09	15,125	1,951	0.41	7,599	3,123	0.66	10,256	2.16
West Virginia	39,513	1,778	1.18	1,135	146	0.10	1,297	533	0.35	2,457	1.64
Wisconsin	147,700	6,647	1.54	9,085	1,172	0.27	10,032	4,123	0.95	11,941	2.76
Wyoming	12,595	567	1.42	547	71	0.18	837	344	0.86	981	2.46
Regions											
Northeast	1,021,543	45,969	1.06	129,429	16,696	0.38	70,098	28,810	0.66	91,476	2.10
Midwest	1,478,463	66,531	1.29	93,929	12,117	0.23	82,299	33,825	0.66	112,472	2.18
South	2,326,316	104,684	1.30	155,332	20,048	0.25	119,889	49,274	0.61	173,996	2.16
West	1,313,635	59,114	1.18	167,851	21,653	0.43	82,262	33,810	0.67	114,576	2.29
U.S. Total	6,139,957	276,298	1.22	546,541	70,514	0.31	354,548	145,719	0.65	492,520	2.18

Source: Nephew, Thomas M., et al. *Apparent Per Capita Alcohol Consumption: National, State, and Regional Trends, 1977–2000.* National Institute on Alcohol Abuse and Alcoholism, Bethesda, Maryland, National Institutes of Health, August 2003.

The individual using an alcohol breath test blows into a device, which computes the person's alcohol blood levels based on the breath sample. The goal of the test is to determine whether the person who appears intoxicated has sufficient alcohol in the breath to qualify as having a blood alcohol level over the legal limit, which is 0.08 for adults in all states. In the case of ZERO-TOLERANCE LAWS for minors, the amount of alcohol on the breath that constitutes a crime is below that allowed among adults. Note that some people who may appear intoxicated have no alcohol in their systems. They may be people with diabetes who are suffering from an incident of severe hypoglycemia (low blood sugar). Some individuals may have Parkinson's disease or other illnesses that cause physical instability that may resemble intoxication.

In many states, refusal to take the alcohol breath tests when a person is stopped by a police officer for drunken driving is equivalent to admitting guilt to illegal intoxication, and the individual's driver's license may be suspended or revoked. In some cases, alcohol breath-test results may be incorrect or inaccurate. For example, if a person has been involved in a car crash that has caused bleeding in the mouth, the alcohol breath-test result can be skewed, as the test is normalized to measure alcohol in the lungs, not alcohol in the blood. In addition, if an individual has taken a drink of alcohol very recently before the test, this action can skew the results because the alcohol in the mouth is interpreted inaccurately as alcohol in the blood.

Ignition Interlock Laws

Many states have ignition interlock laws, which are mandatory alcohol breath-test systems that are incorporated into the ignition of a car. The programs are managed by the courts and the state department of motor vehicles. These laws target individuals with prior convictions for driving while under the influence of alcohol. Only after the individual breathes into the device, and the measurement indicates that the person has either no alcohol or a very low level of alcohol, may the car then be started and operated.

Studies have indicated that ignition interlock laws have been effective in reducing drunken driving; however, according to experts such as Robert Voas and Deborah Fisher, in their article for the National Institute on Alcohol Abuse and Alcoholism, only an estimated 10 percent of drivers who are eligible for such a program agree to have an interlock system installed, preferring, instead, to accept a license suspension. Unfortunately, some individuals continue to drive under the influence of alcohol, even with a suspended driver's license.

A study of the use of interlock devices, performed on 2,273 individuals in Canada previously convicted of driving under the influence of alcohol, was published in the *Journal of Studies on Alcohol* in 2003. The subjects used the interlock system in order to regain their driving privileges. The interlock device was installed for periods ranging from five to 30 months, depending on the prior offenses of the drivers.

In this study, a "fail" test was a breath test that measured an alcohol blood level of 0.04 percent or greater. (In the United States, most state laws on interlock devices use a stricter standard and generally will not allow the car to start if the blood alcohol level is 0.025 or greater.)

The researchers found that 69 percent of the subjects had one or more fail tests in the first five months. However, follow-up on the subjects revealed that only 9 percent were reconvicted of driving under the influence within a four-year period after the interlock device was removed.

In another study, reported in the *American Journal of Drug and Alcohol Abuse,* researchers followed people who had been previously convicted of driving while intoxicated in Greene County, Arkansas. The study group was made up of 315 offenders whose vehicles were equipped with an interlock device and a control group of 312 offenders who had no interlock device.

Within the next three years, 17.5 percent of the offenders in the interlock device group were convicted of driving while intoxicated. In contrast, 25.3 percent of the subjects in the control group were convicted of driving while intoxicated. Thus, the interlock device group had a significantly lower recidivism rate. Said the authors, "The ignition interlock device is not a perfect response, but it may be viewed as appropriate in certain cases. The sentencing judge must weigh the relevant factors. The interlock may be a burden on other family members who may have to share an interlock-equipped vehicle with an offender. It may also be a financial hardship on some offenders and their

families. However the device may also prevent numerous alcohol-related motor vehicle crashes. It provides both incapacitative and rehabilitative functions."

See also DRIVING, IMPAIRED.

Fulkerson, Andrew, et al. "The Breath-Analyzed Ignition Interlock Device as a Technological Response to DWI-Driving While Intoxicated," *American Journal of Drug and Alcohol Abuse,* 2003. Available online. URL: http://www.findarticles.com/p/articles/mi_m0978/is_1_29/ai_101175137/print. Accessed on March 22, 2005.

Margues, Paul, Tippets A., and Voas, R. "Comparative and Joint Prediction of DUI Recidivism from Alcohol Ignition Interlock and Driver Records," *Journal of Studies on Alcohol* 64, no. 1 (2003): 83–92.

Voas, Robert B., and Fisher, Deborah A. "Court Procedures for Handling Intoxicated Drivers," National Institute on Alcohol Abuse and Alcoholism, undated paper. Available online URL: http://www.niaaa.nih.gov/publications/arh25-1/32-42-text.htm. Accessed on March 22, 2005.

alcoholic health problems Medical problems that are caused by the chronic heavy consumption of alcohol and particularly by alcohol abuse and alcoholism. Such problems include CIRRHOSIS (scarring of the liver), heart disease, reproductive problems, and a wide variety of other health issues, including anemia and severe vitamin deficiencies, particularly of thiamine (vitamin B1) and folate. In addition, when a pregnant woman drinks alcohol, even in relatively small amounts, the fetus has a risk of developing FETAL ALCOHOL SYNDROME, which can cause profound and lifelong physical, intellectual, and developmental problems to the child.

Alcoholic Brain Damage

The chronic consumption of alcohol over years can lead to the development of brain damage. This causes such disorders as WERNICKE'S ENCEPHALOPATHY, caused by a severe thiamine deficiency (vitamin B_1), which in turn can exacerbate the brain damage.

According to experts such as Marlene Oscar-Berman and Ksenija Marinkovic in their article on alcoholism and the brain for *Alcohol Research & Health,* about half of the alcoholics in the United States are apparently free of permanent cognitive impairments. The other half have impairments that range from mild to severe. Up to 2 million are so impaired that they need fulltime care by others. Some have dementia. Most alcoholics who give up drinking altogether (ABSTINENCE) will show improved functioning.

The extent of the effect of alcohol on the brain depends on many factors. These include how much alcohol has been consumed, how long the person has been drinking, how old the patient is, the individual's genetic background, the general health status of the patient, and whether the patient was exposed to alcohol before birth.

Oscar-Berman and Marinkovic stated, "Neuroimaging research already has shown that abstinence of less than a month can result in an increase in cerebral metabolism, particularly in the frontal lobes, and that continued abstinence can lead to at least partial reversal in loss of brain tissue."

The Development of Cancers

Alcoholism has been linked to some forms of cancers, particularly colorectal cancer, esophageal cancer, and stomach cancer. In addition, some studies have shown a link between alcohol consumption and the development of breast cancer.

According to Vinzenzo Bagnardi and his colleagues in their article on alcohol consumption and the risk of cancer in *Alcohol Research & Health*, statistically significant increased risks for cancer associated with alcohol consumption have also been found with cancer of the rectum, liver, and ovaries. If individuals who drink also smoke (as many do), they further increase their risk for developing cancer of the upper digestive and respiratory tract.

Heart Disease

Coronary heart disease is not generally a problem for most females until after menopause because of the apparent protective factor of estrogen. However, after menopause occurs, at around age 45–50 years (the onset of menopause varies greatly), females face the same risk of coronary heart disease as males. Chronic alcohol consumption further increases the risk of a heart attack. The risk is also worsened or improved related to blood cholesterol levels.

Damage to the Reproductive System

ALCOHOLISM can affect the menstrual cycle and impede or impair the normal development of puberty in a prepubertal individual. It can also cause infertility in women. If women do become pregnant and continue to drink during their pregnancy, the child may be born with fetal alcohol syndrome. Some studies indicate that alcoholism may impede the male reproductive system as well. Some reproductive problems in men are related to the development of neuropathy causing penile dysfunction. Others are the direct effect of alcohol causing temporary impotence.

Damage to the Digestive System

Alcoholism can cause serious damage to the liver and the pancreas, causing CIRRHOSIS, FATTY LIVER DISEASE, AND ALCOHOLIC HEPATITIS. Chronic heavy drinking that has also lead to excessive vomiting may lead to the development of Mallory-Weiss syndrome, which causes mild to heavy internal bleeding because of a tear that occurs at the location where the esophagus joins the stomach.

Liver damage leads to a multitude of other serious health problems. For example, in many cases, liver damage causes abnormal/inadequate blood clotting throughout the body. In addition, the damaged liver may deteriorate further, such that the venous flow through the liver is decreased because as the liver shrinks or scars, the vessels within the liver become very tight and small. As a result, the backflow of blood occurs, and this condition can then result in swollen veins in the esophagus (the food tube that connects to the stomach). The esophageal veins are fragile and can rupture in response to minor trauma (such as vomiting). When inadequate clotting is combined with the bleeding from ruptured esophageal veins, the patients may die rapidly from blood loss (exsanguination).

A severe loss of thiamine due to chronic alcoholism can lead to Wernicke's encephalopathy. This life-threatening condition can cause coma and even death if untreated.

Impaired Resistance to Infections/ The Immune System

Studies indicate that alcoholism impairs the immune system and causes people who are alcoholics to be more prone to illnesses and infections as well as some forms of cancer. How and why this occurs is not known, although scientists have theories. For example, it is known that alcohol stimulates the hypothalamic-pituitary-adrenal (HPA) axis, which could result in a dampening of the immune response to disease. It is also known that in some studies, alcohol given to female rats affected their production of white blood cells, although why this occurred is not known.

One theory is that in males, prolonged alcohol exposure leads to increased production of glucocorticoids, which in turn leads to a suppressed immune system. There are also theories to explain how alcohol could suppress the immune system in women. In one pathway, prolonged exposure could lead to decreased estrogen, which then leads to a suppressed immune system. In another pathway, prolonged exposure to alcohol leads to increased production of glucocorticoids (as with males) and a suppressed immune system.

Authors Elizabeth J. Kovacs and Kelly A. N. Messingham concluded in their article in *Alcohol Research & Health,*

> "Taken together, these studies show clearly that there are dramatic suppressive effects of both acute and chronic alcohol exposure on inflammation and immunity, regardless of gender. This results in decreased ability of the immune system to fight infections and tumors. The decrease in immunity after consumption of larger quantities of alcohol is in marked contrast to the effects of very low levels of some alcoholic beverages (such as a single glass of red wine), which contain immunosuppressive antioxidants. By depressing estrogen levels, chronic or acute alcohol exposure may cause females to lose the important boost to the immune system that estrogen normally provides. This could act additively or synergistically with an elevation in immunosuppressive glucocorticoids (through activation of the HPA axis) to attenuate immune response, thus leading to a weakened ability to fight infections and tumors.

> "Finally, although chronic alcohol exposure causes liver damage in both males and females, it takes less alcohol and shorter periods of consumption to raise the risk of liver damage for females than for males. Like the observed gender differences in alcohol-induced immune suppression, this effect may involve the combined effect of stimulating glucocorticoid production and inhibiting estrogen production."

Harm to Bone Health

Alcoholics have reduced bone mineral density and an increased risk of fractures, probably due to the loss of balance from intoxication. Decreased bone mineral density increases the risk for osteoporosis, particularly among postmenopausal women. Male alcoholics also have a chronic problem with low bone density.

Emotional Problems and Eating Disorders

Alcohol abuse and alcoholism are associated with short-term or long-term emotional or psychiatric disorders that may be severe, such as depression or anxiety disorders. For example, eating disorders are often associated with alcoholism, including such eating disorders as ANOREXIA NERVOSA or BULIMIA NERVOSA, according to analysis of research published in 2002 in *Alcohol Research & Health.*

According to the authors, the relationship between bulimia nervosa and alcohol use disorders is probably an indirect result of other psychiatric disorders, such as depression or POSTTRAUMATIC STRESS DISORDER. Some studies have shown that women with substance use disorders and bulimia nervosa have higher rates of impulsivity and anxiety than other women.

See also ALCOHOL POISONING; BINGE DRINKING; CANCER; CARCINOGENS; DELIRIUM TREMENS; DETOXIFICATION; HALLUCINATIONS; HEPATITIS; LIVER.

Bagnardi, Vincenzo, et al. "Alcohol Consumption and the Risk of Cancer: A Meta-Analysis," *Alcohol Research & Health* 25, 4 (2001): 263–270.

Emanuele, Mary Ann, M.D., Frederick Wezeman, and Nicholas V. Emanuele, M.D. "Alcohol's Effects on Female Reproductive Function," *Alcohol Research & Health* 26, 4 (2002): 274–281.

Grilo, Carlos M., Rajita Sinha, and Stephanie S. O'Malley. "Eating Disorders and Alcohol Use Disorders," *Alcohol Research & Health* 26, 2 (2002): 51–160.

Kovacs, Elizabeth J. and Kelly A. N. Messingham. "Influence of Alcohol and Gender on Immune Response," *Alcohol Research & Health* 26, 4 (2002): 257–263.

Lieber, Charles S., M.D. "Alcohol and Hepatitis C," *Alcohol Research & Health* 25, 4 (2001): 245–254.

Lieber, Charles Saul, M.D. "Medical Disorders of Alcoholism," *New England Journal of Medicine* 333, 16 (October 19, 1995): 1,058–1,065.

Martin, Peter R., M.D., Charles K. Singleton, and Susanne Hiller-Sturmhofel. "The Role of Thiamine Deficiency in Alcoholic Brain Disease," *Alcohol Research & Health* 27, 3 (2003): 134–142.

Minocha, Anil, M.D. and Christine Adamec. *The Encyclopedia of Digestive Diseases and Disorders.* New York, N.Y.: Facts On File, Inc., 2004.

Oscar-Berman, Marlene and Ksenija Marinkovic. "Alcoholism and the Brain: An Overview," *Alcohol Research & Health* 27, 3 (2003): 125–133.

Register, Thomas C., J. Mark Cline, and Carol A. Shively. "Health Issues in Postmenopausal Women Who Drink," *Alcohol Research & Health* 26, 4 (2002): 299–307.

Sampson, H. Wayne. "Alcohol and Other Factors Affecting Osteoporosis Risk in Women," *Alcohol Research & Health* 26, 4 (2002): 292–298.

alcoholic hepatitis   A severe form of liver disease in which patients are symptomatic, with abdominal pain, nausea, vomiting, weakness, and fever. They are also at risk for developing infections because their immune systems are often compromised. Chronic heavy drinking and alcoholism can lead to FATTY LIVER DISEASE, which may proceed to alcoholic hepatitis and then finally to CIRRHOSIS, which is the most serious form of liver damage. In addition, obese patients also need to lose weight. (Often, ending drinking will help patients lose weight since most forms of alcohol are high in empty calories; it is also thought that alcohol slows the basal metabolic rate.)

People with alcoholic hepatitis must stop drinking immediately to avoid any further damage to their liver and in an attempt to prevent a further progression to cirrhosis. In many cases, the individual cannot handle this task alone and may require inpatient DETOXIFICATION treatment.

According to Dr. Menon and colleagues in their article on alcoholic liver disease for *Mayo Clinic Proceedings,* "The most important factor in both short-term and long-term survival of patients with alcoholic liver disease is abstinence from alcohol. Patients who recover from alcoholic hepatitis and maintain abstinence may evidence continuing improvement in clinical sequelae [results] and laboratory variables for as long as 6 months. Continued alcohol use is detrimental, with a 7-year survival rate of 50% in those who continue to drink alcohol compared with an 80% survival

rate in those who discontinue alcohol intake." The authors warn that survival is also affected by the presence of cirrhosis (a more advanced state than fatty liver disease). Patients with advanced alcoholic cirrhosis can survive only with a liver transplant.

See also ALCOHOLIC HEALTH PROBLEMS; ALCOHOLISM; HEPATITIS; LIVER.

Narayanan Menon, K. V., M.D., Gregory J. Gores, M.D., and Vijay H. Shah, M.D. "Pathogenesis, Diagnosis, and Treatment of Alcoholic Liver Disease," *Mayo Clinic Proceedings* 76, no. 10 (2001): 1,021–1,029.

Alcoholics Anonymous (AA)   The key organization in the United States and other countries that provides self-help and support to individuals who are addicted to alcohol. Alcoholics Anonymous was cofounded in 1935 by a man known as Bill W., a stockbroker in New York and another known as Dr. Bob S., a surgeon from Akron. Both suffered from severe alcoholism that was not responsive to treatment. Bill W. developed his own plan that emphasized sobriety and then met with Dr. Bob S., who reportedly found the idea that alcoholism was a disease to be a revelation. The two men resolved to share their concepts with others. Today the self-help organization has grown to an estimated 2 million members worldwide, including about 1 million members in the United States, an estimated 96,000 members in Canada, and members in many other countries.

Bill W. wrote the initial textbook for the organization. It describes the philosophy and methods. The textbook also emphasizes the TWELVE STEPS of recovery from alcoholism.

The only membership requirement is that the member agrees to stop drinking altogether, because Alcoholics Anonymous strongly supports ABSTINENCE (complete avoidance of alcohol). AA does not charge dues. The organization relies on groups of anonymous members to provide assistance and support to each other.

See also AL-ANON; ALATEEN; ALCOHOLISM; RECOVERY; TWELVE STEPS.

For further information about the organization, contact:

Alcoholics Anonymous World Services, Inc.
Grand Central Station
P.O. Box 459
New York, NY 10163
(212) 870-3400
http://www.alcoholics-anonymous.org

alcoholism An addiction to alcohol. Alcoholism is also known as alcohol dependence. Alcoholism has a profound effect on millions of people worldwide, including people who are alcoholics as well as their family members and others who depend on them. In 2002, the NATIONAL INSTITUTE ON ALCOHOL ABUSE AND ALCOHOLISM (NIAAA) reported that approximately 7.9 million people in the United States were alcoholics, or 3.8 percent of the population (down from an estimated 4.4 percent in 1992).

In another estimate and according to a study released by the Substance Abuse and Mental Health Services Administration, Office of Applied Studies, based on information released in 2004, in considering state averages of alcohol dependence (addiction), the nationwide average statewide percentage of alcoholism for individuals ages 12 years and older for 2002 was 3.50 percent of the population. (See table at right for ages and states.)

Few studies are available of alcohol-dependent populations in other countries. However, a 2001 report, from the World Health Organization, *Alcohol in the European Region—Consumption, Harm and Policies*, provided some data. According to this source, in 1998, 4.9 percent of males in Germany and 1.1 percent of females were alcoholics. Rates were much higher in other countries. The highest reported rate was in Finland, with a rate of 17 percent for men and 6 percent for women, followed by Croatia, with an alcoholism rate of 15 percent for men and 8 percent for women. For some countries, the rates for alcoholism were not broken down by gender; for example, the rate was simply given as 2.0 percent each for Bulgaria and Spain and 1.2 percent (the lowest reported rate) for the Netherlands.

Indicators of Alcoholism

According to the NIAAA in the United States, alcoholism is characterized by three or more of the following indicators:

PERCENTAGES REPORTING PAST YEAR ALCOHOL DEPENDENCE AMONG PERSONS AGES 12 YEARS AND OLDER, BY AGE GROUP AND STATE IN THE UNITED STATES: 2002

State	All Ages Estimate	Age 12–17	Age 18–25	26 or Older
Total	3.50	2.13	7.00	3.08
Alabama	3.20	2.08	5.61	2.92
Alaska	4.01	2.14	7.98	3.74
Arizona	3.75	2.82	7.31	3.25
Arkansas	3.33	2.78	6.27	2.89
California	3.47	1.59	6.09	3.27
Colorado	4.22	2.38	8.37	3.75
Connecticut	3.16	1.73	6.68	2.85
Delaware	3.65	1.23	8.70	3.09
District of Columbia	5.20	2.24	7.80	4.95
Florida	2.97	1.84	6.61	2.60
Georgia	3.88	1.86	5.42	3.89
Hawaii	3.44	1.99	7.43	2.98
Idaho	3.82	3.42	7.22	3.19
Illinois	3.57	2.53	6.79	3.15
Indiana	3.33	2.36	7.27	2.74
Iowa	3.25	3.26	7.24	2.50
Kansas	3.24	2.43	6.80	2.68
Kentucky	3.16	2.50	6.07	2.73
Louisiana	4.20	2.56	7.70	3.75
Maine	2.95	2.17	7.41	2.39
Maryland	3.60	1.59	6.19	3.48
Massachusetts	3.75	2.36	7.68	3.29
Michigan	4.26	2.28	7.92	3.91
Minnesota	3.47	2.48	7.83	2.83
Mississippi	3.77	1.54	5.09	3.84
Missouri	3.13	1.93	7.92	2.45
Montana	3.99	4.76	9.42	2.92
Nebraska	4.21	2.81	8.91	3.52
Nevada	3.35	2.66	5.72	3.07
New Hampshire	3.74	2.62	8.67	3.13
New Jersey	3.06	1.82	7.32	2.62
New Mexico	4.35	2.77	10.23	3.51
New York	3.84	2.31	6.64	3.57
North Carolina	3.69	2.10	6.43	3.43
North Dakota	4.20	4.52	8.88	3.19
Ohio	3.46	1.62	8.31	2.88
Oklahoma	3.07	2.12	6.92	2.46
Oregon	3.12	1.83	7.60	2.53
Pennsylvania	2.79	2.16	6.76	2.23
Rhode Island	4.13	2.59	11.96	2.90
South Carolina	4.07	1.85	7.31	3.79

State	All Ages Estimate	Age 12–17	Age 18–25	26 or Older
South Dakota	4.22	3.90	9.19	3.31
Tennessee	3.12	2.37	6.39	2.67
Texas	3.32	1.85	6.73	2.89
Utah	3.62	1.88	7.03	2.94
Vermont	3.38	2.96	7.90	2.68
Virginia	3.95	2.91	7.96	3.44
Washington	3.05	1.73	7.19	2.54
West Virginia	2.83	3.20	5.62	2.34
Wisconsin	3.82	2.98	9.39	2.94
Wyoming	4.00	2.81	9.30	3.19

Source: Wright, D. *State Estimates of Substance Use from the 2002 National Survey on Drug Use and Health.* Department of Health and Human Services Publication No. SMA 04-3907, NSDUH Series H-23. Substance Abuse and Mental Health Services Administration, Office of Applied Studies, Rockville, Md.: August 2004.

- A TOLERANCE to alcohol (more alcohol is needed to achieve intoxication than in the past)

- WITHDRAWAL symptoms (when alcohol is not consumed, physical symptoms occur, such as nausea, sweating, and shakiness)

- Use of the substance in a larger quantity than intended

- The persistent desire to cut down or to control the use of alcohol

- A significant amount of time spent on obtaining, using, or recovering from alcohol

- Drinking that occurs to avoid the symptoms of withdrawal

- Neglect of an individual's normal social, occupational, or recreational tasks

- Continued use of alcohol despite physical and psychological problems of the user

Patients with Alcoholism

In general, males are more likely to become alcohol dependent than females, although some women are also alcoholics. In the 12-month prevalence and trends report discussed in a 2004 issue of *Drug and Alcohol Dependence,* statistical comparison data was based on the National Institute on Alcohol Abuse and Alcoholism's 2001–02 National Epidemiologic Survey on Alcohol and Related Conditions and the NIAAA 1991–92 National Longitudinal Alcohol Epidemiological Survey. Each survey had greater than 42,000 subjects.

Researchers found that about 5 percent of males were alcoholics, compared with 2 percent of females. At some age ranges, certain male racial groups had the highest rates of alcoholism. For example, between the ages of 18–29 years, nearly 16 percent of Native Americans were alcoholics, followed closely by 15 percent of white males of the same age. Among females, Native American women ages 18–29 had the highest percent of alcoholics (nearly 8 percent), followed by white women of the same age (about 6 percent).

Many people need treatment for their alcoholism. According to the *2002 National Survey on Drug Use and Health,* 1.5 million people received treatment for their alcohol use in 2002. However, an estimated 17.1 million people needed treatment. The reasons for their nontreatment are unknown. It is known that many alcoholics adamantly deny that they have a problem and refuse treatment. Thus this is clearly one factor in nontreatment.

Causes of Alcoholism/Genetic Studies

Scientists have studied the causes of alcoholism for many years, including possible genetic links, ties to depressive psychiatric patterns, and many other possibilities. Saying that alcoholism is a complex and multifactorial illness is probably fair.

Many studies strongly indicate a genetic predisposition to alcoholism. Both twin and adoption studies have shown that children raised apart from their biological relatives have an increased propensity to drink in patterns that are more like their birthparents' behavior than that of their adoptive parents. At the same time, other studies have also shown that adopted adults are also *less* likely to be alcoholic than their biological siblings who were reared by their biological parents, thus indicating that environment, as well as heredity, plays a role in the development of alcoholism.

In a large study of greater than 1,000 alcoholic subjects and their families called the Collaborative Study on the Genetics of Alcoholism, described in a 2002 issue of *Alcohol Research & Health*, the researchers sought to find genetic, psychological, electrophysiological, and physiological traits of the participants. They found several key linkages. For example, they found evidence for a genetic linkage in sibling pairs on the traits of alcoholism and depression, located on chromosome 1. They also found evidence of a possible genetic link to alcohol dependence on chromosome 4.

It is important to understand that a genetic predisposition does not automatically doom a person to become an alcoholic. Most people do not become alcoholics, with or without such a predisposition. A predisposition indicates only an increased risk of becoming an alcoholic. Thus, even if a person is born to two alcoholic parents, he or she will not necessarily become an alcoholic, although the risks for this person are increased over individuals who are born to other families with nonalcoholic parents, both because of genetics and environment. Some people develop alcoholism when their parents are not alcoholics and when no one else in the family has any apparent problems with alcoholism or drinking.

Family Members of Alcoholics

Life with an alcoholic can be very difficult for family members. They are at risk for both neglect and abuse. Attempts to help the alcoholic stop drinking are frequently futile. Such attempts may include taking the car keys to prevent the individual from going out to drink (which is not the same thing as taking the keys to prevent an already intoxicated person from driving, which *is* an advisable act) or pleading with him or her not to drink.

Some behaviors that are meant to be helpful may instead have the unwanted effect of making it more possible for the alcoholic to continue drinking. Such "enabling" acts may include helping to care for the alcoholic during a hangover, calling in sick to an employer for the alcoholic, lending money when the alcoholic has none, and speaking on his or her behalf in court when the individual is arrested for a crime related to drinking.

Some experts recommend that family members take the following steps:

- Stop covering up for the alcoholic. Many family members make constant excuses for the alcoholic as well as literally cleaning up after them. Experts recommend that the alcoholic be allowed to experience the full consequences of

his or her drinking, even though these consequences may be painful for family members as well.

- Arrange an INTERVENTION. Talk to the alcoholic when he or she is sober after an alcohol-related problem, such as an argument or a car crash, has occurred. Consider a group intervention. This approach involves a group of people confronting the alcoholic with the effects of his or her behavior. An intervention should be used only with the help of a trained health care professional.

- State results and provide consequences. Tell the alcoholic that you want him or her to get help and describe what you will do if he or she does not get help for the alcohol problem. Explain that you will do this not as a punishment but as a protection for yourself and the family. However, no ultimatums should be delivered that are not acted on if the alcoholic person does not seek help. Follow through on them.

- Obtain information from the local community. Find out what resources are in your area. Locate the local ALCOHOLICS ANONYMOUS meeting place.

- Ask a friend to help you talk to the alcoholic person. A recovering alcoholic or another person who is nonjudgmental may be a good choice.

- Find support for yourself. Living with an alcoholic can be extremely difficult for family members to cope with. Organizations such as AL-ANON can help. Family members may also need counseling for DEPRESSION.

Diagnosis and Treatment of Alcoholism

Many experts ask individuals to self-evaluate using the CAGE questionnaire, which asks the following questions:

- Have you ever felt the need to **C**ut down on your drinking? (C)

- Have you ever felt **A**nnoyed by criticism of your drinking? (A)

- Have you ever had **G**uilty feelings about your drinking? (G)

- Have you ever taken a morning **E**ye opener? (E)

If a person answers "yes" to even one of the CAGE criteria, then this suggests that the individual needs to be evaluated for alcoholism. If the person answers "yes" to two or more questions, the person is likely an alcoholic. However, one problem with the CAGE questions is that they do not distinguish between the past and present use of alcohol, and thus a recovering alcoholic may also respond positively to two or more questions.

Physicians diagnose alcoholism on the basis of answers to medical history questions as well as on the patient's physical appearance and the results of laboratory tests. For example, the patient may deny having a problem with alcohol yet he or she presents in the doctor's office with bloodshot eyes and tremors. Routine liver function tests may show elevated levels, and a liver scan may show an enlarged liver. These are possible indicators of alcoholism.

If there is an acute problem and the alcoholic patient is undergoing WITHDRAWAL—particularly when he or she is in the state of DELIRIUM TREMENS and has severe symptoms, such as HALLUCINATIONS, mental confusion, seizures and dehydration—the patient should be admitted to the hospital for treatment and monitoring. This is especially true if individuals are ELDERLY, because in such cases, their lives are in danger. Withdrawal from alcohol can be especially dangerous for the long-term elderly alcoholic patient, although detoxification under medical monitoring is advisable.

Alcoholism can be difficult to treat, but many patients have recovered from this problem. Millions of patients have benefited from joining self-help groups, most prominently Alcoholics Anonymous, a group that actively promotes ABSTINENCE from alcohol.

Some patients benefit from medication therapy, such as from ANTABUSE (disulfiram), an aversive drug that causes copious vomiting if any alcohol is consumed. NALTREXONE is a newer drug that has been found by many to be effective in treating alcoholism. Some patients improve with ANTIDEPRESSANTS. Anticonvulsants are often used, such as carbamazepine, particularly to help with withdrawal symptoms from alcohol.

Patients with alcoholism also need psychological counseling to overcome distortions in their thinking about themselves and other people. Many patients with alcoholism benefit from residential treatment.

Alcoholism and Psychiatric Disorders

Many patients with alcoholism have other illnesses, such as DEPRESSION, ANXIETY DISORDERS, and BIPOLAR DISORDER. Both the psychiatric problem and the alcoholism must be treated. If not, the alcoholism (or the psychiatric problem) may resolve but then other addictive behaviors or psychiatric problems are likely to develop, and the cycle will begin again.

Psychiatric problems are common   In a table of an overview of the comorbidity (coexistence) of psychiatric disorders with alcoholism in a 2002 issue of *Alcohol Research & Health,* based on the National Comorbidity Survey in 1996 and the Epidemiologic Catchment Study in 1990, the researchers showed that in a one-year period, 29.2 percent of patients with alcoholism had mood disorders. They also calculated the odds ratio to be 3.6. This means that a person with alcohol dependence was 3.6 times more likely to suffer from a mood disorder than a person who was not an alcoholic. Most of the risk of a mood disorder lay with major depressive disorder, or 27.9 percent of the 29.2 percent.

The researchers also found that over one year, 36.9 percent of alcoholic patients had a risk of suffering from anxiety disorders, and the calculated risk ratio was 2.6 (see table at top of page 18). The anxiety disorders were further divided into generalized anxiety disorder, panic disorder, and posttraumatic stress disorder. The researchers found that for alcoholics, 11.6 percent had a risk of developing generalized anxiety disorder, and their odd ratio was 4.6. Thus, they had nearly five times the risk of the nonalcoholic person of developing generalized anxiety disorder.

Researchers also found that psychiatric problems were significantly greater for people with alcoholism than for people with alcohol abuse. For example, 29.2 percent of alcoholics had a problem with mood disorders, but the rate of mood disorders among those with alcohol abuse was 12.3 percent. That is about the same rate as found in the general population.

As can be seen from the table on page 18, people with alcoholism have a high rate of posttraumatic stress disorder, and nearly 8 percent of alcoholics have this problem. Whether mental illness causes

PREVALENCE OF PSYCHIATRIC DISORDERS IN PEOPLE WITH ALCOHOL DEPENDENCE (ALCOHOLISM)

Comorbid Disorder	One-Year Rate (Percent)	Odds Ratio
Mood disorders	29.2	3.6
Major depressive disorder	27.9	3.9
Bipolar disorder	1.9	6.3
Anxiety disorders	36.9	2.6
Generalized anxiety disorder	11.6	4.6
Panic disorder	3.9	1.7
Posttraumatic stress disorder	7.7	2.2
Schizophrenia	24	3.8

Source: Petrakis, Ismene L., M.D., et al. "Comorbidity of Alcoholism and Psychiatric Disorders," *Alcohol Research & Health* 26, 2 (2002): 81–89.

alcoholism or whether alcoholism triggers mental illness is unknown. In the case of SCHIZOPHRENIA, a thought disorder characterized by delusions (false beliefs) and confused thinking, one of the entries on Table II, individuals with schizophrenia may consume alcohol in an attempt to self-medicate troubling thoughts.

Depression   Research has indicated that prior alcohol dependence increased the risk for major depressive disorder more than fourfold. Often it is not clear, however, whether SUBSTANCE ABUSE is the driving factor in depression or if undiagnosed depression leads some individuals to drink in an attempt to self-medicate their symptoms. In a study described in a 2002 issue of the *Archives of General Psychiatry*, the researchers discussed their findings on 6,050 former drinkers. They found that prior alcohol dependence increased the risk of developing subsequent major depressive disorder by more than four times.

The researchers said, "These findings, in conjunction with other findings that depression during abstinence is a risk factor for relapse, suggest that treatment for depression should not be withheld from alcoholics in stable remission on the assumption that any depressions in such individuals are due to protracted intoxications or withdrawal effects."

Bipolar disorder   Patients with bipolar disorder, also known as manic depressive disorder or manic depression, are often alcohol abusers or alcoholics.

The National Institute of Mental Health's Epidemiologic Catchment Area study in 1990 demonstrated that about 61 percent of patients with bipolar I disorder had a lifetime diagnosis of a substance use disorder (an alcohol or drug use disorder). In addition, 39 percent of patients with bipolar II disorder had an alcohol use disorder. The researchers also found that mania in bipolar I disorder and alcohol use disorders were 6.2 times more likely to occur than would be expected by chance.

The reason for the comorbidity (co-occurrence) of alcoholism and bipolar disorder may be that some psychiatric disorders, such as bipolar disorder, are risk factors for substance abuse. Alternatively, people with untreated bipolar disorder may be more likely to abuse alcohol during manic episodes in an attempt to self-medicate, either to prolong pleasurable states or to sedate their mania. Studies indicate that patients with bipolar disorder and alcoholism may do better when treated than alcoholic patients with other mood disorders. Treatment includes medications such as lithium and valproate (Depakote).

Eating disorders   Patients with alcoholism have an increased risk for eating disorders such as ANOREXIA NERVOSA, BINGE EATING DISORDER, and BULIMIA NERVOSA, according to research reported by Carlos M. Grilo and colleagues in a 2002 issue of *Alcohol Research & Health*. Cognitive behavioral therapy may be effective in treating both the alcoholism and the eating disorder. This form of therapy helps the patient challenge irrational ideas they hold about themselves and their lives and replace them with realistic ideas and new coping skills.

Medication may be very important for alcoholics with psychiatric problems   Alcoholics who also have psychiatric problems may especially need to have medication considered in their cases, according to Dr. Petrakis and colleagues. One reason is that they may have great difficulties finding and using self-help groups. "For example, people with pronounced paranoia or negative symptoms (e.g., social and emotional withdrawal) may be uncomfortable in a group setting or with a treatment approach that includes confrontation."

In addition, patients with psychiatric problems are often familiar with and accepting of taking medications for their illness. Patients with psychiatric problems may also find it difficult to complete assignments or treatments that depend on cognitive behavioral therapy because slowed thinking caused by depression or other psychiatric problems impede their thinking.

A few studies have been done on the use of disulfiram (Antabuse) and patients with comorbid conditions. However, some older clinical reports indicated that high doses of the drug may have triggered psychotic symptoms. Most doctors are still concerned about using the drug with patients because of these reports.

Naltrexone is a more modern medication used to treat alcoholics, and it has also been used in patients with mental illnesses and alcoholism. According to Dr. Petrakis and colleagues, a chart review of naltrexone on 72 patients with major psychiatric illnesses, including schizophrenia, bipolar disorder, schizoaffective disorder, and alcohol dependence, suggested a good clinical response to naltrexone.

Antidepressants are sometimes used to treat patients with alcoholism and mood disorders, particularly selective serotonin reuptake inhibitors (SSRIs). These drugs affect the production and/or the absorption of serotonin, a neurotransmitter. Fluoxetine (Prozac) is one example of an SSRI, and there are many others.

BENZODIAZEPINES may be helpful with this population, especially among patients with anxiety disorders. However, benzodiazepines also have abuse potential. Consequently, physicians must prescribe them carefully and prudently. In particular, benzodiazipines should not be prescribed to anyone with a history of past abuse with this drug. Benzodiazepines are also used to help patients with their detoxification from alcoholism.

To locate a drug or alcohol treatment facility on the Internet, go to the Substance Abuse and Mental Health Services Administration at http://findtreatment.samhsa.gov/facilitylocatordoc.htm.

See also ALATEEN; ALCOHOL; ALCOHOL ABUSE; ALCOHOL/ALCOHOL CONSUMPTION; ALCOHOLIC HEALTH PROBLEMS; ALCOHOLIC HEPATITIS; ALCOHOL POISONING; ANTABUSE; BINGE DRINKING; CIRRHOSIS; CODEPENDENCY; COLLEGE STUDENTS; DRIVING WHILE INTOXICATED/DRIVING UNDER THE INFLUENCE; DUAL DIAGNOSIS; FATTY LIVER DISEASE/STEATOSIS; FETAL ALCOHOL SYNDROME; HEPATITIS; TEENAGE AND YOUTH DRINKING; TWELVE STEPS.

For further information on alcoholism, contact the following organizations:

Al-Anon
1600 Corporate Landing Parkway
Virginia Beach, VA 23454
(888) 425-2666 (toll-free)
http://www.al-anon.org

Alcoholics Anonymous
Grand Central Station
P.O. Box 459
New York, NY 10163
(212) 870-3400
http://www.alcoholics-anonymous.org

National Association for Children of Alcoholics (NaCoa)
11426 Pike
Suite 100
Rockville, MD 20852
(888) 55-4COAS (toll-free)
http://www.nacoa.net

National Council on Alcoholism and Drug Dependence (NCADD)
20 Exchange Place
Suite 2902
New York, NY 10005
(800) 622-2255 (toll-free)
http://www.ncadd.org

National Institute on Alcohol Abuse and Alcoholism (NIAAA)
6000 Executive Boulevard, Wilco Building
Bethesda, MD 20892
http://www.niaaa.nih.gov

Adamec, Christine and William Pierce. *The Encyclopedia of Adoption.* New York, N.Y.: Facts On File, Inc., 2000.

Bierut, Laura Jean, M.D. "Defining Alcohol-Related Phenotypes in Humans: The Collaborative Study on the Genetics of Alcoholism," *Alcohol Research & Health* 26, 3 (2002): 208–213.

Book, Sarah W., M.D. and Carrie L. Randall. "Social Anxiety Disorder and Alcohol Use," *Alcohol Research & Health* 26, 2 (2002): 130–135.

Drake, Robert E., M.D. and Kim T. Mueser. "Co-Occurring Alcohol Use Disorder and Schizophrenia," *Alcohol Research & Health* 26, 2 (2002): 99–102.

Galvan, Frank H. and Raul Caetano, M.D. "Alcohol Use and Related Problems Among Ethnic Minorities in the

United States," *Alcohol Research & Health* 27, 1 (2003): 87–94.

Garbutt, James C., M.D., et al. "Pharmacological Treatment of Alcohol Dependence," *Journal of the American Medical Association* 281, 14 (April 14, 1999): 1,318–1,325.

Grant Bridget F., et al. "The 12-Month Prevalence and Trends in DSM-IV Alcohol Abuse and Dependence: United States, 1991–1992 and 2001–2002," *Drug and Alcohol Dependence* 74, no. 3 (2004): 223–234.

Grilo, Carlos M., et al. "Eating Disorders and Alcohol Use Disorders," *Alcohol Research & Health* 26, 2 (2002): 151–160.

Hasin, Deborah S. and Bridget F. Grant. "Major Depression in 6050 Former Drinkers: Association with Past Alcohol Dependence," *Archives of General Psychiatry* 59 (September 2002): 794–800.

Kosten, Thomas R., M.D. and Patrick G. O'Connor, M.D. "Management of Drug and Alcohol Withdrawal," *New England Journal of Medicine* 348, no. 18 (May 1, 2003): 1,786–1,795.

Li, Ting-Kai, M.D. "The Genetics of Alcoholism," *Alcohol Alert,* National Institute on Alcohol Abuse and Alcoholism, 60 (July 2003).

O'Connor, Patrick G., M.D. and Richard S. Schottenfeld, M.D. "Patients with Alcohol Problems," *New England Journal of Medicine* 338, no. 9 (February 26, 1998): 592–602.

Petrakis, Ismene L., M.D., et al. "Comorbidity of Alcoholism and Psychiatric Disorders," *Alcohol Research & Health* 26, no. 2 (2002): 81–89.

Rehn, Nina with Robin Room and Griffith Edwards. *Alcohol in the European Region—Consumption, Harm and Policies.* World Health Organization Regional Office for Europe, 2001.

Schneider, Robert K., M.D., James L. Levenson, M.D., and Sidney H. Schnoll, M.D. "Update in Addiction Medicine," *Annals of Internal Medicine* 134, (2001): 387–395.

Shivani, Ramesh, M.D., Jeffrey Goldsmith, M.D., and Robert M. Anthenelli, M.D. "Alcoholism and Psychiatric Disorders: Diagnostic Challenges," *Alcohol Research & Health* 26, no. 2 (2002): 90–98.

Sonne, Susan C. and Kathleen T. Brady, M.D. "Bipolar Disorder and Alcoholism," *Alcohol Research and Health* 26, no. 2 (2002): 103–108.

alcohol laws Statutes setting limits for who may consume alcohol and under what conditions. Each state in the United States has its own laws on alcohol consumption, although all states ban drinking for individuals younger than age 21. The state laws vary on the legal definition of what BLOOD ALCOHOL LEVEL constitutes driving while intoxicated, also

known as driving under the influence. Some states use a Breathalyzer test to determine whether an individual is legally intoxicated. In some states, if a person who is suspected by law enforcement officials of exceeding the legal limit for alcohol while driving refuses to take a blood or breath test, then he or she is assumed guilty.

State laws vary regarding establishments that may serve alcohol, the licenses that must be obtained from facilities that serve alcohol, and many other aspects of alcohol provision and consumption. In some states, the state itself sells all alcohol.

See also ALCOHOL BREATH TESTS; DRIVING, IMPAIRED; DRIVING WHILE INTOXICATED/DRIVING UNDER THE INFLUENCE; ETHANOL.

alcohol poisoning Refers to the very heavy consumption of alcohol over such a short period that the liver is unable to metabolize the alcohol rapidly enough and the individual may die. An individual with alcohol poisoning may have a blood alcohol level as high as 0.4, which is five times the legal limit for operating a motor vehicle in states throughout the United States.

An estimated 300 people died of alcohol poisoning in 1998 in the United States, including 245 males and 55 females. Experts report that individuals who are at the greatest risk for alcohol poisoning are males ages 35–54 years.

About 2 percent of alcohol poisoning deaths occur to individuals under age 21 according to Young-Hee Yoon and colleagues in their 2003 article for *Alcohol Research & Health*. Hispanic males and non-Hispanic black males have the highest risk of suffering from alcohol poisoning. Among females, non-Hispanic black females have the greatest risk of alcohol poisoning, although the overall risks are low for females. Divorced or widowed males and females have higher risks of alcohol poisoning than married or never-married individuals.

Accidental alcohol poisoning was a contributing cause of death in an additional 1,158 cases, including 965 males and 193 females. (See table on page 21.)

Some cases of alcohol poisoning occur on college campuses. Students frequently engage in BINGE DRINKING, imbibing very large quantities of

DEATHS FROM ACCIDENTAL ALCOHOL POISONING AS THE UNDERLYING OR CONTRIBUTING CAUSE, BY SEX, UNITED STATES, 1996–1998

	All Races, Both Sexes	All Races, Male	All Races, Female
Accidental alcohol poisoning deaths, underlying cause			
1998	300	245	55
1997	342	266	76
1996	308	246	62
Annual average	317	252	64
Accidental alcohol poisoning deaths, contributing cause			
1998	1,158	965	193
1997	1,104	931	173
1996	967	799	168
Annual average	1,076	898	178
Accidental alcohol poisoning deaths, multiple causes			
1998	1,458	1,210	248
1997	1,446	1,197	249
1996	1,275	1,045	230
Annual average	1,393	1,151	242

Source: Yoon, Young-Hee, et al. "Accidental Alcohol Poisoning Mortality in the United States, 1996–1998," *Alcohol Research & Health, NIAAA's Epidemiological Bulletin No. 40,* 113.

alcohol as a part of a fraternity or sorority ritual or on other occasions or to impress their peers.

See also ALCOHOL BREATH TESTS; ALCOHOL/ALCOHOL CONSUMPTION; ALCOHOLISM; ALCOHOL LAWS; BLACKOUTS, ALCOHOLIC; COLLEGE STUDENTS; DRINKING GAMES; TEENAGE AND YOUTH DRINKING.

Yoon, Young-Hee, et al. "Accidental Alcohol Poisoning Mortality in the United States, 1996–1998," *Alcohol Research & Health* 27, no. 1 (2003): 110–118.

American Psychiatric Association   National organization of psychiatrists (medical doctors who practice psychiatry). Some psychiatrists treat patients who are addicted to drugs and/or alcohol, while others concentrate on patients with emotional problems or issues not complicated by addictions.

For further information, contact:

American Psychiatric Association
1400 K Street NW
Washington, DC 20005
(202) 682-6000
http://www.psych.org

American Psychological Association   A scientific and professional organization with more than 150,000 members and the largest association of psychologists in the world. Psychologists may counsel patients with a variety of addictive behaviors.

For further information, contact:

American Psychological Association
750 First Street NE
Washington, DC 20002
(202) 336-5500
http://www.apa.org

amphetamine psychosis   A usually temporary but severe psychotic condition that is induced by the excessive use of AMPHETAMINES. Continuous heavy use of amphetamines for a week or more can induce a state of extreme psychosis in some individuals. This causes delusions, visual and auditory hallucinations and persecutory delusions, and can also lead individuals who are in this state to commit acts of violence. The symptoms of amphetamine psychosis may be indistinguishable from paranoid SCHIZOPHRENIA, which is why a drug screening is needed to test for amphetamines as part of the diagnosis. A similar psychotic state can sometimes be triggered by the abuse of METHAMPHETAMINES or COCAINE.

When the effects of the amphetamines wear off within a day or two after washout (no more amphetamines are taken), the individual usually recovers from the psychosis. However, according to experts, some individuals (about 5–15 percent) will not recover and instead will remain in a psychotic state.

Those patients who are most likely to remain psychotic were usually addicted to amphetamines prior to their psychotic breakdown. Many also took very high doses of amphetamines prior to the onset of their psychotic breakdown and experienced psychiatric symptoms before they ever began using amphetamines. It is also possible that the amphetamine abuse may have somehow triggered an underlying and preexisting psychiatric problem.

Patients who are diagnosed with an amphetamine psychosis usually need to be hospitalized in a psychiatric facility because they are a danger to themselves and to others. Psychiatrists may administer antipsychotic medications and BENZODIAZEPINES to counter the psychotic symptoms. Some experts recommend the administration of ascorbic acid to speed up the kidney's elimination of the amphetamines from the body.

In a study of a population of prisoners in England and Wales, researchers found a link between the early use of drugs (before age 16) such as cocaine or amphetamine and the subsequent development of psychosis, reporting on their findings in the *British Journal of Psychiatry.* Another risk factor for psychosis was prior drug dependence (addiction).

In this study of 503 prisoners (of whom 78 percent were male and 83 percent were white), about 10 percent of the prisoners were diagnosed with a psychotic disorder. This level of psychosis is about 20 times higher than normally expected in the general population. According to the researchers, "Early use of cocaine and amphetamines almost triples the risk of psychosis in addition to the effect exerted by drug dependence."

The researchers speculated that perhaps individuals with a predisposition to mental illness are more likely to use drugs in adolescence or that there may be a "period of special vulnerability to psychosis." The researchers also looked at the risk for psychosis and alcohol abuse, as well as opioids and heroin, but did not find such a linkage.

See also DUAL DIAGNOSIS; PSYCHIATRISTS; PSYCHOTIC BREAK.

Department of Mental Health and Substance Dependence, Management of Substance Dependence Review Series, *Systematic Review of Treatment for Amphetamine-Related Disorders.* Geneva, Switzerland: World Health Organization, 2001.

Farrell, M., et al. "Psychosis and Drug Dependence: Results from a National Survey of Prisoners," *British Journal of Psychiatry* 181, no. 5 (2002): 393–398.

amphetamines Central nervous system stimulants. Amphetamines may be taken orally, smoked, or injected. First synthesized in the late 1930s, amphetamines are prescribed schedule II drugs under the CONTROLLED SUBSTANCES ACT.

Originally used extensively as DIET PILLS because of their appetite-suppressing qualities, physicians are discouraged from prescribing amphetamines for that purpose in the United States today. According to the National Institutes of Health, when used for this purpose, amphetamines may be dangerous to health.

The peak of amphetamine abuse occurred in the United States and other countries in the 1960s. However, amphetamines are still abused by significant numbers of individuals in the 21st century and continue to be dangerous drugs when abused.

According to Dr. Ellinwood and his colleagues in their article on chronic amphetamine use and abuse, an amphetamine epidemic became a problem in Japan in the 1950s when leftover amphetamine supplies from World War II that had been created for soldiers in combat fatigue situations were freely given out to the general population. When the negative effects of these amphetamines were observed on people, sanctions were applied. In the 1980s, a second-wave epidemic occurred in Japan, based on illegally manufactured METHAMPHETAMINE.

In the United States, the first heavy use of amphetamines occurred in the 1960s and ended in the 1970s with production controls and governmental limitations. In the 1980s, illegally manufactured methamphetamine became a factor in the United States as it did in Japan and other countries.

Some truckers, athletes, and college students have also used amphetamine drugs in order to remain alert. Some have become addicted to them.

A controversial use of amphetamines has been to give them to military combat pilots from the United States in wartime situations. Some experts believe this is dangerous because of the addictive nature of the drugs. Others believe that as long as the drugs are taken over the short term and carefully monitored, they are safe enough to use for this purpose. Amphetamines were commonly used by soldiers during World War II, and their military "kitbags" contained Benzedrine tablets. At that time, it was unknown that amphetamines could be harmful or addictive.

Legal Uses of Amphetamines

Some forms of amphetamines are used for medical purposes in the United States. For example, amphetamines are used to treat individuals with ATTENTION DEFICIT HYPERACTIVITY DISORDER (ADHD). Dexedrine is an example of a legally prescribed amphetamine for ADHD.

Experts report that individuals with ADHD typically do not experience the EUPHORIA or rush from the drug that is felt by those who do not have

ADHD. Instead, if the drug is effective for them, over time individuals with ADHD experience an improved ability to concentrate and focus, and they are less distractible and less restless.

Short-Term and Long-Term Effects of Amphetamines

Over the short term, amphetamine use may cause a feeling of euphoria, increased confidence, and greater energy (unless the individual has been diagnosed with ADHD). Patients may experience decreased appetite and increased heart rate. Side effects from the drug may include fatigue, depression, and anxiety. Some patients experience an increased appetite.

The excessive and long-term abuse of amphetamines may lead to aggression, irritability, and even an AMPHETAMINE PSYCHOSIS that can be difficult to distinguish from schizophrenia. (Some experts believe that an underlying schizophrenia may have been triggered by the use of the drug.)

Indications of Amphetamine Dependence/Addiction

Although not everyone who takes amphetamines develops a problem with the drug, some people do abuse amphetamines or become addicted to them. Some indications of a problem with an addiction to amphetamines are as follows:

- Difficulty sleeping
- Serious loss of appetite
- Loss of sex drive
- Paranoid thoughts and behavior
- Problems with missing work or school
- Participation in uncharacteristic and risky behavior
- Inability to cut back or stop taking the drug
- Use of high doses of the drug in a bingelike fashion

Withdrawal from Amphetamines

When individuals are addicted to amphetamines, withdrawal can be difficult and should be done only under a doctor's care. The emergency room of a hospital is not the best place to withdraw from drugs, although it is the place where some addicted individuals are delivered by concerned family members and friends when the health of the ill person is clearly in jeopardy. Some withdrawal symptoms from amphetamines may include:

- Shakiness
- Nausea and vomiting
- HALLUCINATIONS
- Seizures
- Severe anxiety
- Insomnia
- Heavy sweating
- Increased pulse rate
- Excessive sleepiness
- DEPRESSION

Numbers in Emergency Treatment for Amphetamine Abuse

When individuals abuse amphetamines, they may require urgent medical attention. In 2002, according to the Drug Awareness Warning Network, which is information provided by emergency room hospitals nationwide in the United States, an estimated 21,644 total emergency room visits were caused by amphetamines. This number was up from 18,555 visits in 2001 and also sharply up from earlier years.

What is responsible for this increase in amphetamine abuse is unknown. However, some experts speculate that the increase may have been due to users of methamphetamine. The toxicology finding of amphetamine in the emergency room does not differentiate between amphetamine and methamphetamine.

Illegally derived methamphetamine was the primary substance of abuse in more than 80 percent of 98,000 SUBSTANCE ABUSE treatment admissions in 2001 in the United States, according to the Office of Applied Studies in a 2004 *DASIS Report*. It was also the identified factor in 17,696 emergency department visits in 2002. (There is also a legal use of methamphetamine hydrochloride [Desoxyn] for treatment of ADHD.)

Treatment for Amphetamine Dependency

Individuals addicted to amphetamines will need to undergo withdrawal from the drug. Physicians may help them through the process with ANTIDE-PRESSANTS, sedatives, and other medications. Self-help groups such as NARCOTICS ANONYMOUS help many people overcome the problems that led to their addiction. Some patients need an inpatient treatment program.

See also DRUG ADDICTION; DUAL DIAGNOSIS; EMERGENCY TREATMENT.

Cami, Jordi, M.D. and Magi Farre, M.D. "Drug Addiction," *New England Journal of Medicine* 349, no. 10 (September 4, 2003): 975–986.

Ellinwood, Everett H. M.D., George King, and Tong H. Lee, M.D. "Chronic Amphetamine Use and Abuse," Available online. URL: http://www.acnp.org/g4/GN401000166/CH162.htm Downloaded on June 2, 2004.

Substance Abuse and Mental Health Services Administration. *Emergency Department Trends from the Drug Abuse Warning Network, Final Estimates 1995–2002.* DHHS Publication No. (SMA) 03–3780. Rockville, Md.: Office of Applied Studies, July 2003.

anabolic steroids   Prescribed drugs that are based on synthesized male hormones.

Anabolic steroids have a variety of legitimate medical uses. Physicians may prescribe them to patients who have such diverse conditions as a delayed puberty, a low red blood cell count, a loss of testicle function, or a general physical deterioration caused by surgery or illness. Illegal anabolic steroids are abused, primarily by males wishing to increase their muscle mass. It is unknown how steroidal supplements cause an increase in muscle mass.

According to the DRUG ENFORCEMENT ADMINISTRATION (DEA), the most commonly abused anabolic steroids are Deca-Curabolin, Curabolin, and Winstrol, as well as Equipoise, a veterinary drug. The DEA says that some steroid abusers become addicted, although the number of addicts is unknown.

Taking anabolic steroids for nonmedical purposes is illegal, and abuse and addiction can cause serious long-term health problems. The Anabolic Steroids Control Act of 1990 categorized anabolic steroids as Schedule III SCHEDULED DRUGS under the CONTROLLED SUBSTANCES ACT because of their addiction potential.

Despite this, the National Institute on Drug Abuse has estimated that more than a half million students in the eighth and 10th grades have used anabolic steroids. Other studies, such as the Substance Abuse and Mental Health Services Administration's National Household Survey on Drug Abuse, have shown that nearly 1.1 million Americans have used anabolic steroids.

Users may obtain the drugs illegally from physical trainers or from mail-order houses or Internet outlets. Some steroids are illegally diverted from pharmacies, while others are synthesized in clandestine laboratories in the United States and other countries. Anabolic steroids are also smuggled in from other countries, such as Mexico and European countries. The drugs may be marketed as quick and easy ways to build up muscle mass or even to lose weight quickly, while the dangerous side effects are minimized or not mentioned at all.

Reasons for Anabolic Steroid Abuse

Many people take illegal steroids to improve their athletic performance and/or their muscle mass. However, some individuals abuse anabolic steroids because they have a behavioral syndrome (muscle dysphoria) in which the individual has a distorted view of his or her appearance; for example, the male may view himself as weak and small, despite his average or above-average muscular appearance. The female may see herself as flabby and fat, although she may be muscular and lean.

Some people abuse steroids because they wish to protect themselves better and think that a more muscular body will deter others from attacking them. They may have been sexually abused in the past. According to the National Institute on Drug Abuse, one series of interviews with male weightlifters who were also steroid abusers revealed that 25 percent had memories of childhood physical or sexual abuse. Another study of female weightlifters found that twice as many of the women who had been raped were using steroids, compared to weightlifters who did not abuse steroids. Most of the women who had been raped said they increased their bodybuilding dramatically after the rape. These women believed if they were more muscular, they could discourage further attacks.

Some adolescents abuse anabolic steroids as part of a pattern of high-risk behaviors, such as not wearing a motorcycle helmet, drinking and driving, and abusing other illegal drugs.

Forms of Illegal Anabolic Steroids

The drug can be administered orally or by intramuscular or subcutaneous injection as well as by pellet implantation under the skin or in transdermal patches or gels. When the drug is abused, it is generally taken orally or by injection. According to the DEA, individuals who abuse anabolic steroids may ingest from one to 100 times the normal therapeutic dose of the drug. Even more dangerous, abusers may take several different anabolic steroids at the same time.

Possible Consequences of Anabolic Steroid Abuse

Men abusing anabolic steroids may experience early balding, shrunken testicles, and gynecomastia (abnormal breast development). They may also lose their sexual drive and experience lowered levels of male hormones and diminished sperm production.

Women who abuse anabolic steroids may develop increased facial hair growth, decreased breast size, and a permanently deepened voice. They may also experience changes in their menstrual cycles.

Anabolic steroids may impair fertility in both men and women. The drug may also cause mood swings, including mania that can lead to violent behavior. Users may also suffer from DEPRESSION, delusions, and impaired judgment. In addition, they may experience problems with hypertension and high blood cholesterol levels that can lead to cardiovascular problems, such as stroke and heart attack. Severe acne is another side effect of anabolic steroid abuse.

Other physical side effects of the abuse or addiction of anabolic steroids include the risk of liver disease. The risk of contracting a sexually transmitted disease from sharing of needles, such as the human immunodeficiency virus or other bloodborne diseases, is also increased.

When adolescents abuse anabolic steroids, they may disrupt their normal bone growth and development. As a result, they may attain a shorter height than they would have achieved without the steroids.

See also ATHLETES; TEENAGE AND YOUTH DRUG ABUSE; VIOLENCE.

Drug Enforcement Administration, Office of Diversion Control. *Steroid Abuse in Today's Society: A Guide for Understanding Steroids and Related Substances.* U.S. Department of Justice, March 2004. Available online. URL: http://www.deadiversion.usdoj.gov/pubs/brochures/steroids/professionals/. Accessed on June 15, 2004.

National Institute on Drug Abuse. *Anabolic Steroid Abuse,* NIH Publication number 00-3721, Washington, D.C., National Institute on Drug Abuse, revised April 2000.

anorexia nervosa A severe eating disorder in which the individual's body mass index (BMI) is deliberately reduced to less than or equal to 17.5 kg/m². (The average healthy person has a BMI within the range of 19–24 kg/m². Most physicians have tables in which individuals can look up their height and weight to determine their BMI, and these tables are also available at many Web sites online.) Anorexia nervosa is one of several eating disorders, including BULIMIA NERVOSA and BINGE EATING DISORDER. An estimated 5 million Americans have an eating disorder.

Patients with anorexia nervosa mistakenly perceive that they are obese (despite the fact that they are very underweight). As a result, they severely limit their food intake in an obsessive and addictive manner. If not treated, the patient can actually starve to death. When death occurs, it generally comes from heart failure, severe electrolyte imbalances, or SUICIDE. Some studies have shown that patients who suffer from both anorexia nervosa and ALCOHOLISM have the greatest risk for suicide. Many patients develop malnutrition and other severe medical problems.

Patients with anorexia nervosa exhibit an unusual form of an addiction in which rather than performing an act, their compulsion is to refrain from performing an act, which is eating. They are obsessed with not eating and with achieving an unreasonably low weight. Often, if that weight is attained, the patient then sets an even lower weight as a new goal. Thus the desired weight can never be achieved because it is always changing. In this way, anorexia nervosa can be viewed as an addictive disorder.

Some patients with anorexia nervosa may realize that they are exhibiting irrational behavior but feel helpless and/or unwilling to stop it. Other patients do not believe that they have a problem at all and instead assume that everyone else around them is wrong. They may believe that others are purposely trying to make them fat when they try to induce the anorexic to eat.

Risk Factors for the Development of Anorexia Nervosa

Most patients with anorexia nervosa are female, in about a 10 to one or 20 to one ratio, female to male. Anorexia nervosa is not common and occurs in only about 1 percent of all women. When it occurs, anorexia nervosa characteristically starts in the midteens, but the behavior may occur earlier in life or later.

Athletes, both male and female, are at risk for developing anorexia nervosa because of the heavy emphasis on weight in many sports. In one study, 35 percent of female athletes in college and 10 percent of male athletes were considered at risk for developing anorexia nervosa. Professional dancers, actors, and models also have an increased risk for developing anorexia nervosa because of the importance to their professions of looking very thin.

It is commonly believed that the typical person with anorexia nervosa is an upper middle class white teenage girl; however, researchers have found that anorexia nervosa cuts across race and socioeconomic status. It is true, however, that white teenage girls appear to be the most weight-obsessed group, compared with the other ethnic or racial groups.

People with anorexia nervosa usually have a problem with perfectionism, low self-esteem, and rigid belief structures. As many as half may be clinically depressed. Some patients may be diagnosed with BIPOLAR DISORDER. They may also respond to stress by initiating anorexic behavior, which becomes an ingrained behavior pattern. Some studies have shown that people with anorexia nervosa have a high rate (up to 69 percent of patients) of obsessive compulsive disorder. This may partially explain the person's obsessive thoughts about food and the compulsion to lose weight. Other psychiatric disorders may also be present.

Some researchers have associated childhood sexual abuse with the development of eating disor-

ders. Bulimia nervosa is more commonly associated with childhood sexual abuse than is anorexia nervosa.

Signs and Symptoms of Anorexia Nervosa

Some indications of anorexia nervosa are as follows:

- Excessive weight loss
- Refusal to be weighed
- Excessive exercising
- Withdrawal from social activities, especially those associated with food
- Amenorrhea (absence or cessation of menstruation) in females who have begun menstruating and delayed onset of the first menses in preadolescent girls
- Unexplained fatigue
- Changes in eating habits, such as peculiar preoccupations with types of foods or colors of foods
- Obsessive focus on body weight and body shape

These signs and symptoms may also indicate another serious medical problem is present. Only a medical doctor can assess whether some other underlying problem is causing them. It is important for a person with such indicators to be evaluated by a physician.

Anorexia Nervosa Compared with Bulimia Nervosa

Bulimia nervosa is another eating disorder, with similarities to anorexia nervosa. However, instead of restricting their food intake, people with bulimia eat large quantities of food in a binge and then self-induce vomiting. They often abuse laxatives as well. This is described as a binge-purge cycle. As many as a third of bulimic patients originally had anorexia nervosa that later developed into bulimia nervosa.

Patients with eating disorders such as anorexia nervosa, bulimia nervosa, and binge eating disorder need medical care from experienced psychiatrists as well as from nutritionists and other specialists. In some cases, they require hospitalization in a specialized facility to help them overcome their addictive behaviors. However, as with all addictions, an ACKNOWLEDGMENT OF ADDICTION as a true problem that they need to work on is an essential factor in successful treatment.

Eating Disorders and Use of Alcohol, Illegal Drugs, and Tobacco

Some researchers have found a link between individuals with anorexia nervosa or bulimia nervosa and alcohol abuse or alcoholism as well as the use of illegal drugs and tobacco. According to *Food for Thought: Substance Abuse and Eating Disorders*, a 2003 report by the National Center on Addiction and Substance Abuse at Columbia University, researchers have found that teenage girls with eating disorders have about a five times greater risk than others of abusing alcohol or illegal drugs. When stated another way, girls with eating disorders have about a 50 percent risk of alcohol or drug abuse versus a 9 percent risk of girls of the same age who do not have an eating disorder.

Girls with bulimia nervosa are more likely to abuse drugs and alcohol than girls with anorexia nervosa. However, anorexics may abuse cocaine or psychostimulants for their appetite-suppressing qualities.

Teenage girls sometimes smoke to control their appetites and refuse to give up smoking because they fear gaining weight. Studies have shown, however, that there is no significant difference between the body mass index of teenagers who smoke and the body mass of those who have never smoked. One study showed that teenagers who began smoking experienced weight gain.

According to the *Food for Thought* report, "Girls and young women who smoke to suppress their appetite are a potential group of new nicotine addicts, making females who are concerned about their weight particularly vulnerable targets for the tobacco industry."

Other frequently abused substances that are used by people with eating disorders, according to this report, are alcohol, emetics (drugs that cause vomiting), laxatives, caffeine, appetite suppressants, diuretics (also known as water pills because they increase urination), heroin, and cocaine.

Health Consequences of Anorexia Nervosa

The health consequences of anorexia nervosa are very serious. Many girls and women with anorexia nervosa develop osteoporosis. They also suffer from hair loss, dehydration, and atrophy of muscles. Breast tissue, too, may atrophy in females with anorexia nervosa. The most serious potential consequence is death; this risk is 12 times higher for young women with anorexia nervosa compared with the risk of their peers.

Males with anorexia nervosa may experience decreased levels of testosterone. Anorexic preadolescent boys may have delayed puberty.

One sign of medically concerning anorexia nervosa is the appearance of a downy layer of hair (lanugo). The body manufactures this in order to keep the body warm enough.

Diagnosis and Treatment of Anorexia Nervosa

Diagnosing anorexia nervosa in early cases may be very difficult before the individual has lost significant weight. However, early diagnosis is always best so that treatment can be initiated.

Doctors need to take a complete medical history and perform a physical examination of the patient to rule out any other medical problems that may be present. Several endocrine or hormonal diseases may cause substantial changes in weight. For example, Addison's disease, a disease of the adrenal glands, may cause severe weight loss. Type 1 diabetes (insulin dependent) will also induce a major weight loss. Thus, doctors need to rule out these diseases and other possible causes of the patient's symptoms.

If physicians suspect anorexia nervosa, they will order a test of electrolytes, which may often be out of balance if the patient has abused diuretic drugs or laxatives. Cortisol blood levels may be elevated with anorexia nervosa. Scans of bone loss will indicate bone density abnormalities in as many as 50 percent of patients with anorexia nervosa. Experts report that bone loss can occur in young anorexic women as early as six months from the onset of the anorexic behavior. This is another reason why obtaining treatment as early as possible is so urgent, before the illness causes serious and sometimes irreversible damage.

Treatment can be very difficult. Many patients do not accept that they have a problem. Acknowledgment is an essential part of any successful therapy. Even when patients realize that they have a problem, they may still find it difficult or impossible to resume normal eating.

Involuntarily hospitalizing a patient in order to save her life may become necessary. Eventually, though, she (or he) will leave the institution and the behavior will recur unless the patient accepts that treatment is needed and is able to comply with treatment recommendations. Individual therapy is essential, and family therapy may also be indicated.

The primary goal of treatment is to encourage the patient to gain weight. Antidepressant medications such as fluoxetine (Prozac), which tends to decrease appetite, are not used in severely anorexic patients, although other psychiatric drugs may be very helpful.

In individuals with anorexia nervosa, weight gain must be monitored to avoid excessive edema, possible heart failure, and even suicide. Electrocardiograms, regular tests for serum electrolyte levels, and psychiatric attention are all necessary. Patients may need to reside in a hospital or residential facility until they are deemed well enough to leave. Once discharged, they will need to be monitored on an outpatient basis. Some organizations and facilities specialize in treating patients with anorexia nervosa and other eating disorders.

Female patients who are estrogen deficient because of their anorexia may be treated with estrogen therapy. Multiple vitamin supplements will be necessary to replenish essential vitamins, such as B12 and folate, which are frequently depleted through self-starvation.

See also DIET PILLS; OBSESSIVE-COMPULSIVE DISORDER.

For further information on anorexia nervosa, contact the following organizations:

Anorexia Nervosa and Related Eating Disorders, Inc.
P.O. Box 5102
Eugene, OR 97405
(503) 334-1144

National Association of Anorexia Nervosa and Associated Disorders
P.O. Box 7
Highland Park, IL 60035
(847) 831-3438
http://www.anad.org

Osteoporosis and Related Bone Diseases National Resource Center
2 AMS Circle
Bethesda, MD 20892
(800) 624-BONE or (202) 223-0344

Becker, Anne E., M.D. "Eating Disorders," *New England Journal of Medicine* 340, 14 (April 8, 1999): 1,092–1,098.
Grilo, Carlos M., Rajita Sinha, and Stephanie O'Malley. "Eating Disorders and Alcohol Use Disorders," *Alcohol Research & Health* 26, 2 (2002): 151–160.
National Center on Addiction and Substance Abuse at Columbia University. *Food for Thought: Substance Abuse and Eating Disorders.* New York: National Center on Addiction and Substance Abuse at Columbia University, December 2003.
Klump, K. L., et al. "Genetic and Environmental Influences on Anorexia Nervosa Syndromes in a Population-Based Twin Sample," *Psychological Medicine* 31 (2001): 737–740.

Antabuse (disulfiram) An oral drug that has been used since about the mid 1950s and that is still used by some experts today to treat ALCOHOLISM. Antabuse has also been used to treat patients addicted to cocaine. The drug may be used by patients in residential treatment centers or with outpatients living at home. Antabuse prevents the liver from its normal metabolizing of alcohol and results in a toxic buildup of acetaldehyde, which experts believe cause the drug's prominent side effects of severe nausea and vomiting. These effects occur when a patient taking the drug consumes any amount of alcohol. In addition to severe vomiting, if patients taking Antabuse also ingest alcohol, they may experience the following side effects:

- Blurred vision
- Chest pain
- Dilation of blood vessels leading to skin flushing and a sharp drop in blood pressure
- Headache (severe)
- Rapid heartbeat
- Weakness

Nearly all physicians who prescribe Antabuse also recommend therapy for the patient as well as support groups such as ALCOHOLICS ANONYMOUS.

The patient must be committed to ABSTINENCE from all alcohol for this drug to be effective. In addition, experts report that the drug appears to be most effective in individuals who have jobs and who also have others who provide them with emotional support, such as family members. If patients fear losing their jobs or fear that their partners will leave them if they continue drinking, they may also be good candidates for Antabuse therapy. Some courts may require that patients take Antabuse as a condition of child visitation or as part of a sentence for committing a crime.

Monitored Antabuse is frequently required in legal/criminal situations. Individuals taking monitored Antabuse must personally come to a pharmacy where the Antabuse is given in liquid form, and is taken in the presence of the pharmacist. This ensures that individuals are compliant with the prescribed medication and that they will, in fact, have profound negative reactions to the use of even small quantities of alcohol.

Because they do not wish to tell everyone that they are taking this drug, some people who take Antabuse tell others that they are severely allergic to alcohol, which will induce extreme vomiting. This information is often sufficient to cause restaurant staff as well as friends and family members to heed the warning and avoid giving the person any foods or fluids that contain alcohol. (Although there are still some people who seem to think that "just a little" alcohol could not make a difference. In the case of Antabuse, even very small amounts of alcohol result in severe reactions.)

Other patients who use Antabuse tell some people that they are on a medication that causes severe vomiting if they ingest even a tiny amount of alcohol, such as cooking alcohol or wine. Whatever the means used to convey the information, it is essential that patients taking Antabuse inform people who provide them with food or fluids that the patient cannot tolerate even the tiniest amount of alcohol.

Pros and Cons of Antabuse Therapy

Supporters of the use of Antabuse to treat alcoholics believe that the patient will eventually develop a lasting aversion to alcohol as a result of the repeated vomiting that results from any alcohol consumption. They also believe that when patients know that they cannot drink without suffering severe consequences, they can more easily avoid alcohol and it also helps them greatly with abstinence.

Often abstinence is extremely difficult for people with alcoholism, and an enforced abstinence may be best for some patients. In addition, the use of monitored Antabuse can actively allow the legal system to prevent recurrent offenders from drinking and driving.

On the negative side, many patients refuse to take any medication on a regular basis (such as their high blood pressure medications, and so forth). They are even less likely to take a medication that immediately incurs severe consequences, such as Antabuse. Some patients may do better on another prescribed medication, such as NALTREXONE.

Other Medical Problems

If a doctor is considering Antabuse, patients should be sure to tell the doctor if they have any of the following illnesses, which may be exacerbated by the use of Antabuse:

- Asthma or lung diseases
- Diabetes
- Any seizure disorder
- Heart or blood vessel diseases
- Hypothyroidism (low thyroid levels)
- Skin allergies
- Kidney disease
- Liver disease or cirrhosis of the liver
- Severe MENTAL ILLNESS, such as depression or any other psychiatric problem

Starting Antabuse

Before patients start taking Antabuse, they first need to review carefully with their doctors what they have ingested for the past 12 hours to ensure that nothing with any alcoholic content was consumed since recent past consumption will induce side effects when Antabuse is taken. If patients are unsure what products contain alcohol, they should ask their doctors.

Most patients take the drug in the morning. If it makes them sleepy, though, patients may take it in the evening before bedtime. Antabuse must be taken at the same time every day. If patients stop taking the drug, they should still avoid alcohol for at least 14 days after ending the Antabuse because it has residual effects for as long as two weeks.

Even if the patient does not drink any alcohol while taking Antabuse, some side effects may occur, such as diarrhea or a garlic or tin taste in the mouth. Some patients find that the drug makes them feel tired. In general, the side effects tend to decrease after the patient takes Antabuse for several weeks and the body adapts to it. Doctors should also periodically check the patient's blood to ensure that liver function is within the normal range.

Antabuse should be stored away from damp places including the bathroom medicine cabinet because heat or moisture can cause the drug to break down.

Medication Interactions and Other Chemicals

In addition to the inability of patients taking Antabuse to tolerate any alcohol, some medications can interact negatively with Antabuse. For example, patients taking phenytoin (Dilantin), an antiseizure drug, may need to have their dosages changed while taking Antabuse. Patients taking anticoagulants (blood thinners) may also need their medication dosage adjusted, because Antabuse can increase the effect of the anticoagulants and thus cause too much thinning of the blood. Some medications should be avoided altogether, such as metronidazole (Flagyl).

Patients taking Antabuse should be very careful with products that contain alcohol that are applied to the skin, such as rubbing alcohol, aftershave lotions, colognes, and perfumes. These topical products may not cause vomiting but are likely to cause headache, nausea, and itching. The patient can test the product on a small area of the skin for two hours. If no redness or itching and no other ill side effects occur, then this product may be safe to use in limited amounts.

Some products containing alcohol may induce vomiting among patients taking Antabuse. Some studies have shown that beer in shampoo or alcohol in shaving lotion was sufficient to induce the vomiting response in patients who had taken Antabuse, even though these products were used on the head or face rather than being ingested. As a result, it is very important for patients who take Antabuse to read the labels of all food and nonfood products very carefully. They should also avoid many household products. For example, the smell of paint can induce a toxic reaction in a person taking Antabuse.

Side Effects to Watch Out For

Patients taking Antabuse should immediately contact their doctors if any of the following warning signs are noted:

- Eye pain or vision changes
- Yellowing of the eyes or skin
- Numbness and tingling or pain in the hands and feet
- Dark urine
- Mood changes
- Light-colored or grayish stools
- Severe stomach pain

Emergency Identification Is Essential

Every person who is taking Antabuse should wear an emergency medical bracelet or necklace as well as carry an emergency information card. The emergency bracelet or necklace is very important because often emergency personnel do not have time to search for an emergency identification card in a wallet or a purse, but they will notice an emergency bracelet or necklace that is worn on the injured or ill person.

The emergency identification bracelet or necklace should state that the patient is taking Antabuse so that the emergency staff will not administer any alcohol-based products, which are very commonly used in emergency situations and especially so when the person is unconscious or incoherent. Even the alcohol that is rubbed on the skin to start an intravenous line could be dangerous to the patient who is on Antabuse. The emergency medical bracelet or necklace should also include the name and phone number of the patient's physician as well as a relative or other person who should be contacted.

Once the emergency staff knows that the patient is taking Antabuse, they can then search for an emergency identification card or contact the patient's doctor for instructions. The emergency identification card can usually be obtained from the manufacturer and will provide guidelines on what types of products are safe and not safe to use with a patient who is taking Antabuse.

Antabuse Used to Treat Cocaine

In 2004 the National Institute on Drug Abuse (NIDA) issued a press release stating that a study funded by the NIDA found that individuals addicted to cocaine were able to reduce their use of the drug by taking Antabuse. The most effective use of Antabuse came when the drug was combined with providing patients with cognitive-behavioral therapy, a form of "talk" therapy that teaches patients new ways of acting and responding to their environments.

See also ALCOHOLIC HEALTH PROBLEMS; BEHAVIOR MODIFICATION; CAMPRAL; DETOXIFICATION; NALTREXONE.

Manisses Communication Group, Inc. "The Role of Antabuse (Disulfiram) in the Treatment of Alcohol Use Problems," *Behavioral Healthcare Tomorrow: Addiction Professional* Supplement (May/June 2003). Available online. URL: http://www.manisses.com/FreeReports/reports/Antabuse.pdf. Accessed July 1, 2004. 1–8.

National Institute on Drug Abuse. *NIDA Study Finds Alcohol Treatment Medication, Behavioral Therapy Effective for Treating Cocaine Addiction.* Press release from the U.S. Department of Health and Human Services, March 2, 2004.

antianxiety medications See BENZODIAZEPINES.

antidepressants Prescribed medications used to treat DEPRESSION. Some experts believe that large numbers of individuals who are depressed may be unconsciously attempting to self-medicate their depression or other psychiatric problem by taking illegal or prescribed drugs or alcohol or by exhibiting other addictive behaviors. If the underlying psychiatric disorder can be diagnosed and treated with medication and/or psychotherapy, the individual should be better equipped to overcome these addictive behaviors.

When patients are undergoing withdrawal, particularly from drugs such as COCAINE or AMPHETAMINES, they may become severely depressed. Antidepressants may be necessary in treating these individuals.

Antidepressants are not addictive substances, and they may be useful in treating addicted individuals. For example, bupropion (Wellbutrin) has been clearly shown to have beneficial effects on individuals who are addicted to nicotine. In addition, many antidepressants are useful in managing the aftereffects of addictions and WITHDRAWAL.

See also BIPOLAR DISORDER; DUAL DIAGNOSIS; SMOKING CESSATION; ZYBAN.

antismoking laws State, federal, county, or city laws or ordinances that regulate if, when, and where smoking may occur. Many states have passed laws limiting smoking to outside of buildings. All states ban the sale of cigarettes to minors under the age of 21 years. Many states have passed laws banning smoking in enclosed areas, such as inside offices, malls, or restaurants. Federal laws prohibit smoking on commercial flights within the United States and ban smoking within airport terminals except in specified smoking areas. Laws also ban or control the content of advertising, such as laws against advertising cigarettes in television commercials.

See also MASTER SETTLEMENT AGREEMENT; SMOKING CESSATION; SMOKING AND HEALTH PROBLEMS.

anxiety disorders Emotional illnesses that dominate an individual's life with overwhelming, crippling, chronic anxiety and fear that may grow progressively worse. According to the National Institute of Mental Health (NIMH), more than 19 million adults (about 13 percent of the population) in the United States suffer from anxiety disorders. Children and adolescents may also develop anxiety disorders that usually continue into adulthood.

Studies have shown that people with anxiety disorders are more likely to develop addictive behaviors such as smoking and/or abusing drugs and alcohol. In an article in a 2000 issue of the *Journal of the American Medical Association,* a study indicated that smoking during adolescence appeared to trigger the development of anxiety disorders in adulthood, suggesting that substance usage may also cause anxiety disorders.

Types of Anxiety Disorders

There are several different primary anxiety disorders. These include panic disorder, OBSESSIVE-COMPULSIVE DISORDER (OCD), POSTTRAUMATIC STRESS DISORDER

(PTSD), phobias, and general anxiety disorder (GAD).

Panic disorder   Panic disorder is diagnosed by a psychiatrist when a patient has occurrences of extreme fear that suddenly occur for no apparent reason and when the person is under no real threat. Patients with panic disorder may experience physical symptoms, such as chest pain, abdominal pain, dizziness, and a fear of dying. According to the NIMH, about 2.4 million people in the United States suffer from panic disorder. Panic disorder often first develops in late adolescence or early adulthood. There appears to be a strong genetic component to the development of panic disorder.

Obsessive-compulsive disorder   OCD is characterized by repeated and unwanted thoughts and/or by compulsive behaviors and rituals that the individual feels compelled to perform, such as repeatedly counting things or washing his or her hands. According to the NIMH, about 3.3 million people in the United States have OCD. The first indicators of OCD often appear in childhood or adolescence. There appears to be a strong genetic component to OCD, and ongoing clinical trials should uncover additional genetic evidence.

Often other illness are present that appear related to OCD and that may also have a genetic basis. One example is Tourette's syndrome, an illness characterized by involuntary movements, tics, and vocalizations.

Some preliminary evidence from the NIMH indicates that streptococcal bacterial infection in some young people may lead to the development of OCD. Treatment of the infection in these few cases apparently improves the OCD. These "overnight"-onset OCD illnesses have been termed pediatric autoimmune neuropsychiatric disorders associated streptococcal infections or PANDAS. In addition, a few cases of OCD appear tied to a genetic vulnerability that is also associated with the development of rheumatic fever.

Posttraumatic stress disorder   PTSD refers to symptoms that occur after an individual personally experiences an extremely traumatic event, such as a rape or child abuse, or witnesses the effects of extreme violence during a war or a natural disaster. The person may suffer from recurring nightmares and flashback memories of the distressing events. He or she may also experience DEPRESSION, anger, numbing of emotions, distractibility and easy startling, such that the person jumps dramatically at a minor touch or sound that would not bother others.

The NIMH estimates that 5.2 million people in the United States have PTSD. This disorder can occur at any age since it is driven by situations that the individual experiences.

Phobias   Phobias are severe, persistent, and irrational fears. They may be related to a fear of a specific thing or to a fear of a more general situation. For example, a social phobia can lead to an extreme avoidance of social activities due to disabling fears. Social phobias often develop in childhood or adolescence. According to the NIMH, an estimated 11.5 million people in the United States suffer from phobias.

Generalized anxiety disorder   GAD refers to an exaggerated and constant worry and tension about normal everyday events that occur in life. The person with GAD expects the worst of nearly every situation but actually has little reason to do so. It is not a mere pessimistic or negative outlook. Instead, it is a case of expecting an impending doom almost constantly but for no valid reason.

GAD may be accompanied by headache, nausea, fatigue, and muscle tension. The NIMH estimates that about 4 million people in the United States have generalized anxiety disorder. GAD may occur at any time in the life span. According to the NIMH, though, the risk for the onset of this disorder is highest in childhood and middle age.

Patients with Anxiety Disorders

In general, women are more likely to be diagnosed with most anxiety disorders than men by about two to one. However, in the case of OCD and social phobias, men and women are equally at risk.

Anxiety Disorders and Substance Abuse

The use and abuse of substances are common among patients with anxiety disorders, as shown in the table on page 33. For a comparison basis, the total population's SUBSTANCE ABUSE percentage is provided as well as the percent of the abusers among the patients who were diagnosed with a major depressive disorder.

PAST-YEAR SUBSTANCE USE (PERCENT) BY MENTAL SYNDROME, U.S. POPULATION, AGE 18 AND OLDER, 1996

Substance	Total Adult Population	Major Depressive Episode	Generalized Anxiety Disorder	Agoraphobia ***	Panic Attack
Cigarettes	33.2	50.4	55.5	47.0	49.2
Alcohol (heavy use) *	18.9	23.6	23.0	14.3	20.1
Any illicit drug	10.1	20.6	14.4	15.7	19.9
Psychotherapeutics **	2.9	7.8	4.9	7.7	8.6
Cocaine	1.9	5.0	4.4	2.0	4.0

* Heavy alcohol use is defined as being "drunk" or "very high" on three or more days in the past year.
** Psychotherapeutics refer to the nonmedical use of any prescription-type stimulant, sedative, tranquilizer, or analgesic. It does not include over-the-counter medications.
*** Agoraphobia is an anxiety disorder that is an extreme fear of being in places or situations where loss of control might occur. The individual may actively restrict his or her social interactions as a result.
Source: Rouse, Beatrice A., ed., Web-mounted version prepared by Rick Albright. *Substance Abuse and Mental Health Services Administration (SAMHSA) Statistics Source Book, 1998.* Available online. URL: http://www.whitehousedrugpolicy.gov/publications/pdf/98samhsa2.pdf. Accessed on May 15, 2004.

Agoraphobia is a general dread of having a panic attack and losing control in a public setting. The anticipatory dread can lead to an individual being unable to drive anywhere. It may also prevent a person from entering grocery stores. In extreme cases, a person may be completely unable to leave home.

As can be seen from the table, patients with GAD have a high abuse rate of cigarettes, alcohol, and all other substances, as do patients with panic attack and agoraphobia. For example, 18.9 percent of the total adult population in 1996 in the United States were heavy alcohol abusers, according to this data. Among people with GAD, the rate of heavy drinkers was 23 percent.

In reviewing the use of illicit drugs, 10.1 percent of the general population had abused drugs. Among patients with panic attacks, however, the rate was 19.9 percent, nearly double. Rates of illicit drug use were also higher among patients with agoraphobia (15.7 percent) and GAD (14.4 percent).

Compulsive Gambling

Some studies indicate that patients with compulsive gambling problems are more likely also to have anxiety disorder. However, sample sizes in the studies have been small.

Treatments for Anxiety Disorders

Antidepressants and medications called antianxiety medications or benzodiazepines are often used to treat patients with anxiety disorders. Some examples of benzodiazepine medications are alprazolam (Xanax), lorazepam (Ativan), clonazepam (Klonopin), and diazepam (Valium). Some patients with anxiety disorders are treated with ANTIDEPRESSANTS. Some patients may need several medications because one drug is not sufficient. Antidepressants are often used as the primary treatment for anxiety disorders, and benzodiazepines are used as adjunct or temporary treatments until the antidepressants take effect.

Psychotherapy can help individuals to learn to change their thinking patterns. Cognitive behavioral therapy has been shown to be helpful in many anxiety disorders as have hypnosis, relaxation exercises, and biofeedback. Exposure therapy, or desensitization, is also used for specific phobias. With exposure therapy, the individual is gradually exposed to the feared object or experience until he or she builds up the ability to face it without feelings of panic or excessive fear.

In patients with anxiety disorders in addition to addictive illnesses, both the anxiety disorder and the addiction should be treated simultaneously.

See also ANXIETY DISORDERS; BENZODIAZEPINES; BIPOLAR DISORDER; DUAL DIAGNOSIS; GAMBLING, PATHOLOGICAL; MENTAL ILLNESS/PSYCHIATRIC PROBLEMS; PSYCHOTIC BREAK.

For further information on anxiety disorders, contact the following organizations:

Anxiety Disorders Association of America
8730 Georgia Avenue
Suite 600
Silver Spring, MD 20910
(240) 485-1001
http://www.adaa.org

National Institute of Mental Health
Office of Communications and Public Liaison
6001 Executive Boulevard
Room 8184, MSC 9663
Bethesda, MD 20892
(888) ANXIETY (888) 826-9438
http://www.nimh.nih.gov

Black, Donald W., M.D. and Trent Moyer. "Clinical Features and Psychiatric Comorbidity of Subjects with Pathological Gambling Behavior," *Psychiatric Services* 49, 11 (November 1998): 1,434–1,439.

Johnson, Jeffrey G., et al. "Association Between Cigarette Smoking and Anxiety Disorders During Adolescence and Early Adulthood," *Journal of the American Medical Association* 284, 18 (November 8, 2000): 2,348–2,351.

Lasser, Karen, M.D., et al. "Smoking and Mental Illness: A Population-Based Prevalence Study," *Journal of the American Medical Association* 284, 20 (November 22/29, 2000): 2,606–2,610.

Office of Communications and Public Liaison. *Anxiety Disorders Research Fact Sheet*, Bethesda, Md.: National Institute of Mental Health, August 1999.

athletes Individuals who actively participate in sports as professionals, semiprofessionals, or as high school or college students. Some athletes exhibit addictive behaviors, and they abuse drugs, alcohol, and other addictive substances. Some professional athletes may abuse ANABOLIC STEROIDS in an attempt to boost their physical performance faster than they believe could be achieved with exercise and diet. Athletes also have a higher risk than nonathletes of developing eating disorders such as ANOREXIA NERVOSA or BULIMIA NERVOSA. Some athletes have died from heart attacks or other illnesses caused or exacerbated by drugs that they have taken to enhance their physical performance.

Some athletes also become involved in betting on sports and may develop a problem with compulsive GAMBLING, which may be against the rules of their sport and can be harmful to their careers. Some athletes can become addicted to exercise, leading to what is thought to be a form of anorexia nervosa.

Athletes in High School

In a study published in a 2001 issue of *Adolescence*, author Adam H. Naylor studied drug use patterns among 1,500 high school athletes and nonathletes in 15 public high schools in Massachusetts. Male students represented 51 percent of the sample, and 74 percent of the students had participated in sports during the past year. The researchers asked the students about their use of major pain medications, AMPHETAMINES, anabolic steroids, androstenedione, BARBITURATES, and creatine. They also asked students about their use of alcohol, tobacco, MARIJUANA, and other drugs.

The drug use patterns of the athletes and of the nonathletes had some significant differences. For example, the athletes were significantly less likely to smoke cigarettes: 44 percent of the nonathletes smoked, while 36.1 percent of the athletes smoked. The athletes were also significantly less likely to use psychedelic drugs. Among the nonathletes, 18.1 percent reported taking psychedelic drugs, but the percentage of athletes using them was 9.8 percent. The athletes also had a significantly lower rate of cocaine use. Among the nonathletes, 7.2 percent had used cocaine, while the athletes had a usage rate of 3.1 percent.

In one area, however, the athletes had a higher risk of taking drugs and that was with creatine, a nutritional supplement. Among the nonathletes, only 4.4 percent had used creatine. Among the athletes, however, 10.4 percent reported taking the drug. Apparently, the athletes clearly believed the drug would improve their athletic performance while other drugs would impair their performance. Interestingly, however, many recreational substances were used about equally by athletes and nonathletes. Anabolic steroids were used by both the athletes and nonathletes, as were alcohol and pain medication. Steroids were sometimes used by nonathletes who were attempting to lose weight or improve their body proportions.

See also COLLEGE STUDENTS; EXERCISE ADDICTION/DEPENDENCE.

Naylor, Adam H. "Drug Use Patterns Among High School Athletes and Nonathletes," *Adolescence* 36, 144 (Winter 2001): 627–639.

attention deficit hyperactivity disorder (ADHD)

Developmental disorder in which an individual has scattered and unfocused thinking as well as problems with impulsivity, forgetfulness, disorganization, procrastination, and inattentiveness. Such individuals have difficulty completing tasks and are frequently losing items. Some people with ADHD are hyperactive, while others are largely inattentive but are not hyperactive. The level of impairment ranges from mild to severe. Individuals with ADHD, particularly those who are untreated, may have a greater risk for addictive behaviors, although experts disagree on this subject.

Patients with ADHD are usually diagnosed by psychiatrists or psychologists. There are three primary subtypes. In the primarily inattentive subtype, the patient has difficulty with organization, attentiveness, and task completion. In the primarily hyperactive/impulsive subtype, the individual is hyperactive and has difficulties with self-control and impulse control. In the combined subtype, the person has symptoms of impulsivity, restlessness, and inattention.

An estimated 3–7 percent of children in the United States suffer from ADHD. Boys are diagnosed with ADHD about three times more frequently than girls. Some experts believe that girls may be underdiagnosed with ADHD because they are more likely to express the primarily inattentive form of ADHD rather than the hyperactive form. Inattentiveness causes less of a problem to teachers and to other adults than hyperactive and boisterous behavior, and thus inattentiveness is less noticed. Yet inattentive girls (and boys) with ADHD also have problems with distractibility, disorganization, impulsivity, and other features of ADHD and need help as well.

Adults with ADHD

In the past, it was generally accepted that children outgrew their ADHD at some time during adolescence, although why this view was so widely accepted is unclear. However, it is now actively disputed. Many experts believe that at least half of the children who are diagnosed with ADHD will continue to suffer from their symptoms of ADHD into adulthood and to need medication and/or therapy. On the other hand, many individuals with ADHD were never diagnosed in their childhood and instead, receive a diagnosis of ADHD for the first time in adulthood. Such late diagnoses frequently occur when their own children are diagnosed with ADHD and these adults note that they have (and have always had) the same symptoms that are being treated by the child's doctor. Other adults hear about adult ADHD on television advertisements or talk shows and subsequently receive a first-time diagnosis for symptoms that they have had for many years.

Adults with ADHD may have problems such as multiple, undesired job changes as well as chronic problems in personal relationships due to procrastination and forgetting. They may have experienced financial setbacks because of failure to pay bills or meet other financial obligations. Some adults with ADHD receive numerous traffic tickets, primarily for speeding. In general, most adults with ADHD have normal or above-normal intelligence. Nonetheless, some are working in career fields that appear to be at a level lower than their intelligence would warrant, often because they failed to complete a training program or to graduate from college due to their ADHD symptoms.

ADHD and Addictive Behaviors

Substance abuse problems are common among undiagnosed adults with ADHD. Some studies indicate that such individuals are more likely to exhibit addictive behaviors than their peers without the illness, particularly with regard to abusing alcohol, tobacco, and illegal drugs.

Some studies have indicated that adolescent males with ADHD who have substance use problems (with drugs and/or alcohol) are at greater risk for attempted SUICIDE than their peers.

According to Dr. Timothy Wilens in his article for the *Journal of Clinical Psychiatry,* his studies have shown that the age of onset of substance abuse is younger among adults with ADHD (19 years) than among those who do not have ADHD (22 years).

Some experts believe that undiagnosed patients with ADHD, both adolescents and adults, may use alcohol and drugs, especially AMPHETAMINES, in an unconscious attempt to self-medicate their ADHD symptoms. They may also do so to cope with other psychiatric problems they may have, such as underlying depression or anxiety disorders.

Medication for ADHD May Prevent Substance Abuse

Of importance is that some studies indicate that addictive behaviors appear more likely to occur among individuals who are *not* receiving medication for their ADHD. For example, a study of adolescents with ADHD, reported in *Pediatrics* in 1999, demonstrated that teenage boys with ADHD who were treated with medications for their ADHD had about the same rate of substance abuse as adolescent boys without ADHD. However, among those who were *not* taking medication, the rate of substance abuse was significantly higher.

In this study, funded by the National Institute of Mental Health and the National Institute on Drug Abuse, researchers at Massachusetts General Hospital, the Harvard School of Public Health, and Harvard Medical School examined the substance-abusing records of 56 adolescent boys who were diagnosed with ADHD and who were also receiving medication over the course of four years. The researchers also viewed the substance-abusing records of 19 boys with ADHD who did not take medication. In addition, the researchers looked at 137 boys who did not have ADHD, and they considered the presence or absence of substance abuse in these boys.

The researchers found that 75 percent of the nonmedicated boys with ADHD had a substance abuse problem versus only 25 percent of the medicated boys with ADHD. The substance abuse record for the boys who did not have ADHD was 18 percent, close to the abuse statistic for the medicated boys with ADHD. As a result, for at least some patients with ADHD, appropriate medication may apparently serve as a protection against substance abuse.

Generally a mental health professional, such as a psychiatrist or a psychologist, makes the determination of whether ADHD is present in a patient. Additionally, the psychiatrist (or another physician, such as a pediatrician) determines which medication (if any) is indicated.

If Patients with ADHD Are Substance Abusers

When adolescents or adults who are newly diagnosed with ADHD already have a substance abuse problem, this can present a dilemma to physicians. They may be reluctant to prescribe stimulant medications to these patients. The doctors' concerns are well-founded, according to most experts.

According to Dr. Wilens, when adult patients with ADHD are known to have current substance use problems, these patients need both addiction therapy and psychotherapy as well as medication for the ADHD. Dr. Wilens suggests that the first priority should be to treat the substance abuse disorder.

If the substance use disorder is treated first, writes Dr. Wilens, then the patient is more likely to remain in treatment. The next priority is then to determine the level of any existing psychiatric problem. According to Dr. Wilens in another article, published in *Alcohol Health & Research World*, youths with both ADHD and an alcohol or other drug problem often have juvenile BIPOLAR DISORDER or conduct disorder (a disorder in which the individual consistently violates societal rules and laws). Many patients with ADHD also suffer from depressive disorders.

When another psychiatric problem is present in addition to ADHD, the doctor must decide which problem is more debilitating for the patient: the other psychiatric problem or the ADHD. The problem that is more burdensome must then be treated. Thus, if the patient suffers from both depression and ADHD and the depression is more extreme, then generally an antidepressant is indicated along with psychotherapy. Once the depression is under control, the doctor can begin to help the patient deal with the symptoms of ADHD.

Interestingly, some antidepressants work well in treating both depression and ADHD. For example, bupropion (Wellbutrin) is approved by the Food and Drug Administration for the treatment of depression. However, many physicians also find it effective in treating the symptoms of ADHD, especially in adults. Other medications also serve a dual function. According to Wilens, some tricyclic antidepressants, such as desipramine and imipramine, have been shown to reduce the symptoms of ADHD significantly.

Some drugs that are specifically indicated for the treatment of ADHD are also used as adjunct medications to assist in the treatment of depression. The psychostimulants used to treat ADHD have been shown to improve patient response to antidepressants in those who are considered to have treatment-resistant depression.

If patients have no other psychiatric problems and only ADHD symptoms need to be treated, a good initial choice of medication for those with substance use problems is either atomoxetine hydrochloride (Straterra) or bupropion. These drugs are not addicting nor are they stimulants. There is little likelihood of "diversion," or of the patient selling the drug or giving it away to others. In contrast, patients with known addiction problems who are immediately given SCHEDULED DRUGS such as methylphenidate (Ritalin), or amphetamine (Dexedrine) may be tempted to abuse the drugs or to sell them to others who abuse them.

If atomoxetine or other nonstimulants are not effective, however, and ADHD symptoms continue to be troublesome, a slow and careful progression to stimulants may be in order. A stimulant with low abuse risk is methylphenidate, according to Dr. Wilens. However, diversion is an issue of concern among patients who have substance abuse problems. Extended-release stimulants may reduce this risk. Patients with substance abuse problems who are prescribed stimulants should be subjected to random drug tests by their prescribing physicians or treatment programs.

In a small study reported in a 2002 issue of the *Journal of Addictive Diseases* of 11 patients with ADHD who were also addicted to cocaine and who received treatment with divided doses of bupropion, researchers found good treatment compliance and retention. "Patients reported significant reductions in attention difficulties, hyperactivity and impulsivity. Self-reported cocaine use, cocaine craving, and cocaine positive toxicologies, also decreased significantly." Although the number of patients in this study was small, the results were encouraging.

Therapy for Patients with ADHD

Psychotherapy is also important for many patients with ADHD, for whom medication alone is insufficient. Twelve-step programs may not work as well for patients with ADHD since adults with ADHD often have trouble following such programs. Instead, individual therapy, particularly cognitive-behavioral therapy (CBT) may work well with adults with both substance abuse problems and ADHD. Very simply, CBT is a form of therapy in which patients are trained to challenge irrational and negative thoughts and replace them with rational and positive thoughts.

Many patients with ADHD also do well with a form of therapy called "coaching." In this therapy, they are cued when they are behaving in ways that are disturbing to others, such as failing to focus or talking too much in a group situation.

See also PSYCHIATRISTS.

For more information on ADHD, contact the following organization:

National Resource Center on AD/HD
Children and Adults with Attention-Deficit/
    Hyperactivity Disorder (CHADD)
8181 Professional Place
Suite 150
Landover, MD 20785
Toll-free: (800) 233-4050
http://www.help4adhd.org and
http://www.chadd.org

Elia, Josephine, M.D., Paul J. Ambrosini, M.D., and Judith L. Rapoport, M.D. "Treatment of Attention-Deficit-Hyperactivity Disorder," *New England Journal of Medicine* 340, no. 10 (March 11, 1999): 780–788.

Biederman, Joseph, et al., "Pharmacotherapy of Attention-deficit/Hyperactivity Disorder Reduces Risk for Substance Use Disorder," *Pediatrics* 104, 2 (August 1999). Available online: URL: http://pediatrics.aappublications.org/cgi/reprint/104/2/e20?maxtoshow=&HITS=10&hits=10&RESULTFORMAT=1&author1=biederman%2C+J&andorexacttitle=and&andorexacttitleabs=and&fulltext=adhd&andorexactfulltext=and&searchid=1118671772331_6583&stored_search=&FIRSTINDEX=0&sortspec=relevance&fdate=1/1/1998&journalcode=pediatrics. Downloaded on July 1, 2004.

Kelly, Thomas M., Jack R. Cornelius, and Duncan B. Clark. "Psychiatric Disorders and Attempted Suicide Among Adolescents with Substance Use Disorders," *Drug and Alcohol Dependence* 73, no. 1 (2004): 87–97.

Levin, Frances, R., M.D. "Bupropion Treatment for Cocaine Abuse and Adult Attention-Deficit/Hyperactivity Disorder," *Journal of Addictive Diseases* 21, no. 2 (2002): 1–16.

Wilens, Timothy E., M.D. "AOD Use and Attention Deficit/Hyperactivity Disorder," *Alcohol Health & Research World* 22, no. 2 (1998): 127–130.

Wilens, Timothy E., M.D. "Impact of ADHD and Its Treatment on Substance Abuse in Adults," *Journal of Clinical Psychiatry* 65, supplement 3 (2004): 38–45.

barbiturates A specific category of medications, generally including those prescribed to sedate patients or used to prevent seizures. Some barbiturates have analgesic (painkilling) qualities. Barbiturates are derived from barbituric acid and slow down the central nervous system.

Some barbiturates are classified as SCHEDULED DRUGS under the CONTROLLED SUBSTANCES ACT, such as drugs containing butalbital. They are categorized in this manner because their continued use could lead to a physical and/or psychological need for the drug as well as a need for a higher dose to achieve the same effect. If a person develops an addiction to barbiturates, the WITHDRAWAL from them can cause nausea, vomiting, and seizures. Patients taking barbiturates who wish to withdraw from them are generally tapered off to increasingly lower doses of the drug to avoid serious withdrawal side effects.

It is very dangerous for individuals who are taking barbiturates to consume alcohol at the same time, and doing so could lead to an ACCIDENTAL OVERDOSE. However, sometimes barbiturates are used by experienced physicians to limit the symptoms of patients who are undergoing distressing withdrawal symptoms from alcohol.

See also DETOXIFICATION.

battered partners Married or cohabiting individuals who are physically or sexually abused by their partners. Often alcohol and/or illegal drugs underlie or accelerate the abuse. In the worst case, HOMICIDE may result. COCAINE or ALCOHOL ABUSE is behind many domestic violence incidents.

See also CHILD ABUSE AND NEGLECT; CODEPENDENCY; ENABLERS; METHAMPHETAMINE; SUICIDE; VIOLENCE.

beer A very popular alcoholic beverage made of fermented grain and hops. Beer is the fourth most popular liquid beverage in the United States, after soft drinks, coffee, and milk. It is also a popular beverage throughout the world.

In 2000, beer represented 56 percent of all alcoholic beverages consumed in the United States, according to the NATIONAL INSTITUTE ON ALCOHOL ABUSE AND ALCOHOLISM. In terms of the alcohol (ETHANOL) content of beer, 12 ounces of beer is roughly equal to 5 ounces of wine and to 1.5 ounces of 80-proof distilled spirits.

A common belief is that a person cannot become addicted to beer and instead can become addicted only to hard liquor, such as bourbon, gin, or other alcoholic beverages. However, this belief is wrong. Some people drink large quantities of beer and become alcoholics.

People who are addicted to beer typically have central obesity (a large stomach), with more fat in the stomach than on other places in the body. A markedly distended belly may also mean that individuals have developed fatty liver disease, one of the results of chronic ALCOHOLISM.

Most beer drinkers are male and young. In considering the state by state per capita (per person) consumption of beer in the United States in 2000, states with the highest consumption in gallons of beer were Nevada (1.79), New Hampshire (1.75), and Montana (1.55). States with the lowest per capita consumption of beer in gallons were Utah (0.77), New York (0.92), and Connecticut (0.94). The average per capita consumption of beer in the United States in 2000 was 1.22 gallons.

See also ALCOHOL/ALCOHOL CONSUMPTION; ALCOHOL LAWS; OVEREATING/OBESITY.

Nephew, Thomas M., et al. *Apparent Per Capita Alcohol Consumption: National, State, and Regional Trends, 1977–2000.* Bethesda, Md.: National Institute on Alcohol Abuse and Alcoholism, National Institutes of Health, August 2003.

behavior modification   Attempts to change an individual's pattern of actions through a system of rewards and consequences. Every parent uses some forms of behavior modification, such as smiles for good behavior and frowns for bad behavior, extra privileges for positive behaviors and withdrawn privileges for negative behaviors. In the case of addictive behaviors, the goal is to attempt to replace the rewarding aspect of the addiction with something else that may be less exciting but still be a positive reward or that may be a negative consequence resulting from exhibiting the behavior. For example, a person attempting to quit smoking might replace cigarettes with NICOTINE REPLACEMENT THERAPY, gradually reducing the levels of nicotine used.

Many techniques can be used to modify behaviors. Some individuals purposely see mental health professionals to help them discover how to modify their own behavior. Society itself also causes behavior modification changes as it creates ANTISMOKING LAWS so that smoking in certain places is no longer socially acceptable or legal.

Mental health professionals disagree among themselves on many issues related to addiction and behavior modification. One area of disagreement, for example, is whether individuals wishing to renounce addictive behaviors should concentrate on gaining insight as to why they are exhibiting these behaviors. Supporters believe that gaining such insight is the first step toward changing behavior. Other experts believe that many addictive behaviors are attained bad habits that need to be unlearned through various means, such as by changing the environment, the peer group with whom the individual associates, and other factors.

Many people support the TWELVE STEPS concept pioneered by Alcoholics Anonymous, which has been adapted for many different groups. Basically, individuals accept that they are addicts with no control over their behavior and that they need the help of the group and an individual sponsor to manage the addiction, which is regarded as a lifelong problem. A variety of behavior modification techniques are used by such groups.

See also PSYCHIATRISTS; SMOKING CESSATION.

benzodiazepines   Medications given to treat anxiety disorders and sleep disorders and occasionally used for other purposes, such as to prevent seizures. At higher doses, they may be used as anesthetics. Some physicians prescribe benzodiazepines for a short period to help alcoholics who are undergoing withdrawal in order to reduce the severity of their symptoms and decrease the risk for seizures and DELIRIUM TREMENS.

Benzodiazepines are central nervous system depressants. They are schedule IV drugs under the CONTROLLED SUBSTANCES ACT. Some individuals abuse or develop an addiction to a benzodiazepine medication. This is most likely to occur among younger people and/or individuals who are addicted to other substances such as ALCOHOL, COCAINE, HEROIN, or METHADONE.

The first benzodiazepines introduced in the United States were chlordiazepoxide hydrochloride (Librium) in 1960 and diazepam (Valium) in 1963. They were initially regarded as a safe alternative to BARBITURATES due to their markedly lower risk of death due to toxicity. However, in the 1970s, experts began to realize that benzodiazepines could also be addictive drugs. Diazepam was an especially highly dispensed drug in the 1960s and 1970s. At its peak in 1973, sales of diazepam in the United States were $230 million, which translates to $1 billion in 2004 dollars.

Some current examples of benzodiazepine medications include alprazolam (Xanax), triazolam (Halcion), lorazepam (Ativan), clonazepam (Klonopin), and estazolam (ProSom). According to Department of Justice reports, alprazolam and diazepam are the most frequently found benzodiazepines in the illicit drug market. However, many people who develop an addiction to benzodiazepines receive prescriptions for the drug.

ROHYPNOL, known primarily as a DATE RAPE DRUG because it is used to subdue unwitting victims, is also a benzodiazepine. However, it is not manufactured legally in the United States.

Psychiatrists may prescribe benzodiazepines as antianxiety medications for generalized anxiety disorder or panic disorder. Other doctors may also prescribe the drugs for a variety of reasons, particularly insomnia. Some doctors prescribe short-term doses of the medication to a patient who knows he or she is about to undergo a stressful situation. For example, patients who must undergo a closed magnetic resonance imaging scan and who know they are claustrophobic may be prescribed one dose of diazepam so that they can manage their anxiety during the scan. Some individuals are prescribed alprazolam to cope with their fear of flying.

Side Effects and Medication Interactions

Benzodiazepines can cause a variety of side effects in patients who take them. The most common effect is sedation. Other side effects may include memory impairment (to the point of amnesia), depression, and emotional blunting. Benzodiazepines should not be used by pregnant women because they can affect the fetus nor should they be used by breast-feeding mothers. Among ELDERLY individuals, benzodiazepine use may increase the risk of falls and sundowning, which is a kind of a late in the day delirium.

Medication interactions can occur with benzodiazepines. A medication interaction refers to the effect of two or more drugs taken at the same time, which can cause the effect of one or both drugs to be boosted, weakened, or changed in some way. Because of their sedating effects, benzodiazepines should not be taken in combination with other drugs that also cause sedation such as opioid pain medications or some over-the-counter allergy medications.

Benzodiazepines should *never* be taken with alcohol because such a combination could lead to a fatal overdose. Benzodiazepines can interact with lithium and can also interact with many ANTIDEPRESSANTS. In addition, benzodiazepines may interact with some antipsychotic medications and antiseizure medicines. Patients should consult with their psychiatrists or medical doctors for further details on possible medication interactions.

Addiction to Benzodiazepines

When addiction occurs, patients should not attempt to perform their own DETOXIFICATION. Instead they must consult with experienced medical professionals. Withdrawal from high doses of benzodiazepines can be dangerous and may cause the development of delirium tremens and even death. If the addiction to the benzodiazepine is also combined with an addiction to alcohol, cocaine, or another substance, treatment is even more difficult. The medical professional must help the patient cope with these multiple addictions. Hospitalization or residential treatment is frequently required until the patient is stabilized.

Short-acting and high-potency forms of benzodiazepines such as alprazolam have the greatest risk of causing dependence and addiction, especially if the patient is taking a high dose of the medication. If such a patient stops taking the drug, WITHDRAWAL symptoms will quickly present, such as an increase in blood pressure as well as increased heart rate and tremor. A sudden stopping of the medication may cause the patient to experience severe effects, such as HALLUCINATIONS, grand mal seizures, and delirium tremens.

Not all benzodiazepines have a CROSS-TOLERANCE. This means that very careful detoxification is necessary with benzodiazepines. For example, many individuals who are receiving detoxification treatment from alcohol or benzodiazepines are treated with chlordiazepoxide (Librium). However, this medication is not 100 percent cross-tolerant with alprazolam. Thus, this treatment can result in a disguised withdrawal that has been associated with sudden cardiac death.

Treatment for several weeks with an anticonvulsant drug such as carbamazepine may be indicated to decrease the severity of the patient's withdrawal symptoms, according to Thomas Kosten and Patrick O'Connor in their article on managing drug and alcohol withdrawal in the *New England Journal of Medicine*.

In a study of patients over age 55 years who were taking benzodiazepines for insomnia and who wished to discontinue treatment, reported in a 1999 issue of the *Archives of Internal Medicine*, researchers found that controlled-release melatonin was effective in helping patients discontinue the benzodiazepine without sacrificing a loss of sleep. In response to the criticism that the researchers were just replacing one drug with another, Doron Garfinkel and colleagues reported that the patients did not develop a tolerance to the melatonin despite prolonged use nor did they develop withdrawal symptoms when it was discontinued.

See also ANXIETY DISORDERS; DUAL DIAGNOSIS; PSYCHIATRIC MEDICATIONS.

Garfinkel, Doron, M.D., et al. "Facilitation of Benzodiazepine Discontinuation by Melatonin: A New Clinical Approach," *Archives of Internal Medicine* 159, no. 20 (November 8, 1999): 2,456–2,460.

Kosten, Thomas R., M.D. and Patrick G. O'Connor, M.D. "Management of Drug and Alcohol Withdrawal," *New England Journal of Medicine* 348, no. 18 (May 1, 2003): 1,786–1,795.

Lance P. Longo, M.D. and Brian Johnson, M.D. "Addiction: Part I. Benzodiazepines—Side Effects, Abuse Risks and Alternatives," Available online. URL: http://www.aafp.org/afp/20000401/2121.html. Downloaded on February 11, 2004.

National Institute on Drug Abuse. *Prescription Drugs: Abuse and Addiction.* National Institute on Drug Abuse Research Report, NIH Publication No. 01-4881. Washington, D.C.: National Institute on Drug Abuse, July 2001.

Shader, Richard I. and David J. Greenblatt. "Use of Benzodiazepines in Anxiety Disorders," *New England Journal of Medicine* 328, no. 19 (May 13, 1993): 1,398–1,405.

Betty Ford Center A SUBSTANCE ABUSE rehabilitation clinic that was cofounded in 1978 by former first lady Betty Ford, wife of President Gerald Ford, and her friend Ambassador Leonard Firestone. Mrs. Ford was unusual in that she publicly acknowledged that she had a serious chemical dependency problem that required treatment at a time when it was considered shameful by many people, particularly women, to admit to having a problem with substance abuse. Mrs. Ford's courageous admission freed many people who struggled with problems with alcohol and drugs to seek treatment for their addictions.

The Betty Ford Center offers treatment for both men and women as well as offering support and education for family members. It is also supportive of 12-step programs such as ALCOHOLICS ANONYMOUS and NARCOTICS ANONYMOUS.

Although the Betty Ford Center has become synonymous with a place where wealthy people go for rehabilitation, according to literature from the center, it provides assistance to people of all income levels. The center provides inpatient treatment, residential day treatment, and outpatient treatment.

See also TREATMENT FACILITIES.

For further information, contact:

The Betty Ford Center
39000 Bob Hope Drive
Rancho Mirage, CA 92270
(760) 773-4100
(800) 854-9211 (toll-free)
http://www.bettyfordcenter.org

binge drinking Imbibing five or more drinks in succession for men and four or more drinks in succession for women. Binge drinking is also known as heavy episodic drinking. In looking at all Americans age 12 and over, as the federal *2002 National Survey on Drug Use and Health* did, an estimated 54 million people engaged in at least one incident of binge drinking in the 30 days prior to the survey in 2002.

Extreme binge drinking can lead to ALCOHOL POISONING, which may be fatal because the liver is unable to metabolize the massive quantity of alcohol that has been ingested. Alcohol poisoning can lead to a BLOOD ALCOHOL LEVEL that is as high as 4.0 percent, which is more than five times greater than the legal intoxication level of 0.08 percent in most states.

Some binge drinkers may suffer from alcoholic BLACKOUTS, in which they can move about and even speak, but later they have little or no memory of what they have done during the blackout episode. Anyone experiencing an alcoholic blackout needs to consider seeking treatment for ALCOHOL ABUSE or ALCOHOLISM. However, some college students and others who are social drinkers have also experienced blackouts. They may not yet have an alcohol abuse problem, but the possibility that a problem exists should at least be considered.

Binge drinking also affects a student's academic performance and grade point average. Said Michael Sullivan and John Wodarski in their overview on studies of binge drinking among college students in *Brief Treatment and Crisis Intervention*, "Practice wisdom, research, and common sense all suggest that binge-drinking behaviors have an adverse impact on school performance."

Demographics of Binge Drinkers

High school and college students are the most likely to engage in binge drinking, in part because of their youth and partly because of peer pressure. According to an April 2003 *Alcohol Alert* from the NATIONAL INSTITUTE ON ALCOHOL ABUSE AND ALCOHOLISM, about 30 percent of seniors in high schools in the United States have engaged in binge drinking.

The situation is even more serious for college students. Nearly half of all college students binge drink, although students at four-year colleges are more likely to be heavy alcohol abusers than students at two-year colleges. Some students live in substance-free residence halls on campus, and living in such a residence is associated with a lower risk of binge drinking. In contrast, alcohol misuse among college students is associated with membership in Greek organizations (fraternities or sororities).

Based on results from one study, 86 percent of fraternity members reported that they were heavy drinkers versus 45 percent of the students who were not members of fraternities. A similar situation was also true for females, and 80 percent of sorority residents reported heavy alcohol abuse compared with only 17 percent among nonsorority members.

Binge drinking is also associated with athletics. College athletes are more likely to be binge drinkers than nonathletes, including both male and female athletes.

Some colleges ban alcohol altogether. Students on these campuses are about 30 percent less likely to engage in binge drinking. Commuters (who travel to school rather than live there) are less likely to binge drink than students who reside on the campus.

State by state   In considering the state-by-state percentages of individuals who have engaged in binge drinking, as reported in a 2003 issue of *Morbidity and Mortality Weekly Report,* the average percentage of binge drinkers for individuals of both sexes in all states and of all ages was 14.6 percent. However, wide variations occurred among the states as well as among different age groups. For example, the percentages of individuals of all ages who had engaged in binge drinking in 2001 were much higher in the following states: Wisconsin (25.7 percent), North Dakota (22.3 percent), and South Dakota (18.5 percent). States that had the lowest percentages of individuals who had engaged in binge drinking were Tennessee (6.8 percent), Kentucky (8.7 percent), and West Virginia (9.4 percent).

In considering the ages of adults (age 18 and over) from state to state who engage in binge drinking, the average in 2001 was 29.5 percent of those who were ages 18–24 years old and 21.6 percent of those who were ages 25–34. The percentages of binge drinking continued to decline by age. (See table on page 44.)

When looking at only people who were ages 18–24 in 2001, the states with the greatest percentages of binge drinkers were North Dakota (49.3 percent), Wisconsin (46.6 percent), and Minnesota (44.0 percent). States and territories with the lowest percentages of young binge drinkers were Utah (12.5 percent), the Virgin Islands (13.4 percent), and Tennessee (14.7 percent).

Gender differences   When considering gender alone, men are much more likely than women to be binge drinkers, although some women also binge drink. Based on data from the 2003 *Morbidity and Mortality Weekly Report* for 2001, 22.7 percent of men had engaged in binge drinking, compared with only 7.1 percent of all women. Considerable state-by-state differences occurred among females engaging in binge drinking. The highest percentages were found in Wisconsin (15.2 percent), Alaska (11.0 percent), and North Dakota (10.9 percent).

Racial differences   Binge drinking also varies by race and ethnicity. For example, according to the findings from *Results from the 2002 National Survey on Drug Use and Health: National Findings,* the largest percentage of binge drinkers was found among American Indians/Alaska Natives (27.9 percent), followed by Native Hawaiians and other Pacific Islanders (25.2 percent), Hispanics (24.8 percent), whites (23.4 percent), and blacks (21.0 percent).

Problems Created by Binge Drinking

People who engage in binge drinking have a greater risk for developing heart disease. In an article in a 2002 issue of *Alcohol Research & Health* by Jurgen Rehm and colleagues, the researchers reported on studies of drinking and heart disease. They have found that binge drinkers have greater risks for major coronary events (such as heart

PREVALENCE OF BINGE DRINKING BY PERCENTAGE OF AGE GROUP, UNITED STATES, BEHAVIOR RISK FACTOR SURVEILLANCE SYSTEM, 2001

State or Territory	Age 18–24 Percent	Age 25–34 Percent	Age 35–44 Percent	Age 45–54 Percent
Alabama	21.0	17.6	13.0	9.0
Alaska	26.5	26.7	20.1	11.3
Arizona	32.2	27.4	20.5	7.9
Arkansas	23.3	16.3	13.4	11.3
California	28.6	20.4	15.0	9.4
Colorado	35.8	26.6	18.0	11.2
Connecticut	30.5	22.0	15.8	9.1
Delaware	33.9	24.7	14.8	12.0
District of Columbia	38.7	23.7	11.7	8.2
Florida	23.9	17.2	15.7	12.0
Georgia	23.3	14.6	14.5	9.0
Hawaii	20.9	15.2	12.9	6.7
Idaho	25.2	18.1	13.8	12.8
Illinois	34.0	28.2	17.1	13.0
Indiana	31.9	17.4	15.8	11.1
Iowa	37.7	25.3	17.4	12.2
Kansas	34.6	22.4	15.7	9.5
Kentucky	18.0	11.6	10.8	6.1
Louisiana	23.0	19.1	16.5	10.3
Maine	34.2	22.1	16.0	13.4
Maryland	23.1	19.8	12.6	8.3
Massachusetts	39.8	28.8	18.5	11.9
Michigan	36.2	26.8	18.5	13.7
Minnesota	44.0	27.5	20.3	14.5
Mississippi	22.5	17.5	12.0	9.9
Missouri	36.4	18.3	15.5	10.1
Montana	35.2	25.4	18.9	13.0
Nebraska	33.9	21.3	15.4	10.2
Nevada	25.5	28.2	19.3	11.9
New Hampshire	32.0	21.4	19.0	10.5
New Jersey	32.1	20.6	15.2	9.1
New Mexico	26.5	22.4	19.4	11.0
New York	34.8	19.7	14.2	9.5
North Carolina	18.6	16.8	10.3	8.0
North Dakota	49.3	32.6	23.4	17.0
Ohio	33.9	25.9	18.4	12.4
Oklahoma	22.5	18.6	10.7	9.1
Oregon	32.6	24.2	14.8	10.7
Pennsylvania	32.9	25.6	19.0	13.0
Rhode Island	32.6	21.0	19.0	9.6
South Carolina	26.5	17.1	13.1	9.8
South Dakota	38.8	32.2	22.0	12.5
Tennessee	14.7	10.7	5.8	6.2
Texas	28.8	19.8	16.7	13.4
Utah	12.5	14.1	11.9	8.4
Vermont	36.7	22.9	17.4	8.7
Virginia	30.1	22.2	15.9	8.3
Washington	30.1	21.4	14.6	14.0
West Virginia	26.4	15.7	9.6	5.8
Wisconsin	46.6	38.7	30.5	19.8
Wyoming	28.8	24.6	17.8	12.8
Guam	21.1	20.5	19.9	16.2
Puerto Rico	14.4	12.4	15.1	9.2
Virgin Islands	13.4	14.5	12.7	12.2
Average for All States	29.5	21.6	16.0	10.9

Source: Centers for Disease Control and Prevention. "State-Specific Prevalence of Selected Chronic Disease-Related Characteristics—Behavioral Risk Factor Surveillance System, 2001," *Morbidity and Mortality Weekly Report* 52, SS-8 (August 22, 2003): p. 33.

attack or coronary death). Studies have also shown a link between stroke and binge drinking.

Binge drinking creates many other problems as well. For example, there is a relationship between binge drinking and causing or being victimized by physical assault or sexual harassment. There are also various unpleasant by-products of a night of binge drinking, which some researchers refer to as "secondhand effects." For example, over half of all college administrators of schools with high levels of excessive drinking report that they have experienced serious problems with property damage and vandalism.

Treatment

Binge drinkers should receive rehabilitative counseling and may also need outpatient or residential treatment. The binge drinking that occurs in youths may become a habit of adulthood and can lead to long-term alcoholism if not treated. Binge drinkers can change their habits and can avoid the many health and emotional problems of individuals who are alcoholics.

See also ALCOHOL/ALCOHOL CONSUMPTION; ALCOHOLIC HEALTH PROBLEMS; COLLEGE STUDENTS; DRINK-

ING GAMES; DRIVING, IMPAIRED; DRIVING WHILE INTOX-
ICATED/DRIVING UNDER THE INFLUENCE; FETAL ALCO-
HOL SYNDROME; TEENAGE AND YOUTH DRINKING.

Centers for Disease Control and Prevention. "State-Specific Prevalence of Selected Chronic Disease-Related
Characteristics—Behavioral Risk Factor Surveillance
System, 2001," *Morbidity and Mortality Weekly Report*
52, SS-8 (August 22, 2003): 33.
National Institute on Alcohol Abuse and Alcoholism.
"Underage Drinking: A Major Public Health Chal-
lenge," *Alcohol Alert*, 59 (April 2003): 1. Available
online. URL: http://www.niaaa.nih.gov/publications/
aa59.htm. Accessed on March 11, 2004.
Rehm, Jurgen, et al. "Alcohol-Related Morbidity and Mor-
tality," *Alcohol Research & Health* 27, no. 1 (2002): 39–51.
Substance Abuse and Mental Health Services Adminis-
tration. *Results from the 2002 National Survey on Drug
Use and Health: National Findings*. Rockville, Md.:
Office of Applied Studies, NHSDA Series H-22,
Department of Health and Human Services Publica-
tion No. SMA 03-3836, September 2003.
Sullivan, Michael and John Wodarski. "Rating College
Students' Substance Abuse: A Systematic Literature
Review," *Brief Treatment and Crisis Intervention* 4, no. 1
(Spring 2004): 71–91.
Task Force of the National Advisory Council on Alcohol
Abuse and Alcoholism. *High Risk Drinking in College:
What We Know and What We Need to Learn. Final Report
of the Panel on Contexts and Consequences*. Washington,
D.C.: National Institute on Alcohol Abuse and Alco-
holism, 2002.

binge eating disorder The episodic and/or
chronic consumption of copious quantities of food,
usually without regard to hunger or appetite, but
often in response to external stress. With binge eating disorder, binge eating occurs at least two days a
week during a six-month period or more. Binge
eating is not associated with fasting, purging (causing oneself to vomit or have diarrhea), or excessive
exercise. Binge eating disorder is an addictive
behavior because it is compulsive, is chronic, and
has negative consequences.

Many binge eaters are overweight or obese,
although some are of normal weight. Occasional
excessive eating, such as overeating a holiday
meal, does not constitute binge eating.

According to the National Institutes of Health,
about 4 million people in the United States are
binge eaters. They are both males and females,
although the disorder is more common in women.
It affects three women for every two men who
have it. People of all races can develop binge eating
disorder.

Binge eating disorder is considered the most
common of the eating disorders, which also
include ANOREXIA NERVOSA and BULIMIA NERVOSA.

The causes of binge eating disorder are not
known but are suspected to be linked to DEPRES-
SION. Whether depression leads to binge eating or
if binge eaters become depressed subsequent to the
onset of the disorder is unclear.

Most people with binge eating disorder are very
upset about their illness and may feel out of control
and angry. If they are also obese, they are at risk for
developing serious illnesses, such as diabetes,
hypertension, gallbladder disease, heart disease,
high blood cholesterol levels, and even CANCER.

Signs and Symptoms
Binge eating disorder may be indicated by at least
three of the following behaviors, according to the
National Institutes of Mental Health:

- Eating much faster than usual
- Eating that continues after the person is full
- Eating when the person is not hungry
- Eating that occurs when the person is alone due
  to embarrassment over the large quantity of
  food consumed
- Feelings of self-disgust, depression, or guilt after
  overeating

Diagnosis and Treatment
Many people with binge eating disorder are ashamed
and embarrassed about their behavior. A careful and
patient physician may be needed to uncover this illness. Physicians may recommend strict dieting for
obese and overweight patients, but people with binge
eating disorder often do very poorly with such diets.
They may decide to skip meals or eat insufficient
meals, interspersed with out-of-control binges.
These patients should be treated by a psychiatrist or
other mental health professional who can address
the emotional elements of binge eating disorder
and help the patient to change the behavior in

combination with attention from a primary care physician and a nutritionist.

Some medications have been shown to be very helpful in patients with binge eating and bulimia nervosa. Some inpatient and outpatient medical facilities also specialize in treating binge eating disorder. Individuals should be able to obtain this information from their psychiatrist.

See also DIET PILLS; OVEREATING/OBESITY.

For further information on binge eating disorder, contact the following organizations:

Academy for Eating Disorders
6728 Old McLean Village Drive
Mclean, VA 22101
(703) 556-9222
http://www.aedweb.org

National Eating Disorder Association
Information and Referral Program
603 Stewart Street
Suite 803
Seattle, WA 98101
(800) 931-2237 (toll-free)
(206) 382-3587
http://www.nationaleatingdisorders.org

National Institute of Mental Health *Eating Disorders: Facts About Eating Disorders and the Search for Solutions.* NIH Publication No. 01-4901, Bethesda, Md.: National Institutes of Health, 2001.

bipolar disorder A serious psychiatric disorder characterized by extremes of moods, including mania and depression. Bipolar disorder is also known as manic depressive disorder or manic depression. Individuals with bipolar disorder may be more likely to exhibit addictive behaviors because of their lack of impulse control when they are in a manic (overly excited) state or because of their extremely low mood state when they are depressed. Some experts believe that some undiagnosed patients with bipolar disorder may use drugs or alcohol in an attempt to self-medicate their psychiatric symptoms. About 1–2 percent of the population in the United States is affected by bipolar disorder.

Forms of Bipolar Disorder

There are two primary forms of bipolar disorder with several subsets of interest to psychiatrists and other mental health professionals. Bipolar I disorder is the more classic form of the illness. It is characterized by manic episodes that may last for at least a week and are followed by depressive periods that may last for two weeks or more. Some patients are so manic that they require hospitalization in order to avoid causing harm to themselves or others. Patients may also have both a mania and a depression simultaneously, which is called a mixed mania. These patients are at greater risk for suicide.

Bipolar II disorder is a less well-defined form of the illness and is typified by hypomania, which is a less severe form of mania than seen with bipolar I disorder. There is a predominance of depression and depressive symptoms. This disorder is less easy to diagnose and to treat than bipolar type I but causes substantial disability in the general population.

Substance Abuse Prevalence with Bipolar Disorder

Large studies of patients with bipolar I disorder have shown that about 61 percent developed a SUBSTANCE ABUSE disorder during their lifetimes, abusing either alcohol or another drug. Another 41 percent had a drug abuse or dependence diagnosis.

Studies of patients with bipolar II disorder revealed that 48 percent developed a substance abuse disorder. Another 21 percent had a drug or alcohol dependency.

Mood disorders that occur earlier in life, such as during adolescence, may have a different outcome than those that occur at younger ages. According to a report from the National Center on Addiction and Substance Abuse at Columbia University on pathways to substance abuse among girls and young women ages 8–22 years old, "Children who develop mood disorders, such as bipolar disorder, during their teen years are almost nine times likelier to develop a substance use disorder compared to those whose mood disorder emerges earlier in childhood."

Some studies have shown that alcoholism and other forms of substance abuse in patients with bipolar disorder predict a more severe clinical course. Whether there is a cause and effect relationship is not clear. Substance abuse may trigger bipolar episodes. The substance abuse may cause other brain changes that are harmful to the person with bipolar disorder. The bipolar disorder in some individuals may be of sufficient severity to worsen the addictive behaviors. Finally, the substance abuse problem may be independent from the MENTAL ILLNESS.

In alcohol treatment programs, individuals with bipolar disorder can do markedly better when the bipolar disorder is appropriately treated compared with alcoholic patients without bipolar disorder. This finding is related to the theory that patients with bipolar disorder may have been using alcohol in some way to manage their psychiatric symptoms. Once these symptoms are appropriately treated, the alcohol abuse is also more treatable.

Medications for Bipolar Disorder

Medications are the treatment of choice for most patients with bipolar disorder. These medications are often referred to as MOOD STABILIZERS. The two key medications used to treat most patients with bipolar disorder are lithium and valproate (Depakote, Depakene). Lithium has been the accepted treatment for bipolar disorder for many years. However, some studies indicate that it may not work as well as other drugs for patients with a substance abuse problem.

Valproate is an anticonvulsant drug that was approved by the Food and Drug Administration to treat the mania associated with bipolar disorder. In considering patient compliance with taking their medicine, studies have shown that alcoholic and drug-abusing patients are more compliant with valproate than with lithium, possibly because lithium has more side effects, particularly weight gain.

Other anticonvulsants that have been used to treat bipolar disorder include carbamazapine (Tegretol), topiramate (Topamax), and lamotrigine (Lamictal).

Another drug used more recently is NALTREXONE. It has been shown to be effective in treating patients with both alcoholism and psychiatric problems such as depression and bipolar disorder.

Some doctors have treated bipolar patients with substance abuse problems with antipsychotic drugs, such as olanzapine (Zyprexa).

Residential Treatment for Bipolar Patients with Alcoholism or Drug Abuse

Some treatment facilities specialize in the treatment of individuals with both psychiatric and addictive disorders. These DUAL-DIAGNOSIS programs have expertise in diagnosing and treating individuals whose psychiatric illness complicates the treatment of an addictive disorder. DEPRESSION, ANXIETY DISORDERS, SCHIZOPHRENIA, and bipolar disorder must be treated simultaneously with any addictive disorder to maximize the response to treatment and prevent RELAPSE.

Bipolar Disorder and Smoking

Patients with bipolar disorder are also significantly more likely to be smokers. In a study that compared patients with no mental illness to patients with bipolar disorder and other psychiatric diagnoses, published in a 2000 issue of the *Journal of the American Medical Association,* researchers found that patients with bipolar disorder had very high rates of smoking. About 69 percent were current smokers. Among the population with no mental illness, only 22.5 percent were current smokers.

The bipolar respondents also apparently had the greatest difficulty with smoking cessation. They had the lowest quit rates of smoking of all the populations, or 16.6 percent. The quit rate for individuals with no mental illness was 42.5 percent. Interestingly, the smoking quit rate was also higher for patients with other psychiatric diagnoses, such as panic disorder (41.4 percent), major depression (38.1 percent), and dysthymia, a form of depression (37.0 percent). It may be uniquely difficult for patients with bipolar disorder to stop smoking, although they should certainly try. They are at risk for the same illnesses as others who are chronic tobacco users, such as LUNG CANCER and EMPHYSEMA.

Bipolar Disorder and Other Addictive Behaviors

Patients with bipolar disorder may be more prone to developing problems with compulsive GAMBLING, particularly when they are in manic stages of the illness.

Patients with bipolar disorder may also have problems with COMPULSIVE SHOPPING and CREDIT CARD OVERSPENDING to the extent that they create severe financial hardship for themselves and their families. They may also exhibit dysfunctional sexual behavior, similar to that of a sex addict.

Said Dr. Francis Mark Mondimore in his book on bipolar disorder,

"The feelings of exuberance and overconfidence that characterize mania can lead to several patterns of behavior typical of the manic state: spending sprees, sexual promiscuity, and overuse of alcohol and other intoxicating substances.

"Spending sprees can be extravagant and financially catastrophic, because the manic person has no concern for where the money will come from when the bills come due. The increased sexual feelings of this stage of mania may lead to infatuations and even betrothals."

Virtually any addictive behavior is more likely to be a problem for the person with bipolar disorder. However, treatment can enable many people with the illness to lead normal lives.

See also MOOD STABILIZERS; PSYCHIATRIC MEDICATIONS; PSYCHIATRISTS; PSYCHOTIC BREAK.

Lasser, Karen, M.D., et al. "Smoking and Mental Illness: A Population-Based Prevalence Study," *Journal of the American Medical Association* 284, no. 20 (November 22/29, 2000): 2,606–2,610.

Mondimore, Francis Mark, M.D. *Bipolar Disorder: A Guide for Patients and Families.* Baltimore, Md.: Johns Hopkins University Press, 1999.

Sokhkhah, Ramon, M.D. and Timothy E. Wilens, M.D. "Pharmacotherapy of Adolescent Alcohol and Other Drug Use Disorders," *Alcohol Health & Research World* 22, no. 2 (1998): 122–126.

Sonne, Susan C. and Kathleen T. Brady, M.D. "Bipolar Disorder and Alcoholism," Available online. URL: http://www.niaaa.nih.gov/publicatons/arh26-2/103-108.htm Downloaded on May 19, 2004.

blackouts, alcoholic An experience of extreme intoxication that induces a partial or total amnesiac state in which the person is incapable of remembering some or all of the behavior or events that occurred while he or she was in that condition. The period when the person is in that state may range from minutes or hours to as long as several days, depending on the individual and the circumstance.

Many people confuse passing out with blackouts, but the two circumstances are distinctly different. Alcoholic blackouts do not involve a loss of consciousness. Rather than falling asleep, as many extremely intoxicated people do, the individual who is experiencing an alcoholic blackout may talk to others, move about, and act in many complex ways, including driving a car, arguing with other individuals, having unprotected sexual

intercourse with acquaintances or strangers, and performing other behaviors. However, the next day, the person has little or no memory of what has transpired. The individual may wake up in an unfamiliar bed, very disoriented and confused. The person may seek out others to help him or her piece together what happened.

Alcoholic blackouts may occur among individuals with severe alcohol abuse problems or alcoholism. They were first identified based on a survey of members of ALCOHOLICS ANONYMOUS by E. M. Jellinek in his studies in the mid 1940s, and it was assumed that people who had blackouts were alcoholics. Some experts such as Aaron M. White now say that alcoholic blackouts may occur to social drinkers as well, especially under certain conditions, such as extremely heavy drinking that occurs over a very short period. However, experts agree any person who has experienced even one alcoholic blackout needs to reevaluate his or her drinking habits and consider whether treatment is indicated.

Researchers report that drinking heavily is generally not sufficient to cause an alcoholic blackout. Alcoholic blackouts are usually caused by very heavy drinking that is also combined with other behaviors, such as drinking on an empty stomach and gulping down alcohol very rapidly. Each of these behaviors together contributes to elevate the individual's BLOOD ALCOHOL LEVEL very rapidly. Research has shown a direct link between a rapidly rising blood alcohol level and an alcoholic blackout.

Partial and Total Blackouts

Researcher Aaron White describes alcoholic blackouts in his article in a 2003 issue of *Alcohol Research & Health.* According to White, research has indicated that some alcoholics experiencing blackouts cannot remember anything that happened while they were intoxicated, which White calls "en block blackouts." These blackouts are in contrast to fragmentary blackouts, in which the drinker can later remember some parts of what occurred to them when they are cued by others, but their memory is still very spotty.

Social Drinkers and Blackouts

White says that the evidence that social drinkers can experience blackouts is clear, although often ignored, while the problem that alcoholics experience with blackouts has been emphasized instead. White says that in one study, 33 percent of first-year medical students reported having at least one blackout, and most were inexperienced drinkers who drank too much and too fast. In addition, in a study of over 2,000 Finnish men, 35 percent reported at least one blackout in the year before the survey was conducted.

Said White, "Blackouts are much more common among social drinkers than previously assumed and should be viewed as a potential consequence of acute intoxication regardless of age or whether one is clinically dependent upon alcohol."

College Students

Blackouts may be more common among college students than previously known. This may occur partly because many are social drinkers and also because some college students have problems with alcohol abuse and alcoholism. Some college students engage in BINGE DRINKING, which may make them at greater risk for experiencing alcoholic blackouts.

In a survey of 772 undergraduates performed by White and his colleagues, reported in the *American Journal of American College Health*, 51 percent who had ever consumed alcohol said they had blacked out at some point. Among students who consumed alcohol two weeks before the survey, 9.4 percent said that they had experienced a blackout during that time.

These blackouts sometimes led to risky behaviors. Some students reported that they later discovered that they had participated in acts they did not recall, such as unprotected sexual intercourse, driving a car, committing vandalism, and other acts. The researchers discovered that 30.4 percent of the females and 36.0 percent of the males with a history of blackouts at some time in their lives found out that during a blackout they had insulted someone. In the case of an unintended expenditure of money, 20.4 percent of females and 35.4 percent of males reported this behavior. In the case of having unprotected intercourse, 4.2 percent of the females and 8.5 percent of the males reported this behavior. As for unwanted intercourse, 5.8 percent of the females and 4.3 percent of the males reported this experience occurred during a black-

out. Although it seems hard to imagine, 1.6 percent of the females and 3.7 percent of the males reported driving a car during an alcoholic blackout. None of the students reported being arrested during their blackouts.

Greater numbers of blackouts indicate a substance abuse problem. According to White's study, students who had three or more blackouts in college also had lower grade point averages than other students, and they had started drinking at earlier ages than their peers. In addition, they drank frequently during their senior year of high school and were more likely to have heard others voice concern to them about their drinking.

Some students were so frightened by their experience with an alcoholic blackout that they resolved to give up drinking altogether. This is generally truer for females than for males.

Blackouts and the Brain

The mechanism of how alcohol affects memory and causes an alcoholic blackout is complex. White explains, "Alcohol disrupts activity in the hippocampus [a part of the brain] via several routes—directly, through effects on hippocampal circuitry, and indirectly, by interfering with interactions between the hippocampus and other brain regions. The impact of alcohol on the frontal lobes remains poorly understood, but probably plays an important role in alcohol-induced memory impairments." Neuroimaging techniques developed in the future may be able to provide further information on how alcohol causes or contributes to memory impairments.

See also ALCOHOLIC HEALTH PROBLEMS; ALCOHOLISM; ALCOHOL POISONING; COLLEGE STUDENTS.

White, Aaron M. "What Happened? Alcohol, Memory Blackouts, and the Brain," *Alcohol Research & Health* 27, no. 2 (2003): 186–196.
White, Aaron M., David W. Jamieson-Drake, and H. Scott Swartwelder. "Prevalence and Correlates of Alcohol-Induced Blackouts Among College Students: Results of an E-Mail Survey," *Journal of American College Health* 51, no. 3 (2002): 117–131.

blood alcohol levels   Refers to a measurement of the amount of alcohol in the bloodstream and also one way to determine if a person is legally intoxicated. A blood alcohol level of 0.10 percent is equal to 0.10 grams of alcohol per 100 milliliters of blood.

As a rule of thumb, in terms of alcohol content, 12 ounces of beer is equal to 5 ounces of wine and to 1.5 ounces of 80-proof distilled spirits. When stated another way, one drink is equivalent to 0.54 ounces of alcohol, which is about the same amount of alcohol found in a glass of wine, a can of beer, or a shot of distilled spirits. (ETHANOL is the alcohol in alcoholic beverages and the substance that causes intoxication. It is only part of the beer, wine, or spirits, which also include water, flavoring, and other items.)

Blood alcohol levels are individually affected by a person's body weight and the individual's ability to absorb and metabolize alcohol. In general, a 170-pound man who has four drinks on an empty stomach would have the same blood alcohol level as a 137-pound woman who has three drinks on an empty stomach: about 0.08 percent. In 2000, Congress ordered all states to lower their blood alcohol levels for legal intoxication to 0.08 percent by 2004 or risk losing a portion of federal highway construction funds. The goal is to reduce the number of fatalities caused by alcohol abuse.

Among individuals with ALCOHOL POISONING, who drink massive quantities of alcohol over very short periods, their blood alcohol level may be as high as 0.4 percent. This is five times the legal intoxication limit.

Zero-Tolerance Laws

If the individual who is drinking and driving is under age 21, that person is subject, in all states, to ZERO-TOLERANCE LAWS. These state that virtually any amount of blood alcohol above zero is grounds for arrest.

Blood Alcohol Levels and Fatalities

The higher that an individual's blood alcohol levels are beyond zero, the greater the risk for death from a fatal car crash. For example, as can be seen in the table at top right, males ages 16–20 years old (the highest risk group) with blood alcohol levels between 0.02 and 0.049 have a five times greater chance of dying in a crash than if alcohol were not present.

The risk rises with the blood alcohol level. If it increases to between 0.10 and 0.149 in this same

THE INCREASED RISK OF DEATH AS BLOOD ALCOHOL LEVELS RISE

Multiplies the Chance of Being Killed in a Single-Vehicle Crash By:

Driver's Blood Alcohol In This Range						
	Males			Females		
Ages	16–20	21–34	35+	16–20	21–34	35+
0.02–0.049	5	3	3	3	3	3
0.05–0.079	17	7	6	7	7	6
0.08–0.099	52	13	11	15	13	11
0.10–0.149	241	37	29	43	37	29
0.15+	15,560	572	382	738	572	382

Source: Hingson, Ralph and Winter, Michael. "Epidemiology and Consequences of Drinking and Driving," *Alcohol Research & Health* 27, no. 1 (2003): 63–70.

population, the risk for death is increased 241 times. If the blood alcohol level is 0.15 or greater, the risk is multiplied by 15,560 times for young males when no alcohol is involved, making death from a car crash a high probability. (See the table for risks for females in this age group and for males and females in other age groups.)

Measuring Blood Alcohol Levels

The blood alcohol level can be measured in different ways, such as with a Breathalyzer machine, in which the individual blows into a device and the alcohol in the breath is estimated. Blood alcohol levels can also be measured with a blood test and a urine test.

See also ALCOHOL BREATH TESTS; ALCOHOLISM; BEER; BINGE DRINKING; DRINKING GAMES; DRIVING IMPAIRED; DRIVING WHILE INTOXICATED/DRIVING UNDER THE INFLUENCE.

Hingson, Ralph and Michael Winter. "Epidemiology and Consequences of Drinking and Driving," *Alcohol Research & Health* 27, no. 1 (2003): 63–70.

bulimia nervosa An eating disorder in which the individual consumes copious amounts of food in a binge eating fashion, followed by the inducing of vomiting and/or the use of laxatives or diuretics. According to Dr. Philip Mehler in his 2003 article for the *New England Journal of Medicine*, as the illness progresses further, bulimic patients who have previously self-induced vomiting can discover how to vomit reflexively without any stimulation. (They do not need to stick their fingers down their throat.)

Risk Factors

According to the National Institute of Mental Health (NIMH), from 1–4 percent of females have bulimia nervosa during their lifetime. The average onset of the disorder is around age 18, although it may occur at younger or older ages. Most patients with bulimia nervosa are female, but males represent about 10–15 percent of bulimics. Most patients with bulimia nervosa are not overweight, although in most cases they actively fear gaining weight. Experts believe that many patients with bulimia nervosa initially had anorexia nervosa that later developed into bulimia nervosa.

Patients who have been physically or sexually abused have an increased risk for developing bulimia nervosa as well as for developing problems with SUBSTANCE ABUSE. Some experts believe that as many as 25 percent of all women with bulimia nervosa were sexually abused as children. A severely stressful event other than childhood abuse may also cause the development of bulimia.

Signs and Symptoms of Bulimia

According to the NIMH, the symptoms of bulimia nervosa are as follows:

- Binge eating of excessive food accompanied by a feeling of no control over eating as it occurs
- Inappropriate compensatory behavior to avoid weight gain, such as inducing vomiting or abusing laxatives, diuretics, enemas, or other medications; some patients also fast or exercise excessively
- Binge eating and inappropriate compensatory behaviors that occur at least twice a week for three months
- A self-image that is heavily influenced by the weight and shape of the body

Health Consequences

The health consequences of bulimia nervosa are primarily caused by the method and frequency of purging, in contrast to the key problems of starvation and weight loss that are found with anorexia nervosa. Self-induced vomiting causes oral problems and upper digestive systems. Laxative abuse, in contrast, causes severe constipation and lower gastrointestinal problems.

Self-induced vomiting also causes soreness of the throat and leads to damage to the enamel of the teeth, caused by the acidity of the regurgitated material. Induced vomiting also increases the risk for cavities of the teeth. Most dentists can recognize the consequences of bulimia in a routine dental examination.

The bulimic patient may also have fluid and electrolyte abnormalities. For example, vomiting causes a decrease in the blood levels of potassium and chloride. Urinary levels of sodium, potassium, and chloride are also decreased.

Some patients abuse ipecac, an over-the-counter drug that induces vomiting. Continued ipecac abuse can lead to cardiomyopathy and muscle weakness.

Bulimia Nervosa and Substance Abuse

According to a 2003 report by the National Center on Addiction and Substance Abuse at Columbia University, bulimic individuals are at a high risk for substance abuse. This report states, "In a study comparing anorexic women with bulimic women, women with bulimia nervosa were more likely to have abused amphetamines, barbiturates, marijuana, tranquilizers and cocaine. The heaviest illicit drug use is found among those who binge and then purge (e.g. by vomiting or taking pills) to compensate for the binge eating. Indeed, some bulimics report that they use heroin to help them vomit."

Diagnosis and Treatment

Physicians diagnose bulimia nervosa based on a medical history, physical examination, and laboratory testing. Because most people with bulimia nervosa actively seek to hide their behaviors, and are often successful, and also because they do not have a weight loss, the disorder is difficult for many physicians to diagnose.

If diagnosed or suspected, in addition to being treated by the primary care provider, the patient should see a mental health professional as well, such as a psychiatrist. The psychiatrist can recommend therapy and also order medications as needed, such as antidepressants. Selective serotonin reuptake inhibitors such as fluoxetine (Prozac) have been found effective in treating patients with bulimia nervosa. As of this writing, Prozac is the only drug approved by the Food and Drug Administration for the treatment of bulimia nervosa. Studies have indicated that most patients improve with 60 mg versus 20 mg. Physicians may prescribe other off-label medications, such as other antidepressants. The medication bupropion (Wellbutrin) should not be used at all in patients who binge and purge, due to the risk of seizure.

Treatment of the medical problems caused by bulimia nervosa is vitally important. Patients with acid reflux symptoms can be treated with proton pump inhibitors. Laxative dependence can be difficult to treat. However, exercise, a high-fiber diet, and an increase of fluids can help considerably. Sometimes physicians will also order glycerin suppositories or nonstimulant laxatives such as lactulose until the constipation that occurs without the laxatives abates.

Patients with hypokalemia (low potassium levels) should take oral potassium chloride. Some patients may need to take supplemental potassium for a long period, as needed.

If a patient with an eating disorder is at risk for dehydration, electrolyte imbalance, or death and is also a substance abuser, physicians should first stabilize the patient before addressing the substance abuse issue.

Psychiatric Issues

Mental health professionals are needed to help the patient resolve feelings of anxiety, DEPRESSION, low self-esteem, and other emotional components of eating disorders. In addition, any clinical psychiatric problems should be diagnosed and treated.

Which form of therapy is best is not clear. In a study of 220 patients who were treated with either cognitive behavioral therapy (a therapy in which a patient is trained to recognize and challenge irrational ideas) or interpersonal psychotherapy (in which a patient is trained to have insight over behavior), 30 percent of the cognitive behavioral patients were in remission at the end of five months versus only 6 percent in the psychotherapy group. Other studies have borne out the short-term value of cognitive behavioral therapy versus other therapies. However, if these improvements are sustained over longer periods is unknown.

Most patients with bulimia nervosa are treated on an outpatient basis, and they do not require hospitalization. This is in contrast to many patients who have anorexia nervosa. According to Dr. Philip S. Mehler, "Factors that suggest a need for hospitalization include severe depression, disabling symptoms, purging that is rapidly worsening and has proved refractory to outpatient treatment, severe hypokalemia (plasma potassium level <2.0 to 3.0 mmol per liter) and major orthostatic changes in blood pressure (>30 beats per minute)."

See also ANOREXIA NERVOSA; BINGE EATING DISORDER; DIET PILLS.

For further information on bulimia nervosa, contact the following organizations:

Harvard Eating Disorders Center
Massachusetts General Hospital
15 Parkman Street
Boston, MA 02114
(617) 726-8470
http://www.hedc.org

National Association of Anorexia Nervosa and
   Associated Disorders
P.O. Box 7
Highland Park, IL 60035
(847) 831-3438
http://www.anad.org

National Eating Disorders Association
603 Stewart Street
Suite 803
Seattle, WA 98101
(206) 382-3587
http://www.nationaleatingdisorders.org

Mehler, Philip S., M.D. "Bulimia Nervosa," *New England Journal of Medicine* 349, no. 9 (August 28, 2003): 675–881.

National Center on Addiction and Substance Abuse at Columbia University. *Food for Thought: Substance Abuse and Eating Disorders.* New York: National Center on Addiction and Substance Abuse at Columbia University, December 2003.

National Institute of Mental Health. *Eating Disorders: Facts About Eating Disorders and the Search for Solutions,* NIH Publication No. 01-4901. Bethesda, Md.: National Institutes of Health, 2001.

buprenorphine   A medication used on an outpatient basis to treat opioid addiction under the brand names of Subutex (buprenorphine hydrochloride) and Suboxone (buprenorphine hydrochloride and naloxone). Most patients who are treated with buprenorphine are addicted to HEROIN. However, some are addicted to other opioid substances, such as hydrocodone (Vicodin), oxycodone/acetaminophen (Percocet), oxycodone controlled release (OXYCONTIN), or other narcotics.

Before buprenorphine was available, most patients who sought recovery took METHADONE and had to travel to a clinic as frequently as daily in order to obtain their medication. Some patients sought to undergo DETOXIFICATION on their own, a very dangerous choice. Others obtained their treatment from residential treatment centers.

Although buprenorphine is believed to be less addicting than methadone, physicians who wish to treat patients with buprenorphine outside residential treatment centers must obtain a waiver from special registration requirements under the CONTROLLED SUBSTANCES ACT. Physicians can con-

tact the Center for Substance Abuse Treatment, which is part of the Substance and Mental Health Services Administration (SAMHSA), for further information.

The doctors must meet special criteria under the Drug Addiction Treatment Act of 2000. For example, one qualifying criterion is that the doctor is certified in addiction psychiatry by the American Board of Medical Specialties, while another is that the doctor is certified in addiction treatment by the American Society of Addiction Medicine, among other criteria. Doctors may also be able to register for required courses online that will subsequently allow them to become providers of buprenorphine.

Physicians who are approved receive a special identification number from the DRUG ENFORCEMENT ADMINISTRATION. The doctor may treat no more than 30 patients at a time with buprenophine. Qualified doctors eligible to treat with buprenorphine can be located on the SAMHSA Buprenorphine Physician Locator Web site at http://buprenorphine.samhsa.gov/bwns_locator/index.html.

caffeine A legal stimulant that is present in many substances, such as most soft drinks, coffee, tea, and chocolate. It is estimated that as much as 80 percent of the world population consumes some form of caffeine on a daily or regular basis. Caffeine is often used as a routine part of daily life, although sometimes it is specifically taken to stimulate physical or mental performance. For example, the military has given caffeine to service members in combat to enable them to overcome fatigue and remain alert. Many college students load up on caffeinated beverages before taking their final examinations. Some people believe that giving an intoxicated person large quantities of coffee, is a good idea to counteract the effect of alcohol. However, it is a myth that coffee can counteract or cancel out intoxication.

In large quantities, caffeine can cause a person to become nervous and to suffer from insomnia. However, in most cases, a heavy user of caffeine should not suddenly stop consuming caffeine altogether at once. The sudden lack of caffeine is likely to cause severe headaches and other symptoms of physical withdrawal, such as irritability.

Caffeine acts on the central nervous system. The amount of caffeine in individual items varies greatly. In general, though, a cup of brewed coffee (8 ounces) has about 125 mg of caffeine, while the same amount of iced tea has 60 mg. One can of a caffeinated soft drink has about 40 mg of caffeine. In general, adults receive about two-thirds of their daily consumption of caffeine from coffee, while children receive about half their daily caffeine consumption from soft drinks.

Many people can tolerate about 300 mg of caffeine per day although sleep can be affected by as low a dose as 200 mg of caffeine. Caffeinated beverages and foods containing caffeine should not be consumed within three to four hours before the time when an individual wishes to sleep.

An excess of caffeine (more than 250 mg) can induce restlessness, nervousness, a flushed appearance, and even some psychiatric symptoms such as rambling speech or impaired thinking. In some cases, excessive caffeine intake can induce an ANXIETY DISORDER, which will usually resolve itself when the caffeine is out of the person's system.

Excessive caffeine consumption is dangerous for pregnant women. In a study of 562 women in Sweden who had spontaneous abortions (also known as miscarriages) in the first trimester of pregnancy, more pregnancy losses occurred in women who had ingested at least 100 mg of caffeine per day than in women who had consumed lower amounts.

Some mentally ill people are heavy abusers of caffeine, especially people with SCHIZOPHRENIA or BIPOLAR DISORDER. They may consume large quantities of caffeine in order to combat the sedating effects of the medications that they take.

Chronic heavy consumption of caffeine can lead to a generalized nervousness. It can also cause other medical problems, such as urinary incontinence, bladder pain, and bladder spasms, particularly if the daily intake exceeds 400 mg.

Genetic Aspects of Consumption

As with many other addictive behaviors, the drive to consume caffeine may have a strong genetic link. In a study reported in the *American Journal of Psychiatry* in 1999, researchers studied female twins from the Virginia Twin Registry and analyzed their caffeine consumption. Data was available for nearly 2,000 individual twins. "Heavy use" of caffeine was defined as equal to or greater than 625 mg daily or near daily. The researchers questioned the twins about their consumption of caffeinated coffee, tea, and soft drinks.

The researchers did not find a significant difference between the levels of past-year caffeine consumption of monozygotic (identical) and dizygotic (fraternal) twins. The researchers used self-reports from the twins for their findings. Based on the data, a large percentage of the twins had developed a tolerance to caffeine and some had a toxicity problem with it.

For example, a positive response to the question, "During the time when you consumed caffeinated beverages the most, did you find that you needed to drink a lot more to get the desired effect than you did when you first drank them?" indicated a tolerance problem. A positive response to the question, "During the time when you consumed caffeinated beverages the most, did you ever feel ill or shaky or jittery after drinking caffeinated beverages?" indicated a caffeine toxicity problem. They found that among the monozygotic twins, there was an 11.9 percent toxicity rate and a 14.9 percent tolerance rate. Among the dizygotic twins, there was a 14.0 percent toxicity rate and a 16.4 percent tolerance rate.

The researchers did find an apparent genetic linkage to caffeine use. They said, "Genetic factors appear to substantially influence a woman's vulnerability to caffeine use, heavy use, intoxication, tolerance and withdrawal." They also added, "Our results have implications for the debate over the status of caffeine as a drug of abuse. By demonstrating genetic influences on caffeine tolerance and withdrawal in man, our findings provide evidence in support of the validity of these phenomena."

Positive and Protective Aspects of Caffeine

Interestingly, caffeine has been shown to have some apparent positive or protective aspects. For example, it is frequently used with acetaminophen to treat patients with migraine or tension-type headaches. However, regular use of drugs such as butalbital (Fiorcet, Fiornal) can lead to rebound headaches, which are headaches caused by the medication. In such cases, patients must be tapered off the drug.

Caffeine also has some apparent protective aspects. A study reported in a 1999 issue of the *Journal of the American Medical Association* included about 46,000 men ranging from the age of 40–75 years and with no prior history of gallstone disease. The men with a significantly higher consumption of coffee had a lower risk of developing gallstones than the other men. (It is unknown if this protective factor is present in female coffee drinkers.)

In another study described in a 2000 issue of the *Journal of the American Medical Association*, data was analyzed on the caffeine and coffee consumption of about 8,000 Japanese-American men ages 45–68 years enrolled in the Honolulu Heart Program between 1965 and 1968. The researchers found that a higher coffee and caffeine intake was associated with a lower risk of developing Parkinson's disease. The researchers suggested that it was probably the caffeine rather than anything else in the coffee that was responsible for the results. If this tendency is also present among females or other racial or ethnic groups is unknown.

Cnattingius, Sven, M.D., et al. "Caffeine Intake and the Risk of First-Trimester Spontaneous Abortion," *New England Journal of Medicine* 343, no. 25 (December 21, 2000): 1,839–1,945.

Kendler, Kenneth S., M.D. and Carol A. Prescott. "Caffeine Intake, Tolerance, and Withdrawal in Women: A Population-Based Twin Study," *American Journal of Psychiatry* 156, no. 2 (February 1999): 223–228.

Lande, R. Gregory. "Caffeine-Related Psychiatric Disorders," Available online. URL: http://www.emedicine. com/med/topic3115.htm Downloaded on April 11, 2004.

Ross, G. Webster, M.D. "Association of Coffee and Caffeine Intake with the Risk of Parkinson Disease," *Journal of the American Medical Association* 283, no. 20 (May 24–31, 2000): 2,674–2,679.

Campral (acamprosate calcium) Delayed-release tablet that is used to treat alcoholism, and which was approved by the Food and Drug Administration in 2004 and first used in the United States in 2005. Campral acts on neurotransmitters (brain chemicals) known as glutamates to stabilize them. Some researchers believe overactive glutamates make withdrawal from alcohol difficult. Usually, detoxification from alcohol occurs before Campral is given. Campral is the first new antialcoholism drug introduced in nearly a decade in the United

States. Some physicians may combine Campral with naltrexone, a generic drug used to treat alcoholism. Campral reduces some of the symptoms that make withdrawal from alcohol difficult, such as anxiety, sleep disturbances, and sweating. In the general treatment setting, Campral is also noted to decrease the CRAVING for alcohol, thus decreasing RELAPSE rates and, even when relapse occurs, decreasing the severity of alcohol usage. Unlike Antabuse (disulfiram), Campral does not cause negative reactions when combined with alcohol. The purpose of Campral is to decrease alcohol craving and improve the rates of sobriety in recovering alcoholics.

The drug may cause diarrhea, nausea, and pruritis (itchy skin). Campral should not be used in patients who have kidney insufficiency. Patients who take Campral should be monitored for depression or suicidal thoughts.

See also ALCOHOLISM; ANTABUSE; NALTREXONE.

Saitz, Richard, M.D., "Unhealthy Alcohol Use," *New England Journal of Medicine* 352, 6 (February 10, 2005) : 596–607.

cancer A malignant tumor. Many forms of cancer are curable, and most forms are treatable. However, some cancers are very difficult to treat. Sometimes addictive behaviors increase the risk of developing cancer. For example, smoking cigarettes for many years significantly increases the risk for developing LUNG CANCER and ORAL CANCER. ALCOHOLISM increases the risk for developing colorectal cancer, esophageal cancer, and stomach cancer.

In general, most cancers are treated with surgery. If surgery is not possible because the tumor is not resectable (removable), the physician may choose radiation therapy to try to shrink the tumor so that surgery may be possible. Radiation therapy is also a primary form of therapy for cancer. Chemotherapy is another treatment. Chemotherapy refers to medications that are given to kill cancer cells; some cancers are very sensitive to chemotherapy. Note that in the medical setting, the word *chemotherapy* can also be used to refer to the medications used to treat other medical conditions, but in the treatment of cancer, this term is generally used to describe cell-killing drug treatment.

Fear of Addiction

Some doctors report that some patients who have advanced cancer and/or their families are reluctant for the patient to take narcotic painkillers because they fear that the patient may become addicted to the narcotics. However, according to the National Cancer Institute (NCI) in their report on substance abuse issues in cancer, substance abuse is very rare among patients with cancer. The report explained that generally patients with no past history of substance abuse are not at risk for developing such problems when taking opioids or related drugs to control their pain. Even cancer patients with a past history of substance abuse can usually be given narcotics under strict controls.

According to the NCI, "At one time it was assumed that many addictions originated from the use of drugs prescribed for pain." As a result, says the NCI, patients were undertreated for pain and to some extent, this problem still occurs today. The NCI says, "Patients and some health care professionals continue to have unfounded fears that opioid use for controlling cancer pain may become addictive when a more significant problem is the undertreatment of pain."

Yet conversely, because it has been proven that cancer patients have been able to use opioids for long-term pain effectively without developing an addiction, the NCI says that the risks and benefits of opioids in other long-term pain conditions should be reassessed. They state, "Three studies of over 24,000 patients without drug addiction histories who were being treated for burn, headache, or other pain [with opioids], found opioid abuse in only 7 patients."

However, the use of opioids for pain management in other chronic pain disorders is controversial among physicians. Even government agencies sometimes seem to be on opposing sides of this issue.

Former Substance Abusers with Cancer

Some patients who have recovered from alcohol or drug abuse in past years and who later develop cancer may be fearful of taking opiates for pain because they are concerned that they will develop an addiction and all their hard work will be lost. They do not understand that opiates taken for pain do not induce euphoria.

According to the NCI, "The health care provider should help the patient resolve these concerns and assure the patient that use of opioids to control symptoms of progressive disease does not result in the euphoria experienced by opioid abusers who do not have a medical illness." The NCI suggests that for patients who are reluctant to begin opioid therapy but who need narcotics for pain control, the doctor can work with the patient to develop strict guidelines for the use of the drug, which will help to give the patient a sense of control.

Current Substance Abusers with Cancer

Although most cancer patients are not substance abusers nor will they become addicted to opiates that are used to control pain, a small number of people who develop cancer were alcoholics or addicted to drugs before being diagnosed with cancer and they continue to be substance abusers. Such patients are best treated by a team, including one or more physicians, nurses, social workers, and, whenever possible, an expert in addiction medicine.

Physicians may hesitate to prescribe opioids to control pain in a patient who has been known to abuse drugs or alcohol recently. However, the problem with extreme caution can be that prescribing a below-normal dose of medication may result in undertreatment of the pain and consequently can result in causing the patient to seek illegal drugs in order to manage the severe pain. This does not mean that physicians can or should be lax about monitoring such patients. Doctors may choose to use frequent random urine tests for drugs to test for unprescribed or illegal drug use in these patients.

If substance-abusing patients with cancer need to undergo surgery, doctors may choose to admit them to the hospital several days early in order to stabilize their drug use prior to the procedure, according to the NCI. In addition, restrictions can be placed on the number of visitors as well as on packages that visitors are allowed to bring to the patient.

See also CARCINOGENS; MORPHINE; NARCOTICS; OPIATES; PAIN; PAIN MANAGEMENT.

National Cancer Institute. "Substance Abuse Issues in Cancer," Available online. URL: http://www.cancer.gov/cancerinfo/pdq/supportivcare/substanceabuse/patient Downloaded on April 18, 2004.

carcinogens   Substances known to cause or contribute to the development of cancer, such as the NICOTINE, tar, and carbon monoxide that are inhaled when people smoke cigarettes.

carisoprodol (Soma)   A sedating muscle relaxant that may be prescribed for pain. When used on a long-term basis, some patients may develop an addiction to the drug. Some experts also report that carisoprodol is sometimes used by drug abusers in order to prolong the effects of narcotics or BENZODIAZEPINES used illegally or to calm a person who feels excessively jittery from cocaine abuse.

Carisoprodol should not be taken with other central nervous system depressants. Additionally, it should not be taken with alcohol because the combination of drugs could be dangerous or even fatal.

Experts disagree on whether carisoprodol should always be avoided or is rarely appropriate in elderly individuals. Some believe it may be advisable in older, otherwise healthy patients for a short course of pain treatment, such as acute back pain.

Carisoprodol is not a SCHEDULED DRUG at the federal level, but some states have placed it as a Schedule IV drug at the state level (see SCHEDULED DRUGS). Patients with a history of substance abuse may have a problem with this drug. When metabolized in the blood, one of the substances that carisoprodol metabolizes to in the body is meprobamate, which is the cause of drug addiction in some patients.

Addicted patients have a difficult withdrawal from this drug. The most severe withdrawal reactions include seizures and coma, according to a 1993 article in the *American Journal of Drug and Alcohol Abuse.* Individuals who use large doses of carisoprodol over time can also develop psychotic symptoms, paranoia, or mania in response to the carisoprodol and the meprobamate metabolite. As a result of these problems, carisoprodol should be used with caution.

See also PRESCRIPTION DRUG ABUSE; TRAMADOL.

Jordan, Joe, Ann Hamer, and Kathy L. Katchum. "Carisoprodol (Soma) and Sedative Quantities to be Restricted on November 15, 2002," Available online. URL: http://pharmacy.oregonstate.edu/drug_policy/news/4_8/4_8.html. Downloaded on August 13, 2004.

Littrell, Robert A., Therese Sage, and William Miller. "Meprobamate Dependence Secondary to Carisoprodol Use—Soma," Available online. URL: http://www.findarticles.com/p/articles/mi_m0978/is-n1_v19/ai_13497394. Downloaded on August 13, 2004.

celebrities   Individuals who are famous or notorious because of their performance in movies or on television, in athletic events, at concerts, in politics, or in some other manner.

Many celebrities are exposed to a wide variety of addictive substances. Because they may be suddenly wealthy and inexperienced in handling money or because they may fear losing their celebrity status, they may feel extreme stress. To cope with that stress, some celebrities may abuse alcohol or drugs. Others may exhibit such addictive behaviors as chronic GAMBLING, engaging in excessive cosmetic surgery, or engaging in other problematic choices. Some celebrities can develop a sense of being above the law or have an inflated self-esteem that leads to increased problems with impulse control in many areas.

In general, the public appears sympathetic to celebrities who seek to obtain treatment for their addictive behaviors, such as those who obtain treatment from the BETTY FORD CENTER or similar treatment clinics.

See also ATHLETES.

chewing tobacco   See SMOKELESS TOBACCO.

child abuse and neglect   Child abuse is deliberate, human-inflicted injury or harm to a minor child under the age of 18 years, including physical abuse or sexual abuse; neglect is the failure to provide needed care, such as the failure to provide food and shelter. In the case of infants and small children, neglect can lead to fatalities. Individuals addicted to drugs or alcohol are more likely than others to commit crimes of child abuse and neglect. Studies have shown that children who have been physically or sexually abused and/or who have witnessed domestic violence are more likely to attempt SUICIDE as adults than those who have not been exposed to violence.

According to the National Clearinghouse on Child Abuse and Neglect Information, about 6 million children in the United States live with at least one parent who abused alcohol or other drugs in 2003. This organization also reports that an estimated one-third to two-thirds of all child maltreatment cases involve SUBSTANCE ABUSE. Children of substance-abusing parents are more likely to enter the foster care system and are more likely to stay in the system longer than other children.

The Adoption and Safe Families Act (ASFA) of 1997 limits the time that children can stay in foster care and provides for either their return to their families or their placement for adoption. ASFA is enabling many foster children to be adopted who, in the past, would have remained in foster care for their entire childhoods. However, one major problem with state social services agencies working under the ASFA is that they try to reunite children with their biological parents as soon as possible, which may mean returning children to substance-abusing parents who are still in need of treatment.

To explain the problem further, the ASFA requires that parental rights be terminated if the child has been in foster care for 15 of the past 22 months. Finding treatment and having the patient complete treatment within this timeframe can be very difficult. Thus, compliance with ASFA may not occur in the case of children of substance-abusing parents because the termination of parental rights are consequently delayed. Conversely, compliance with the law may occur. In those instances, the family will be broken up, and the children will be placed into adoptive families.

Turbulent Behaviors in the Home

According to data from the National Survey on Drug Use and Health, alcoholism (also called alcohol dependence) or alcohol abuse in a household is linked to a higher percentage of turbulent behaviors in the home. For example, in 2002 in the United States, serious arguments occurred in the households of about 30 percent of people who were alcoholics or alcohol abusers, compared with serious arguments in 18 percent of the households without alcohol problems. In households with alcoholism/alcohol abuse, in about 12 percent of the cases, a spouse or partner hit or threatened to hit someone one or more times. In contrast, hitting behaviors occurred in about 5 percent of the families without alcohol problems, a much lower percentage.

Predicting Maltreatment Recurrence in Child Abuse

Knowing if maltreatment recurrence could be predicted in child protective cases where alcohol and other drugs were involved would be useful. Two researchers sought to identify factors that predicted maltreatment recurrence, reporting on their results in a 2003 issue of *Children and Youth Services Review.*

The researchers collected data from 95 investigations in Illinois that involved alcohol or other drugs as part of the maltreatment allegation. The majority of the subjects were African American (60 percent), and the balance was about evenly split between whites and Latinas. Most families (68 percent) were headed by a single parent. The most common form of maltreatment was neglect (38 percent) followed by substance-exposed infants (37 percent). Physical abuse (7 percent) and sexual abuse (2 percent) were much less frequently found.

The researchers also found several significant factors of predictability that were related to short-term maltreatment recurrence. For example, among families in which protective service workers had initially found that substance abuse was present, the abusers were 13 times more likely to maltreat their children again. Another maltreatment report occurred within 60 days of the first report in 26 percent of the sample with an alcohol or drug problem.

The second predictive factor was whether criminal activity was present. If the protective worker had noted a high risk for such activity in the initial report, these cases were 770 times more likely to recur for maltreatment than cases that were noted as no risk.

Interestingly, protective cases in which the police were not initially involved were 18 times more likely to be referred for maltreatment again.

Assessing Parents in Substance-Abusing Families

Protective service workers sometimes have difficulty assessing families for child abuse and neglect. Workers may be inexperienced in the area of developmental delays, mental and physical health problems, and substance abuse. According to the National Center on Child Abuse and Neglect in their manual on protecting children in substance-abusing families, workers can gain information about substance abuse from parents by asking the following questions:

- How often do you drink beer, wine, liquor?
- How many drinks do you generally have when you are drinking?
- How old were you when you had your first drink?
- When do you tend to want a drink? When alone or with others? If you drink with others, with whom? When bored or when you want to party? When you are angry, frustrated, or stressed?
- What drugs have you tried?
- How often do you use?
- How do/did you use/take it?
- How long have you been using? How long did you use?
- How much do you smoke?
- When do you usually want a cigarette?
- When you were pregnant, what was your drinking/drug use like?
- How does your behavior change when you drink/use?
- How do you feel when you drink/use?
- What impact has alcohol and/or any other drug use had on your own health?
- What legal problems have you encountered as a result of your alcohol and/or drug use?
- How has the use of alcohol and/or other drugs affected your employment?
- How has your use of alcohol and/or other drugs affected your social relationships?
- Has the use of alcohol and/or other drugs resulted in violence or abuse in the home?
- What concerns do you have about your use of alcohol and/or other drugs?

It is also recommended that questions be asked about the impact of substance abuse on other members of the family, including such questions as:

- How do family members view alcohol and/or other drug use?
- Do family members deny use and/or its impact?
- Do family members express worry about the user?

- Do family members feel tense, anxious, or overly responsible?
- Are family members angry with the user?
- Do children in the family exhibit adult behaviors or assume adult parenting roles?

It is also suggested that workers evaluate the parents' awareness of the relationship of their substance abuse and the children's care. Professionals need to consider the following issues:

- If the parents were under the influence when the suspect child abuse or neglect occurred, and this was a contributing factor, do the parents acknowledge this relationship, and are they willing to make the changes necessary to avoid repeated injury or neglect?
- How have the parents provided for their children's needs in situations of relapse? It is helpful to determine whether parents have exercised the judgment to leave their children in the care of responsible relatives or friends, or whether the children have been left with strangers or brought along with the parents into dangerous situations.
- In cases of prenatal substance abuse, how do the parents view the infant's symptoms? Initially, parents may deny that symptoms or developmental problems exist. Although this initial denial can serve as a protective coping mechanism for parents, continual denial may interfere with the parents' obtaining needed services for their children.

See also CHILDREN, EFFECT OF PARENTAL SUBSTANCE ABUSE ON.

Clark, Robin E., Judith Freeman Clark, with Christine Adamec. *The Encyclopedia of Child Abuse,* 2nd ed. New York, N.Y.: Facts On File, Inc., 2000.

Fuller, Tamara L., and Susan J. Wells. "Predicting Maltreatment Recurrence Among CPS Cases with Alcohol and Other Drug Involvement," *Children and Youth Services Review* 25, no. 7 (2003): 553–569.

Kropenske, Vickie, and Judy Howard. *Protecting Children in Substance-Abusing Families.* Washington, D.C.: U.S. Department of Health and Human Services, Administration for Children and Families, National Center on Child Abuse and Neglect, 1994.

Office of Applied Studies. "Alcohol Dependence or Abuse among Parents with Children Living in the Home," *The NSDUH Report,* (February 12, 2004). Available online. URL: http://www.oas.samhsa.gov/2k4/ACOA/ACOA.htm. Accessed on May 2004.

children, effect of parental substance abuse on

The direct and indirect consequences of parental SUBSTANCE ABUSE on their children. The consequences of parental substance abuse are profound and may also be lifelong. Children who see their parents abuse drugs and/or alcohol may grow up to become substance abusers themselves. If they were victims of child abuse, they may also become abusive, should they become parents. However, this cycle can be broken with insight and understanding. The children of alcoholics or drug abusers are not doomed to repeat the mistakes of their parents.

Adverse Childhood Experiences Study

In a large study of 8,613 adults in California, reported in a 2003 issue of *Pediatrics,* the subjects in the Adverse Childhood Experiences (ACE) study were surveyed on problems with childhood abuse, neglect, illicit drug use, household dysfunction, criminality of household members, and mental illness of household members. They also compared the adults' abuse or addiction to drugs with childhood problems. The majority (54 percent) of the subjects were female, and their average age was 55 years.

The researchers found that a higher level of adverse childhood experiences, or ACE score, increased the likelihood of drug abuse or drug addiction by two to four times by the age of 14 years. The elevated risk continued into adulthood. Of those subjects who had no adverse childhood events, 1.3 percent reported ever having a drug problem, and less than 1 percent was ever addicted to drugs. When the person had one ACE, the percent who ever had a drug problem increased to 3 percent and those who were ever addicted to drugs rose to 2.1 percent. With each additional ACE, the risk for drug abuse and addiction rose. For example, when there were five or more ACEs, 12 percent had a drug problem and 9.2 percent had been addicted to drugs.

The authors said, "Because ACEs seem to account for one half to two thirds of serious problems with drug use, progress in meeting the national goals for reducing drug use will necessitate serious attention to these types of stressful and disturbing childhood experiences by pediatric practice."

See also CHILD ABUSE AND NEGLECT; FETAL ALCOHOL SYNDROME; SUICIDE.

Dube, Shanta R., et al. "Childhood Abuse, Neglect, and Household Dysfunction and the Risk of Illicit Drug Use: The Adverse Childhood Experiences Study," *Pediatrics* 111, no. 3 (March 2003): 564–572.

cirrhosis   Dangerous scarring and inflammation of the liver, often caused by ALCOHOLISM but sometimes also caused by viral HEPATITIS, such as hepatitis B or C. In addition, some individuals are alcoholics who have also contracted a form of hepatitis. Thus both their drinking and the hepatitis has harmed their liver. Some forms of hepatitis can be contracted by intravenous drug users through the sharing of contaminated needles. In addition, toxic damage to the liver over long periods of time from the abuse of some common medications such as acetaminophen (Tylenol) can lead to cirrhosis.

Some hereditary disorders such as hemochromatosis (iron overload) and Wilson's disease (copper overload) can also lead to cirrhosis. These illnesses should be ruled out in cases of suspected cirrhosis.

Individuals with cirrhosis also face an increased risk of developing liver cancer.

Symptoms of Cirrhosis

Although symptoms are rare in the early stages, some of the key indicators of cirrhosis are as follows:

- Jaundice (yellowing of the whites of the eyes or the skin, caused by a buildup of bilirubin)
- Nausea
- Fatigue
- An increased sensitivity to drugs that are metabolized by the liver, such as acetaminophen (Tylenol)
- Ascites (fluid buildup in the abdomen)
- An altered mental status (hepatic encephalopathy)

Diagnosis and Treatment

No symptoms usually appear in the early stages of cirrhosis, and liver function tests may continue to show normal values. When the cirrhosis becomes advanced, patients are diagnosed based on their symptoms, laboratory tests of liver function, and sometimes a liver biopsy is in order to verify the diagnosis and the cause. Imaging tests may show scarring of the liver.

Patients who are alcoholics diagnosed with cirrhosis should be hospitalized. During that time, they will undergo DETOXIFICATION from alcohol in order to enforce abstinence as well as to obtain medical treatment for the withdrawal symptoms. These withdrawal symptoms can include seizures, extreme vomiting, diarrhea, and other symptoms related to DELIRIUM TREMENS.

Patients with cirrhosis should be vaccinated against hepatitis A and B if they have not already been exposed to these infections. Contracting hepatitis would cause further liver damage to the already-impaired liver.

In early cases of cirrhosis, if alcoholic patients stop drinking entirely, their liver tissues may regenerate sufficiently to allow for adequate function. The only known cure for advanced liver cirrhosis is liver transplantation. Medical science has advanced to the extent that some patients can receive a portion of a liver from a live donor, rather than relying upon donations from cadavers.

See also ALCOHOLIC HEALTH PROBLEMS; ALCHOLIC HEPATITIS; FATTY LIVER DISEASE/STEATOSIS; LIVER.

Minocha, Anil, M.D. and Christine Adamec. *The Encyclopedia of the Digestive System and Digestive Disorders.* New York, N.Y.: Facts On File, Inc., 2004.

club drugs   A term for drugs that are sold, traded, or given away by patrons at nightclubs. These include drugs such as methylenedioxymethamphetamine or MDMA (ECSTASY), flunitrazepam (Rohypnol), gamma hydroxybutyrate (GHB), KETAMINE, and other illegal substances. Club drugs are also often called designer drugs because they are derived from other drugs; for example, MDMA is derived from METHAMPHETAMINE. These drugs may be very dangerous substances that can cause long-term consequences up to and including memory loss, brain damage, and death.

See also DATE/ACQUAINTANCE RAPE; DATE RAPE DRUGS.

National Institute on Drug Abuse. "Club Drugs," *NIDA InfoFacts,* (January 2004). Available onlinee. URL:

cocaine   A fine white powder that, when ingested, is a central nervous system stimulant. Medically prescribed cocaine is sometimes available and has some limited practical uses that are legal, primarily by physicians who are performing procedures on the eyes, ears, nose, and throat. However, the nonmedical use of cocaine is illegal. Illegal cocaine is often diluted, or cut, with substances such as lidocaine to increase the volume and provide greater profits to the drug dealer. Cocaine is made from the coca leaf grown primarily in Latin America and South America.

Cocaine can be administered intravenously or intranasally (also known as *snorting*). The effects of cocaine ingestion may last from a few minutes to a few hours. Users often report feeling euphoric after taking cocaine. Because it can dampen the appetite, some women have used cocaine to lose weight, which is not a legal use of the drug.

According to the Office of National Drug Policy, Executive Office of the President, in the November 2003 fact sheet on cocaine, there were about 2.7 million chronic users of cocaine in 2000 and an estimated 3 million occasional users of the drug in the United States.

Dangers of Cocaine Use

Cocaine use is dangerous because it can lead to serious long-term health problems and even to psychotic symptoms, such as auditory HALLUCINATIONS and paranoia. In addition, cocaine has been linked to a significant number of fatalities. The use of this drug has also been strongly associated with VIOLENCE and sexual abuse, including rape.

Some studies have shown that violence is particularly likely if both the abuser and the victim are using cocaine. This may occur because when only one person's judgment is impaired by cocaine, the other person may have a chance to escape the situation or resolve it peacefully. However, when both individuals are in an impaired state, the risk of violence is increased because both individuals may be more aggressive and violent than when not under the influence of the drug.

Researchers have identified a dangerous interaction between cocaine and alcohol, which leads to the production of cocaethylene in the liver. This newly created substance is more dangerous because it is more toxic and lasts longer than either cocaine or alcohol by themselves, and it can lead to death.

Many people who are abusers or addicts of cocaine have related problems, such as ALCOHOLISM and pathological GAMBLING.

Health Risks for Cocaine Addicts

Additional risks that cocaine addicts face are as follows:

- Heart attack
- Heart arrhythmia
- Chest pain
- Respiratory failure
- Strokes
- Seizures
- Abdominal pain
- Loss of the sense of smell
- Nosebleeds
- Chronically inflamed and runny nose
- Increased risk for contracting human immuno-deficiency virus (HIV) and acquired immune deficiency syndrome (AIDS)
- Increased risk for contracting HEPATITIS B and C
- Increased risk for contracting sexually transmitted diseases

History of Cocaine Use

According to Joseph F. Spillane, the author of *Cocaine: From Medical Marvel to Modern Menace in the United States, 1884–1920*, cocaine was first introduced in the United States in 1884 and was used as an anesthetic by physicians. At that time, no comparable anesthetic was available for patients who needed to be alert during a surgical procedure. Patients who needed surgery on their eyes, ears, nose, and throat faced excruciating pain from surgery. Cocaine alleviated the pain and enabled surgeons to perform the procedures.

Initially, the coca leaf was primarily imported from the leaves of the *Erythroxylon coca* bush from both Peru and Bolivia. Many of the shipments were of extremely poor quality. The leaves died before the plants arrived in the United States. Later, scientists learned how to create the drug first before shipping it to the end users.

Former president Ulysses S. Grant received the drug for his incurable throat cancer in order to relieve his severe pain. Many doctors believed that they had found a safe and effective substitute for barbiturates.

Doctors also used cocaine as a stimulating tonic as well as a drug to treat colds and hay fever. Cocaine was included in some tooth drops for toothaches. Cocaine was also used to treat an addiction to opiates and sometimes to treat alcoholism and depression (which was known as *melancholia* in the late 19th century). According to Cora Lee Wetherington and Adele B. Roman in their executive summary of *Drug Addiction Research and the Health of Women*, cocaine was an ingredient in Coca-Cola until 1906, when it was replaced with CAFFEINE.

Cocaine was later banned from most general use under the Harrison Narcotic Act of 1914. In 1970, Congress classified cocaine as a Schedule II narcotic under the CONTROLLED SUBSTANCES ACT. In the 1980s, some individuals began using CRACK

COCAINE. This is a chemically altered form of the drug and is smoked.

Demographics of Cocaine Users Today

According to the National Survey on Drug Use and Health, approximately 2 million Americans were cocaine users in 2002. About 28 million people in the United States, age 12 years and older, have tried some form of cocaine at least once in their lifetime. Of this number, 6 million have used crack cocaine. Among high school students, about 2.3 percent of all high school seniors used cocaine in the past month in 2002, which was slightly up from 2.1 percent in 2001.

Males are more likely to use cocaine than females based on the data from the National Survey on Drug Use and Health, or 2.7 percent of high school males, compared with 1.8 percent of females. Whites were much more likely to use cocaine than African Americans, and 2.8 percent of white high school seniors used the drug within the past month compared with 0.2 percent of African-America seniors. (See table below.)

Emergency Treatment for Cocaine Overdoses

Young adults have the greatest risk of experiencing a cocaine-related visit to a hospital emergency

PERCENT USE OF COCAINE IN THE PAST MONTH BY HIGH SCHOOL SENIORS, EIGHTH AND TENTH GRADERS, ACCORDING TO SEX AND RACE: UNITED STATES, SELECTED YEARS, 1991–2002							
	1991	**1995**	**1998**	**1999**	**2000**	**2001**	**2002**
All seniors	1.4	1.8	2.4	2.6	2.1	2.1	2.3
Males	1.7	2.2	3.0	3.3	2.7	2.5	2.7
Females	0.9	1.3	1.7	1.8	1.6	1.6	1.6
White	1.3	1.7	2.7	2.8	2.2	2.3	2.8
African American	0.8	0.4	0.4	0.5	1.0	0.6	0.2
All tenth-graders	0.7	1.7	2.1	1.9	1.8	1.3	1.6
Males	0.7	1.8	2.4	2.2	2.1	1.5	1.8
Females	0.6	1.5	1.8	1.6	1.4	1.2	1.4
White	0.6	1.7	2.0	1.9	1.7	1.2	1.7
African American	0.2	0.4	0.8	0.3	0.4	0.3	0.4
All eighth-graders	0.5	1.2	1.4	1.3	1.2	1.2	1.1
Male	0.7	1.1	1.5	1.4	1.3	1.1	1.1
Female	0.4	1.2	1.2	1.2	1.1	1.2	1.1
White	0.4	1.0	1.0	1.1	1.1	1.1	1.0
African American	0.4	0.4	0.6	0.3	0.5	0.4	0.5

Source: Fried, V. M., et al. *Chartbook on Trends in the Health of Americans. Health, United States, 2003.* Hyattsville, Md.: National Center for Health Statistics, 2003.

COCAINE-RELATED EMERGENCY DEPARTMENT EPISODES, ACCORDING TO AGE AND SEX: UNITED STATES, SELECTED YEARS, 1991–2001, EPISODES PER 100,000 POPULATION

Age and Sex	1991	1995	1996	1997	1998	1999	2000	2001
Both sexes								
12–17 years	10.6	9.3	11.5	16.0	18.8	14.0	18.8	14.5
18–25 years	76.9	76.2	80.1	91.8	88.2	89.5	88.9	85.5
26–34 years	120.5	153.7	166.7	164.5	173.1	161.9	154.6	176.4
35 years and older	26.5	46.0	54.0	57.4	63.2	63.7	67.7	76.2
Males								
12–17 years	9.5	10.5	12.9	15.3	20.7	17.4	16.7	14.3
18–25 years	102.7	98.1	101.9	116.1	115.2	120.5	118.5	112.8
26–34 years	152.8	196.2	212.7	211.3	219.7	195.5	193.8	220.8
35 years and older	40.7	69.2	61.2	85.6	92.2	92.0	97.1	108.0
Females								
12–17 years	11.0	7.8	10.0	16.6	16.7	10.2	20.9	14.5
18–25 years	53.0	54.1	57.5	66.4	61.7	57.7	58.2	55.6
26–34 years	86.1	108.6	118.9	117.0	125.0	127.3	112.9	130.0
35 years and older	13.6	24.8	29.2	31.3	36.6	37.9	40.1	46.6

Source: Fried, V. M., et al. *Chartbook on Trends in the Health of Americans. Health, United States, 2003.* Hyattsville, Md.: National Center for Health Statistics, 2003.

room. The number of episodes increased from 2000 to 2001 for some groups of individuals, particularly those age 26 and older. (See table above.)

As can be seen from the table, in 2001, males ages 12–17 years had about the same level of emergency room visits for cocaine abuse as females (14.3 per 100,000 population for males versus 14.5 per 100,000 for females). After that age, however, the risk for males sharply increased. For example, the rate per 100,000 of emergency room admissions for males ages 18–25 years was 112.8 per 100,000 compared with a rate of 55.6 per 100,000 for females. The rate escalated still further for males ages 26–34 years, or 220.8 episodes per 100,000 for males versus 130.0 per 100,000 for females. As individuals age beyond 34 years, their rate of hospital emergency visits for cocaine abuse sharply drops for both males and females, as seen in the table above.

Cocaine and Social Problems

Many, although not all, users of cocaine come from poverty-stricken neighborhoods where there is little hope for advancement or opportunities to leave the area. Most cocaine users are poorly educated. However, some individuals from affluent backgrounds abuse cocaine, perhaps initially perceiving it as a glamorous drug and a "perk" of their success, and then later becoming addicted to the drug.

Cocaine and Pregnant Women

Women who are pregnant should not use cocaine because it can affect fetal development. For a period of several years during the latter part of the 20th century, some states criminalized the use of cocaine by pregnant women. Women who tested positive for cocaine use after the delivery of an infant were compelled to enter a rehabilitative treatment center. Sometimes their children were taken away from them and placed into foster care for the safety of the child. In some cases, women did not regain custody of their children.

This policy was challenged in a class action lawsuit in 1994, according to George Annas, who is both an attorney and a medical doctor, in his 2001 article for the *New England Journal of Medicine*. The women prevailed in their lawsuit at the U.S. Supreme Court level in 2001.

Symptoms of Cocaine Use

Individuals who use cocaine may experience short-term effects, such as dilated pupils and an increased heart rate, blood pressure, and body temperature. Large amounts of cocaine may induce short-term aggressive or even violent behavior or paranoia. High amounts may also cause the individual to experience muscle twitches, vertigo, and body tremors.

According to the American Psychiatric Association in the *Diagnostic and Statistical Manual of Mental Disorders, Fourth Edition, Text Revision* (otherwise known as the *DSM-IV-TR*), cocaine dependence (which alludes to addiction) can cause psychiatric symptoms, such as DEPRESSION, ANXIETY DISORDER, and, as already mentioned regarding those who ingest large amounts of cocaine, aggressive behavior and paranoia. Some individuals develop cocaine intoxication, which is a severe reaction to the use of cocaine. Initially, the person is euphoric, hyperactive, talkative, grandiose, and restless. There are also physical signs, such as a change in the pulse rate, heightened or decreased blood pressure, and confusion.

Suicide and Cocaine Patients

Some patients who abuse cocaine are at risk for SUICIDE. In a study by Steven J. Garlow, M.D. reported in a 2002 issue of the *American Journal of Psychiatry,* Dr. Garlow discussed his analysis of the records from the medical examiner of patients who had committed suicide in Fulton County, Georgia, between 1994 and 1998. He found that nearly all

(95 percent) of the deceased victims who were positive for cocaine use were male, and the majority (51 percent) were African-American males, while 43 percent were white males. The large majority of the suicide victims were between the ages of 21 and 50 years old.

In another study of 84 cocaine addicts who had attempted suicide (and failed), reported by Alec Roy, M.D. in a 2001 issue of the *American Journal of Psychiatry,* the majority were female with a family history of suicidal behavior. The patients attempting suicide were compared with 130 cocaine-dependent patients who did not attempt suicide. Those who attempted suicide had made 175 attempts, or about two tries per person. They also had a greater use of other substances, such as alcohol and opiates. In addition, they had higher rates of depression and physical disorders than cocaine-dependent patients who did not attempt suicide.

Withdrawal from Cocaine

Because cocaine is a highly addictive drug, a sudden withdrawal is very traumatic and can be fatal. According to the *DSM-IV-TR,* withdrawal from cocaine can cause the individual to experience fatigue, heightened dreams or nightmares, sleep disorders (excessive sleeping or insomnia), an increased appetite, either lethargy or agitation, as well as somatosensory hallucinations of skin crawling or *formication.* Withdrawal should only be

COMPARISON OF LAW ENFORCEMENT AGENCIES IN THE UNITED STATES AND THE PERCEPTION OF COCAINE AND CRACK COCAINE AS THEIR GREATEST THREAT, BY PERCENTAGE, 2001

	New England	New York/ New Jersey	Mid-Atlantic	Great Lakes	Southwest	Florida/ Caribbean	West Central	Pacific	Southeast
Powdered cocaine	15.5	8.9	8.9	11.1	7.9	12.9	3.5	0.7	6.4
Crack cocaine	10.9	20.6	27.0	25.9	14.7	47.8	8.5	2.7	55.3

The New England region: Massachusetts, New Hampshire, Rhode Island, Connecticut, Vermont, and Maine. The New York/New Jersey region: New York and New Jersey. The mid-Atlantic region: Pennsylvania, West Virginia, Virginia, Maryland, and the District of Columbia. The Great Lakes region: northern Illinois and all of Minnesota, Wisconsin, Michigan, Indiana, Ohio, and Kentucky. The Southeast region: Tennessee, North Carolina, South Carolina, Georgia, Alabama, Mississippi, and Alabama. The Southwest region: southern California and all of Arizona, New Mexico, Oklahoma, and Texas. The Florida/Caribbean region: Florida, Puerto Rico, and the Virgin Islands. The West Central region: the southern part of Illinois and all of Montana, North Dakota, South Dakota, Wyoming, Nebraska, Iowa, Utah, Colorado, Kansas, Missouri, and Arkansas. The Pacific region: about two-thirds of California and all of Oregon, Washington, Nevada, and Idaho.
Source: National Drug Intelligence Center. *National Drug Threat Assessment 2003.* U.S. Department of Justice Product No. 2003-Q0317-001, January 2003.

undergone by patients who are under the treatment of a physician who is experienced in treating people addicted to cocaine.

The Distribution of Cocaine

According to the National Drug Intelligence Center in 2003, about 8 percent of state and local law enforcement agencies identified cocaine as their greatest drug of concern in 2001. Some regional differences occurred. For example, a greater percentage of state and local agencies in New England (15.5 percent), the Florida/Caribbean region (12.9 percent), and the Great Lakes (11.1 percent) identified powder cocaine as their greatest drug threat.

In contrast, crack cocaine was viewed as their greatest drug threat by 24.9 percent of state and local law enforcement agencies nationwide in 2001. Marked regional differences occurred in the perception of the threat of crack cocaine. For example, 55.3 percent of law enforcement agencies in the Southeast viewed crack cocaine as their greatest threat, followed by 47.8 percent in the Florida/Caribbean area and 27.0 percent in the mid-Atlantic area. (See table on page 66.)

Some stark regional differences occurred among law enforcement agencies over the perception of crack cocaine as a major threat. For example, crack cocaine was perceived as the major drug threat by 55.3 percent of the law enforcement agencies in the southeastern states, compared with a low of 2.7 percent in the Pacific region. (Methamphetamine was regarded as the greatest drug threat in the Pacific region.)

In their *National Drug Threat Assessment 2003*, the National Drug Intelligence Center estimated that about 28 percent of the cocaine that was illegally produced for world markets was smuggled into the United States in 2001, largely though the Mexico-Central America corridor. The cocaine was then primarily distributed in markets in large cities, such as Atlanta, Chicago, Houston, Los Angeles, Miami, and New York.

Some experts have been concerned that the penalties for smoking crack cocaine are generally stiffer than those for using powdered cocaine. Since many more users of crack cocaine are poor and African American, such policies essentially discriminate against these groups.

Treatment for Cocaine Addiction

Unfortunately, treating cocaine addiction is very difficult. Some researchers have tested the efficacy of alternative remedies, such as acupuncture, with mixed results. Drugs such as naloxone and NALTREXONE have been used to treat cocaine addiction, and some physicians have used disulfiram (ANTABUSE) and bupropion (Wellbutrin). A study released in 2004 reported that disulfiram, more commonly used to treat alcoholics, was effective in some patients who were addicted to cocaine, whether or not the patients were also alcohol abusers.

Many patients may benefit from taking antidepressants because of the low mood caused by withdrawal from cocaine. In addition, some doctors have found that bromocriptine has decreased the craving for cocaine in some patients, helping them to detoxify from the drug as well as to abstain from taking it later. Psychotherapy is an important part of recovery from cocaine addiction.

See also BEHAVIOR MODIFICATION; CRACK HOUSES; DEATH; TEENAGE AND YOUTH DRUG ABUSE.

American Psychiatric Association. *Diagnostic and Statistical Manual of Mental Disorders,* 4th ed., *Text Revision.* Washington, D.C.: American Psychiatric Association, 2000.

Annas, George J., M.D. "Testing Poor Pregnant Women for Cocaine—Physicians as Police Investigators," *New England Journal of Medicine* 344, no. 22 (May 31, 2001): 1,729–1,732.

Brookoff, Daniel, et al. "Testing Reckless Drivers for Cocaine and Marijuana," *New England Journal of Medicine* 331, no. 8 (August 25, 1994): 518–522.

Grisso, Jeanne Ann, M.D., et al. "Violent Injuries Among Women in an Urban Area," *New England Journal of Medicine* 341, no. 25 (December 16, 1999): 1,899–1,905.

Mendelson, Jack H., M.D. and Nancy K. Mello. "Management of Cocaine Abuse and Dependence," *New England Journal of Medicine* 335, no. 15 (April 11, 1996): 965–972.

National Drug Intelligence Center. *National Drug Threat Assessment 2003.* Johnstown, Pa.: U.S. Department of Justice Product No. 2003-Q0317-001, January 2003.

National Institute on Drug Abuse. "NIDA Study Finds Alcohol Treatment Medication, Behavioral Therapy Effective for Treating Cocaine Addiction," Press Release from the U.S. Department of Health and Human Services, March 2, 2004.

Roy, Alec M., M.D. "Characteristics of Cocaine-Dependent Patients Who Attempt Suicide," *American Journal of Psychiatry* 158, no. 8 (August 2001): 1,215–1,219.

Spillane, Joseph F. *Cocaine: From Medical Marvel to Modern Menace in the United States, 1884–1920.* Baltimore, Md.: Johns Hopkins University Press, 2000.

Wetheringon, Cora Lee and Adele B. Roman, ed., *Drug Addiction Research on the Health of Women.* Rockville, Md.: National Institute of Drug Abuse, 1998.

codependency   Refers to an unhealthy relationship in which a person who is closely involved with an alcoholic or addicted person, acts in such a way as to allow the addict to continue the addictive behavior. Codependency can also occur when an individual is addicted to sex or to any form of compulsive behavior. A codependent relationship usually happens between spouses, lovers, or relatives but can also occur between close friends.

The codependent person may seek to hide the consequences of an individual's addiction, such as by calling in sick to a boss when the alcoholic or drug addict is ill from the effects of alcohol or drugs, or by lying to others about the reasons for the addict's behavior. These actions are called enabling, because they actively help addicts to avoid the consequences of their acts and as a result, they enable the addict to continue the addiction.

Experts state that individuals who are codependent may feel that they are saintly or martyrs and that they are giving up their lives to save the addicted person. They may also experience an enmeshment of their personality with the addicted person such that sometimes the codependent person has difficulty in distinguishing what is best for herself or himself as separate from what is best for the addicted individual. Thus, all actions and decisions are subordinated to what will make the addicted person happy or, at least, not angry or upset. This becomes a particular problem if children are involved and when the codependent subordinates the needs of the children to the needs of the addict.

According to Dennis L. Thombs in his book *Introduction to Addictive Behaviors,* second edition, six key characteristics of psychological distress are experienced by most people who are codependents. First, they have low self-esteem. They may have grown up in alcoholic families or families in which they were physically or emotionally abused. Next, codependents have a need to be needed, and they primarily rate their own value based on how well they care for others. The third characteristic is an urge to control or change others, which may seem to be discordant since it does not appear to go along with low self-esteem and the other traits. However, the codependent believes rather grandiosely that he or she has the power to help the addict overcome the problem, far beyond what is realistic for the situation.

Says Thombs, "This may partly explain why some codependent women always seem to end up in dysfunctional relationships with addicted men, and why some women appear to take on unhealthy or impaired men as 'rehabilitation projects.' "

The fourth characteristic that is common to codependent individuals is the willingness to suffer. This is an important trait because suffering will inevitably come with living with an addicted person. Despite the suffering, however, the codependent may feel morally superior to other people who eventually give up on the addicted person. The codependent may feel that he or she really cares, unlike others.

The fifth characteristic is a resistance to change and the belief that leaving the addict is not a consideration. Last, the codependent has a fear of change and the belief that although the current situation is bad, a change in circumstances would be even worse.

Codependent individuals may have conscious or unconscious fears. They may fear that if the addict recovers, they would have to deal with demands with which they are uncomfortable. They may fear being asked to change something about themselves, or they may fear giving up control of the household. They may even fear giving up an addiction of their own.

Organizations like AL-ANON teach people who are codependent to cast off their codependency and let the addicted person take responsibility for his or her actions. These organizations can be of great help to those who discover that they have lost past opportunities with other potential marriage partners, lovers, or jobs because of their codependency. These self-help groups can also help codependent individuals to contemplate the harm that was done to their children as a result of the partner's addiction. In addition, such organizations can offer ongoing advice and support to avoid such behaviors in the future.

See also ENABLERS.

Thombs, Dennis L. *Introduction to Addictive Behaviors,* 2nd ed. New York: The Guilford Press, 1999.

college students Undergraduate or graduate students who are receiving education after graduation from high school. College students, as a group, have a tendency to abuse substances such as alcohol or drugs and may also develop other addictions, such as compulsive GAMBLING. In some cases, the addictions that they developed at a younger age may continue, while in other cases, the behavior develops while they are in college. College students are at particular risk for BINGE DRINKING and ALCOHOL ABUSE. An extreme intake of alcohol over a short period can lead to ALCOHOL POISONING and death.

Students who abuse illegal drugs and alcohol are more likely to engage in violent behavior and engage in risky sexual encounters such as failing to protect against pregnancy or sexually transmitted diseases. They are also more likely to be injured in car crashes or involved in sexual assaults. Some factors mitigate against alcohol abuse. For example, research indicates that favorable attitudes toward religion among college students may decrease the risk of drinking and alcohol-related problems.

Alcohol and College Students

Alcohol is the major addictive behavior for most college students. According to the Alcoholism Task Force on College Drinking in their report *High-Risk Drinking in College: What We Know and What We Need to Learn,* "The Panel found that on many college campuses, heavy drinking is interwoven overtly or subtly throughout the culture of the institution. As a result, students perceive this drinking pattern as the social norm rather than as unhealthy and potentially destructive behavior."

The panel identified several factors that influenced college students' drinking habits, including the following:

- The students' value systems and personalities
- The students' expectations regarding alcohol's effects (whether good or bad)
- Genetic predisposition, often reflected in a family history of alcoholism
- The family background and peers
- The social integration of drinking into college life
- The context in which drinking occurs (on- or off-campus parties, on- or off-campus bars)
- The economic availability of alcohol
- The level of law enforcement

Alcohol Abuse: Comparing College Students to Noncollege Students

Based on survey results from the National Institute on Drug Abuse, in the United States on the prevalence of ever having used drugs or alcohol when asked in 2002, the rate for college students was about the same as use was for their noncollege peers. A majority, 86 percent, of full-time college students used alcohol, compared with 86.4 percent of their peers. (See table on page 70.)

However, when considering the 30-day prevalence, or the use of the substance over the timeframe of the past 30 days, college students were worse abusers of alcohol than their peers who were not in college. (See table at top of page 71.) Nearly 69 percent of college students used alcohol, compared with 60.1 percent of their noncollege age peers, possibly because of the excessive drinking that occurs on many college campuses.

Finally, the most serious use of addictive substances is measured by daily consumption. When taking a look at the daily use of alcohol, college students have a more serious alcohol problem than their peers. (See table at bottom of page 71.) As can be seen from the table, 5 percent of college students were drinking alcohol daily in 2002, compared with 4.3 percent of their peers. In addition, 40.1 percent of college students, compared with 35.4 percent of their peers, engaged in binge drinking (defined as consuming five or more drinks in a row for men and four or more drinks in a row for women in the past two weeks).

Binge Drinking

College students have an escalated risk for engaging in binge drinking. An average of about 40 percent of college students have engaged in binge drinking. Rates among colleges vary dramatically, though, from as low as 1 percent to greater than 70 percent, depending on the particular institution. Because of this prevalence, both the United States Surgeon General and the United States Department of Health and Human Services have identified binge drinking among college students as a major public health problem, especially among males and young adults.

Students at Risk for Heavy Drinking

Studies indicate that binge drinking and alcohol abuse is the heaviest among white male students, followed by Hispanic males and African-American males. Most are younger than age 24. Members of fraternities and sororities who live in residence are heavier drinkers than nonresidents. College athletes are often heavier drinkers than nonathletes. Female binge drinkers have an increased risk of suffering from rape. Studies have shown that 10 percent experienced rape compared with the 3 percent risk of nonbinging female students.

Female (and Male) Drinkers May Underestimate Their Problem

Female heavy drinkers in college are more likely to underestimate their drinking problem, according to *Binge Drinking on America's College Campuses: Findings from the Harvard School of Public Health College Alcohol Study.* This research revealed that of those drinkers who binged three or more times in the past two weeks, 7 percent of the women said they were heavy or problem drinkers, compared with 20 percent of the men who identified themselves

LIFETIME PREVALENCE OF USE FOR VARIOUS TYPES OF DRUGS, 2002: FULL-TIME COLLEGE STUDENTS VS. OTHERS AMONG RESPONDENTS 1–4 YEARS BEYOND HIGH SCHOOL (PERCENTAGES)

	Total		Males		Females	
	Full-time College	Others	Full-time College	Others	Full-time College	Others
Any illicit drug	51.8	62.3	54.3	58.4	50.2	65.3
Any illicit drug other than marijuana	26.9	39.0	30.4	37.6	24.6	40.0
Marijuana	49.5	59.6	51.5	56.4	48.2	62.0
Inhalants	7.7	15.6	9.3	17.0	6.6	14.6
Hallucinogens	13.6	22.2	17.1	22.8	11.3	21.8
LSD	8.6	17.5	8.7	18.0	7.9	17.2
Cocaine	8.2	17.4	9.9	19.2	7.1	16.0
Crack	1.9	6.5	1.4	8.3	2.1	5.2
MDMA (Ecstasy)	12.7	18.7	13.0	19.0	12.6	18.5
Heroin	1.0	2.3	0.9	2.7	1.0	1.9
Other narcotics	10.6	15.5	11.7	18.8	9.9	13.1
Amphetamines, adjusted	11.9	18.6	12.1	17.9	11.7	19.2
Ice	2.0	6.7	1.8	9.6	2.1	4.4
Barbiturates	5.9	11.7	7.1	12.8	5.1	10.8
Tranquilizers	10.7	18.3	11.9	20.0	9.9	17.1
Alcohol	86.0	86.4	85.9	84.2	86.1	88.1

Source: Johnston, Lloyd D., Patrick M. O'Malley, and Jerald G. Bachman. *Monitoring the Future National Survey Results on Drug Use, 1975–2002; Volume II: College Students and Adults Ages 19–40.* National Institute on Drug Abuse, NIH Publication No. 03-5375. Bethesda, Md.: National Institute on Drug Abuse, 2003.

30-DAY PREVALENCE OF USE FOR VARIOUS TYPES OF DRUGS, 2002: FULL-TIME COLLEGE STUDENTS VS. OTHERS AMONG RESPONDENTS 1–4 YEARS BEYOND HIGH SCHOOL, IN PERCENTAGES

	Total		Males		Females	
	Full-time College	Others	Full-time College	Others	Full-time College	Others
Any illicit drug	21.5	26.2	25.1	27.3	19.3	25.4
Any illicit drug other than marijuana	7.8	12.1	8.4	11.7	7.4	12.4
Marijuana	19.7	23.1	23.7	25.2	17.2	21.4
Inhalants	0.7	1.1	0.5	2.2	0.9	0.3
Hallucinogens	1.2	1.6	2.0	2.4	0.7	1.0
LSD	0.2	0.5	0.4	0.9	0.1	0.2
Cocaine	1.6	3.6	2.2	5.3	1.2	2.4
Crack	0.3	0.9	0.1	1.3	0.4	0.6
MDMA (Ecstasy)	0.7	1.9	0.9	2.0	0.7	1.8
Heroin	0.0	Almost 0	0.0	0.1	0.0	0.0
Other narcotics	1.6	2.7	1.4	4.7	1.8	1.2
Amphetamines, adjusted	3.0	3.8	3.2	2.5	2.8	4.7
Ice	0.0	1.8	0.0	2.5	0.0	1.3
Barbiturates	1.7	2.8	2.2	3.0	1.4	2.7
Tranquilizers	3.0	4.8	3.1	4.7	2.9	4.8
Alcohol	68.9	60.1	70.2	65.5	68.0	56.1
Cigarettes	26.7	37.6	30.0	36.3	24.6	38.3

Source: Johnston, Lloyd D., Patrick M. O'Malley, and Jerald G. Bachman. *Monitoring the Future National Survey Results on Drug Use, 1975–2002; Volume II: College Students and Adults Ages 19–40.* National Institute on Drug Abuse, NIH Publication No. 03-5375. Bethesda, Md.: National Institute on Drug Abuse, 2003.

30-DAY PREVALENCE OF DAILY USE FOR VARIOUS USE OF DRUGS, 2002: FULL-TIME COLLEGE STUDENTS VS. OTHERS AMONG RESPONDENTS 1–4 YEARS BEYOND HIGH SCHOOL, IN PERCENTAGES

	Full-time College	Others	Full-time College	Others	Full-time College	Others
Marijuana	4.1	8.7	5.7	10.7	3.0	7.2
Cocaine	0.0	Almost 0	0.0	0.1	0.0	0.0
Amphetamines, adjusted	0.1	0.3	0.2	0.0	0.1	0.5
Alcohol						
Daily	5.0	4.3	7.0	5.3	3.7	3.5
5+ drinks in a row in past 2 weeks	40.1	35.4	50.7	43.8	33.4	29.0
Cigarettes						
Daily	15.9	31.5	16.6	29.5	15.4	33.0
Half-pack or more per day	7.9	21.9	8.7	20.5	7.3	22.8

Source: Johnston, Lloyd D., Patrick M. O'Malley, and Jerald G. Bachman. *Monitoring the Future National Survey Results on Drug Use, 1975–2002; Volume II: College Students and Adults Ages 19–40.* National Institute on Drug Abuse, NIH Publication No. 03-5375. Bethesda, Md.: National Institute on Drug Abuse, 2003.

in this manner. Thus, although denial of problem drinking was prevalent with both genders, the male students were statistically more likely to identify their own problematic drinking pattern.

Emotions Affect Drinking

Other studies have looked at the emotional states of college students and found linkages to other problems. In a study in a 2004 issue of the *Journal of Nervous and Mental Disease,* a researcher surveyed students at 119 colleges nationwide in the United States. She found that students with poor mental health and depression were more likely to be female, nonwhite, and to engage in heavy drinking and in drinking in order to get intoxicated.

Drinking and Driving

Alcohol has an effect on the ability to drive safely. According to the National Highway Traffic Safety Administration, more than 1,400 college students ages 18–24 years died from alcohol-related injuries in 1998. About 80 percent of these deaths occurred in motor vehicle crashes.

Yet many college students continue to drive while drunk or with others who are intoxicated according to the Centers for Disease Control and Prevention. For example, in 1998, more than 2 million of an estimated 8 million college students drove vehicles while under the influence of alcohol, and 3 million students rode with a drinking driver.

In one study of the age of the individual at the time when they were first intoxicated compared with other behaviors, published in a 2003 issue of the *Journal of Studies on Alcohol,* researchers found that students who had been drunk for the first time before they were age 19 were significantly more likely to become heavy drinkers or alcoholics later. They were also more likely to drive after drinking, to ride in a car with a driver who was either drinking or high, and to receive injuries that required medical attention. The subjects who were intoxicated at early ages apparently overestimated their own abilities as to how much they could drink and yet still manage to drive safely.

Said the researchers, "Respondents first intoxicated at younger ages believed they could consume more drinks and still drive safely and legally; this contributed to their greater likelihood of driving after drinking and riding with high or drunk drivers."

Violence and Drinking

Drinking on campus increases the risk for violence. In 1998, an estimated 600,000 college students were assaulted by another student who had been drinking. An estimated 70,000 students were victims of alcohol-related sexual assaults or acquaintance rapes. Half or more of all sexual assaults are associated with alcohol abuse by one or both parties. The actual number of these assaults is estimated to be much higher as they are often not reported because of guilt and shame experienced by the victim.

High-risk Sexual Behavior

Excessive drinking is linked to risky sexual behavior. Alcohol abusers are less likely to engage in safe sex and are at greater risk for contracting a sexually transmitted disease or creating an unplanned pregnancy. Some studies have also shown that students who are heavy drinkers have a two to three times greater likelihood than others of having multiple sex partners in the past month.

Memory Loss

Heavy drinking can cause memory loss (alcoholic blackout), and this is a problem among some college students who drink. In one study of college students, reported in *High-Risk Drinking in College; What We Know and What We Need to Learn,* 54 percent of frequent binge drinkers, 27 percent of occasional binge drinkers, and 10 percent of nonbinge drinkers reported one or more incidents of forgetting where they were or what they were doing while drinking.

Drugs and College Students

Most college students are not heavy drug users although they may experiment with drugs such as MARIJUANA. (See table at bottom of page 71.) According to *Monitoring the Future: National Survey Results on Drug Use, 1975–2002; Volume II: College Students and Adults Ages 19–40,* published in 2003, about 4 percent of college students were daily marijuana users in 2002, and about 4.5 percent of all young adults used marijuana on a daily basis.

As can be seen from the tables, the majority of college students (51.8 percent) have used an illicit drug at some time, compared with 62.3 percent of their peers not in college. Most (49.5 percent) have tried marijuana, followed by methylenedioxy-methamphetamine (ECSTASY) (12.7 percent) and AMPHETAMINES (11.9 percent). In considering the use in the past 30 days (table bottom of page 71.), marijuana is again the most popular drug (after alcohol), and 19.7 percent of college students reported using this drug. It was followed in popularity by COCAINE (1.6 percent).

Tobacco and College Students

As shown from the tables, college students apparently smoke cigarettes at about half the rate of their peers of the same age. Based on the data provided by the National Institute on Drug Abuse, about 16 percent of college students smoke daily, compared with 31.5 percent of their peers. About 8 percent are heavy smokers, compared with nearly 22 percent of their peers of the same age.

However, the results of a 1997 national survey, reported in a 2000 issue of the *Journal of the American Medical Association,* showed a somewhat different picture and, instead, revealed a higher usage of tobacco. This data indicated that college students used forms of tobacco other than cigarettes; for example, they used cigars and SMOKELESS TOBACCO. Among college men in 1997, 8.7 percent, primarily intercollegiate male athletes, used smokeless tobacco. Use of pipe tobacco use, however, was virtually unknown.

In this comprehensive survey, over 14,000 students were queried at 119 colleges in the United States. Nearly half the students (46 percent) had used a tobacco product in the past year, and one-third said they currently used tobacco. Most used cigarettes (29 percent), but many also used cigars (8.5 percent). Many students smoked both cigars and cigarettes.

Gambling and College Students

Some students are compulsive gamblers. In a study reported in a 2004 issue of the *Journal of American College Health,* based on a survey of 1,350 undergraduates at four campuses of Connecticut State University in 2000, the researchers found that 4 percent of the females and 18 percent of the males had gambling behaviors that were problematic. The students identified as problem gamblers also had other behavioral problems and had a greater risk for heavy drinking and regular tobacco and marijuana use. In addition, they were more likely to engage in BINGE EATING. The researchers also found that ATHLETES were at greater risk for gambling problems than nonathletes.

See also BLACKOUTS, ALCOHOLIC; DATE/ACQUAINTANCE RAPE; DATE RAPE DRUGS; DRINKING GAMES; DRIVING, IMPAIRED; DRIVING WHILE INTOXICATED/DRIVING UNDER THE INFLUENCE; SMOKING AND HEALTH PROBLEMS; TEENAGE AND YOUTH DRINKING; TEENAGE AND YOUTH DRUG ABUSE; TEENAGE AND YOUTH GAMBLING; TEENAGE AND YOUTH SMOKING.

Engwall, Douglas, Robert Hunter, and Marvin Steinberg. "Gambling and Other Risk Behaviors on University Campuses," *Journal of American College of Health* 52, no. 6 (May/June 2004): 245–255.

Hingson, Ralph, et al. "Age of First Intoxication, Heavy Drinking, Driving after Drinking and Risk of Unintentional Injury Among U.S. College Students," *Journal of Studies on Alcohol* 64, no. 1 (2003): 23–31.

Johnston, Lloyd D., Patrick M. O'Malley, and Jerald G. Bachman. *Monitoring the Future National Survey Results on Drug Use, 1975–2002; Volume II: College Students and Adults Ages 19–40.* National Institute on Drug Abuse, NIH Publication No. 03-5375. Bethesda, Md.: National Institute on Drug Abuse, 2003.

National Advisory Council on Alcohol Abuse and Alcoholism Task Force on College Drinking. *High-Risk Drinking in College: What We Know and What We Need to Learn: Final Report of the Panel on Contexts and Consequences.* Washington, D.C.: National Institute on Alcohol Abuse and Alcoholism, April 2002.

O'Malley, Patrick M. and Lloyd Johnston. "Epidemiology and Other Drug Use Among American College Students," *Journal of Studies on Alcohol, Supplement* no. 14 (2002): 23–39.

Rigotti, Nancy A., M.D., Jae Eun Lee, and Henry Wechsler. "U.S. College Students' Use of Tobacco Products: Results of a National Survey," *Journal of the American Medical Association* 284, no. 6 (August 9, 2000): 699–705.

The National Center on Addiction and Substance Abuse at Columbia University. *The Formative Years: Pathways to Substance Abuse Among Girls and Young Women Ages 8–22.* New York: Columbia University, February 2003.

Wechsler, Henry. "Binge Drinking on America's College Campuses: Findings from the Harvard School of Public Health College Alcohol Study." Available online. URL: http://www.hsph.harvard.edu/cas/Documents/monograph_2000/cas_mono_2000.pdf Downloaded on June 26, 2004.

Weitzman, Elissa R. "Poor Mental Health, Depression, and Associations with Alcohol Consumption, Harm, and Abuse in a National Sample of Young Adults in College," *Journal of Nervous & Mental Disease* 192, no. 4 (April 2004): 269–277.

Zimmerman, Robert and William DeJong. *Safe Lanes on Campus: A Guide for Preventing Impaired Driving and Underage Drinking.* Newton, Mass.: Higher Education Center for Alcohol and Other Drug Prevention, 2003.

Colombia   A South American country that is a major supplier of illegal drugs abused in the United States and Canada, such as HEROIN and COCAINE. A large proportion of these drugs are smuggled through MEXICO. However, according to the National Drug Control Strategy, released by the White House in 2004, cocaine production in Colombia decreased by about 15 percent from 2001–02. In addition, opium poppy cultivation decreased by an estimated 25 percent. (Heroin is derived from opium poppies.) These are positive indicators for those concerned about addictive drugs.

Heroin poppies also grow in Asian countries such as Afghanistan, which is the world's largest cultivator of poppies as well as the largest producer of opiates. According to the White House report, if all the poppies grown in Afghanistan in 2003 were converted to heroin, this would result in 337 metric tons of heroin. Despite these facts, most of the heroin that is used in North America comes from South America, and Columbia and Mexico together produce less than 20 metric tons combined. This amount is sufficient to meet the illicit demand for heroin in North America.

The DRUG ENFORCEMENT ADMINISTRATION of the United States has offices in cities in other countries, such as Bogotà, Colombia. In 2002, greater than 1.3 metric tons of heroin were seized in South American airports by U.S. federal agents. In addition, about 1.8 metric tons of heroin were seized in 2002 at airports in the United States.

The White House. *National Drug Control Strategy: Update.* Washington, D.C.: Office of National Drug Control Policy, March 2004.

compulsive shopping   The need to purchase items that are usually unnecessary to the buyer and are also often beyond the financial means of the individual as well. Compulsive shopping is an addictive behavior that may affect 2–8 percent of the population in the United States. Most compulsive shoppers are female. Compulsive shopping may be a form of impulse control disorder for many people. Some experts believe that compulsive shoplifting by affluent individuals is a "sister" addictive behavior to compulsive shopping.

The shopping can sometimes take unusual forms. For example, a compulsive shopper may buy the same item in multiple colors or sizes. Some women focus on a particular type of item, such as shoes or handbags; some buy hundreds of the same item. Specific compulsions to buy items such as paper goods or hoarding of purchased items may represent additional features of compulsive shopping. Many individuals with this problem do not ever use the items but find returning them to be difficult from an emotional standpoint.

The availability of credit cards may facilitate compulsive shopping for many people. Spending may not seem as real to compulsive shoppers when they use a credit card as when they pay for items with cash. When the credit card bills become due, the compulsive shopper may be unable to meet minimum monthly payments and go into a panic. Some compulsive shoppers must declare bankruptcy as a last financial resort because they cannot create a plan to pay off the massive debts that they have accrued as a result of their compulsive spending.

Although many people joke about the urge to "shop until they drop," a compulsive shopping problem can be serious. It can cause not only financial hardship for the individual and the family but often leads to the end of marital and other important relationships.

There are some indications that compulsive shopping can be treated with medication. In a 2003 issue of the *Journal of Clinical Psychiatry,* scientists at Stanford University Medical Center reported their findings on 24 people diagnosed with compulsive shopping disorders, including one person who had purchased more than 2,000 wrenches. All of these patients had been compulsive shoppers for 10 years or longer.

The researchers gave some of the patients the antidepressant medication citalopram (Celexa). A significant number of the patients taking the medication experienced improvement and no longer felt compelled to shop compulsively and beyond their financial means. Findings like these may indicate that compulsive shopping has an underlying component of obsessive-compulsive disorder, DEPRESSION, and/or anxiety.

Dr. Lorrin M. Koran, one of the study researchers said in a July 17, 2003 press release from Stanford University Medical Center, "I'm very excited about the dramatic response from people who had been suffering from decades. My hope is that people with this disorder will become aware that it's treatable and they don't have to suffer."

Patients can also be treated with cognitive behavioral therapy in which they are trained to identify and challenge their irrational thoughts related to their addiction. With the help of a skilled and experienced therapist, compulsive shopping and its underlying components of depression, anxiety, or obsessive-compulsive disorder can often be overcome.

See also CREDIT CARD OVERSPENDING; IMPULSE CONTROL DISORDER.

Aboujaoude, Elias, Nona Gamel, and Lorrin M. Koran. "A 1-year Naturalistic Follow-up of Patients with Compulsive Shopping Disorder," *Journal of Clinical Psychiatry* 64, no. 8 (August 2003): 946–950.

Controlled Substances Act   A law passed in 1970 in the United States that is the basis for determining which drugs are classified as SCHEDULED DRUGS, requiring special control by physicians and law enforcement officials. Some scheduled drugs are illegal, such as MARIJUANA, HEROIN, LYSERGIC ACID DIETHYLAMIDE (LSD), and CRACK COCAINE. (The powdered form of COCAINE is lawfully used by some physicians, such as ophthalmologists or otylaryngologists, who sometimes use the drug as an anesthetic to treat conditions of the eyes, ears, nose, and throat.)

Many scheduled drugs are legal if they are prescribed by physicians, although their use is monitored by federal and state agencies. Such drugs include some narcotics and other painkilling drugs, some ANABOLIC STEROIDS, and some sedating drugs, such as BARBITURATES and BENZODIAZEPINES.

Since 1970, some drugs have been added to the scheduled drugs list, such as ECSTASY (methylene-dioxymethamphetamine) and ANABOLIC STEROIDS, among others.

See also DRUG ENFORCEMENT ADMINISTRATION; NARCOTICS; OPIATES.

cosmetic surgery, addiction to   A problem in which a person has repeated unnecessary cosmetic surgery procedures. The patient feels compelled to have surgery to correct real or imagined imperfections. However, once the procedure occurs and if the supposed defect is corrected, the patient finds yet another problem to obsess about and subsequently desires correction of this newfound defect through cosmetic surgery. Both women and men may have this problem, although it is more commonly noted in females.

The Probable Cause of Cosmetic Surgery Addiction: Body Dysmorphic Disorder

Some individuals confuse their appearance with their entire identity. Thus, if they do not believe that they are extremely attractive, they think that they have no personal worth. They may try to hide themselves away from others despite the fact that most people would say that most such individuals had an average or even an above-average appearance.

Experts believe such individuals may have body dysmorphic disorder (BDD), a psychiatric problem in which they cannot see their bodies as they actually are, with both good points and flaws. Instead, they perceive their appearance or some feature of their appearance as extremely ugly or unattractive and much worse than it actually appears to others. Some experts estimate that up to 7 percent of patients who present to cosmetic surgeons have BDD. It is estimated that about 1–2 percent of the population may have BDD, although this estimate may be low.

Some experts believe that BDD is a form of OBSESSIVE-COMPULSIVE DISORDER, while others think it may be a form of eating disorder or delusional disorder. Some patients with this problem also excessively exercise to the point of an apparent EXERCISE ADDICTION.

In its most extreme case, an addiction to cosmetic surgery can be very disfiguring, as with celebrities such as pop singer Michael Jackson. Numerous procedures in the same part of the body can damage the cartilage, skin, and muscle tone, depending on the area operated on. Eventually, no further surgeries can be performed for cosmetic purposes, either because there is not enough tissue or the existing tissue is too badly damaged.

Most reputable plastic surgeons warn their patients ahead of time that elective cosmetic surgery is likely to improve their appearance but is not some magical solution that will make their lives problem free subsequent to the surgery.

Studies

In one unique study, reported in *Psychiatric Bulletin,* psychiatrist David Veale studied 25 patients with BDD who collectively had undergone a total of 46 cosmetic surgery procedures. Of the patients, four had had three procedures, and one patient had had four procedures. The other patients had gone through one or two procedures each. The most unhappy patients were those who had had rhinoplasty (nose surgery) or repeated procedures.

In about half the cases, after the procedure, if the patient was satisfied with the result, the dissatisfaction was transferred to another part of the body. Such patients should avoid cosmetic surgery.

Dr. Veale said, "When patients were dissatisfied with their operation, they often felt guilty or angry with themselves or the surgeon for having made their appearance worse, thus further fuelling their depression and a failure to achieve their ideal. This in turn tended to increase mirror gazing and craving for more surgery."

In nine cases discussed by Dr. Veale, patients who could not afford cosmetic surgery attempted to perform their own surgical procedures at extreme risk. For example, one man who thought the skin on his face was too loose used a staple gun to make it more taut. Fortunately, the staples fell out but the man nearly damaged his facial nerve. Another man used sandpaper to attempt dermabrasion on his skin. One woman used a knife to attempt her own liposuction of the fat on her thighs. One man rode his bicycle into a truck to cause a crash and fracture his jaw because he was unhappy with his chin and thought the crash would enable surgery. At the last minute, he changed his mind, raised his head, and suffered a fractured skull. As might be expected, none of these patients were happy with the outcomes of their own efforts.

According to one author in the *British Medical Journal,* men with BDD are usually unhappy with the results of cosmetic surgery and may become "severely depressed, suicidal, litigious, or even violent towards the treating physician." In addition to or instead of cosmetic surgery, some men attempt to alter their body by taking ANABOLIC STEROIDS.

In another study of patients who had multiple cosmetic surgery procedures, the authors found that factors often related to unhappiness with outcome included youth, male gender, having had previous unsatisfactory cosmetic procedures, and holding unrealistic expectations. In addition, a history of depression, anxiety, or personality disorder were indicators of a patient who would probably be unhappy. Some studies found that BDD predicted poor outcome.

Patients with BDD may also have other disorders, such as depression or obsessive-compulsive disorder. Some may have social phobias.

Treatment

Antidepressants may be helpful for patients with BDD who insist on repeated cosmetic surgery procedures, although such patients may be resistant, insisting that their "ugliness" is a valid problem. Surgeons themselves would be wise to screen such patients ahead of time since they are unlikely to be pleased with the outcome, no matter how effective the surgery.

See also ANOREXIA NERVOSA; ANXIETY DISORDERS; BULIMIA NERVOSA.

Honigman, Robert J., Katharine A. Phillips, and David J. Castle. "A Review of Psychosocial Outcomes for Patients Seeking Cosmetic Surgery," *Plastic Reconstructive Surgery* 113, no. 4 (April 1, 2004): 1,229–1,237.

Phillips, Katharine A., and David J. Castle. "Body Dysmorphic Disorder in Men," *British Medical Journal* 323, no. 7320 (November 3, 2001): 1,015–1,016.

Veale, David. "Outcome of Cosmetic Surgery and 'DIY' Surgery in Patients with Body Dysmorphic Disorder," *Psychiatric Bulletin* 24 (2000): 218–221.

cough syrup   Medication that is taken to treat severe coughs. Cough medicines may contain codeine, an addictive substance. In addition, even over-the-counter cold medications often include alcohol, which can be addictive in some individuals and which consequently are abused by some people. Cough syrups that contain codeine are SCHEDULED DRUGS under the CONTROLLED SUBSTANCES ACT. The reason for this is that continued use of cough syrup with codeine may lead to an addiction.

Some individuals, primarily adolescents and some young adults, abuse over-the-counter cough medicine and cold remedies and may develop a psychological and a physical tolerance to them, needing higher doses to achieve the same effect. They may legally purchase these items, or sometimes they may shoplift them from pharmacies or supermarkets. Some pharmacists keep certain remedies, those they believe or know to be the most likely to be abused, at the pharmacy counter, where they must be specifically requested.

According to the DRUG ENFORCEMENT ADMINISTRATION, some individuals abuse cough syrups not only because of their codeine content but also because they contain a chemical known as dextromethorphan, which is a cough suppressant. Abusers consume large quantities of cough syrup with dextromethorphan for its euphoric qualities. There are also oral tablets of dextromethorphan that are sold legally as cough suppressants and that are sometimes abused.

Large quantities of dextromethorphan may induce HALLUCINATIONS and dissociative effects (a feeling of not being really present) similar to symptoms found with the abuse of KETAMINE. Abuse of dextromethorphan may also induce hyperthermia (a very high fever), nausea and vomiting, abdominal pain, irregular heartbeat, high blood pressure, headache, loss of consciousness, brain damage, and death. In addition, over-the-counter medications that include dextromethorphan frequently contain other ingredients that may be harmful when taken in extremely high doses, such as acetaminophen (Tylenol), decongestants, and antihistamines.

crack cocaine   A highly addictive form of cocaine that is smoked. Crack cocaine is very rapid acting. Users experience a euphoric high within about 10 seconds of smoking it.

This form of cocaine initially became popular in the mid-1980s, and it was called crack because of the crackling sound that is heard when the drug is smoked. Because of the large number of arrests for crack cocaine in the 1980s, the concept and reality of DRUG COURTS were instituted. In these courts, only offenses related to drugs are considered and specific plans are given to offenders. If offenders follow the plan, they stay out of jail. If they do not, they go to jail.

Crack is created by dissolving powdered cocaine with water and either ammonia or baking soda. This substance is boiled until it solidifies, and then it is broken up into chunks of white or off-white rocks. Some users combine crack with HEROIN or marijuana.

Crack cocaine is illegal under the CONTROLLED SUBSTANCES ACT. There are no medical indications for the use of crack cocaine, in contrast to powdered cocaine, which has some legal medicinal uses when administered by physicians.

According to the National Survey on Drug Use and Health, an estimated 6 million people in the United States have used crack cocaine. Among high school students, about 2.3 percent of all high school seniors used cocaine in the past month in 2002, which was slightly up from 2.1 percent in 2001.

In general, the possession or selling of crack cocaine is punished more severely than the possession of powder cocaine. Some experts feel this is a form of discrimination since minorities and individuals who are poor are more likely to use crack than powdered cocaine.

Effects of Crack

As with cocaine abuse, there are many side effects and health risks associated with the use of crack cocaine. The drug may cause increased blood pressure, heart rate, and body temperature (hyperthermia) as well as an elevated risk of seizures and heart attack. In addition to these risks, crack cocaine users may also develop severe respiratory problems, such as shortness of breath and lung trauma. Smoking crack cocaine can also lead to major behavioral changes and may cause users to develop aggressive and/or paranoid behavior.

In the past, it was assumed that "crack babies" (infants born to mothers addicted to crack) would inevitably be seriously learning disabled, hyperactive, and otherwise harmed or damaged for life.

Research so far on such children has not borne out these extreme fears.

Crack Cocaine Use Among Patients Admitted for Treatment

According to a 2003 *DASIS Report* (from the Drug and Alcohol Services Information System), in 2000, crack cocaine was the primary drug of abuse for 14 percent of adult females who were admitted to substance abuse treatment programs nationwide in the United States. (This data was drawn from the Treatment Episode Data Set [TEDS], which is a compilation of data on the demographic traits of individuals who are admitted for substance abuse treatment.)

In addition, of all the women who were admitted to a treatment center for cocaine dependency, 77 percent were users of crack cocaine. About half of the women had been smoking cocaine for more than 10 years. The average age of women entering treatment was 35 years old. The majority (58 percent) were African American, followed by whites (32 percent) and Hispanics (5 percent).

Most of the women (81 percent) who entered treatment also abused other substances as well. An estimated 50 percent abused alcohol and 29 percent abused MARIJUANA.

See also COCAINE; CRACK HOUSES; CRIME; PROSTITUTION.

Drug and Alcohol Services Information System. "Women in Treatment for Smoked Cocaine: 2000," *The DASIS Report,* September 26, 2003. Available online. URL: http://www.oas.samhsa.gov/2k3/FemCrack/FemCrack. htm. Downloaded March 1, 2004.

crack houses   The name for sites where individuals illegally buy and sell CRACK COCAINE. Crack houses are usually in poor neighborhoods where there is little or no police surveillance, and the police are either distant from the area or reluctant to enter it because of the high crime rate and risk of violence.

See also COCAINE.

crank   See METHAMPHETAMINE.

craving   Intense and often overpowering desire to perform a behavior. Craving is an essential aspect of every form of addiction. It precedes the act, often increasing in intensity until the individual engages in the addictive behavior, whether the behavior is smoking, drinking alcohol, using illegal drugs, or engaging in another addiction. A craving is temporarily satisfied when the individual engages in the addictive behavior; however, it recurs again and again among addicted individuals.

See also ACKNOWLEDGMENT OF ADDICTION; RECOVERY.

credit card overspending   Spending to the limit on one's credit cards despite an inability to pay the amounts that are charged. Many addicted individuals get into trouble with credit card overspending for a variety of reasons. They may have spent all or most of their money on their addiction, whether it is to alcohol, drugs, GAMBLING, or other addictions, and turn to their credit cards as a last means to finance their addictive behaviors.

Individuals who overspend on their credit cards may have psychiatric problems, such as BIPOLAR DISORDER. They may also have a problem with COMPULSIVE SHOPPING. Many individuals with such problems cannot pay their bills and, consequently, must turn to family members for help. Ultimately, many must file for bankruptcy.

See also IMPULSIVITY.

For further information on credit card overspending, contact the following organization:

Debtors Anonymous
P.O. Box 920888
Needham, MA 02492
http://www.debtorsanonymous.org

crime and addiction   An illegal act that is associated with one or more addictive behaviors. A crime may be a felony, such as a HOMICIDE (murder), a sexual assault, or other serious types of crime, or it may be a misdemeanor, which is a lesser crime, such as shoplifting an inexpensive item. CHILD ABUSE is also a criminal act. Individuals addicted to drugs or alcohol are more likely than others to commit crimes of child abuse as well as other crimes.

Using illegal drugs is itself a crime that is punishable and can lead to jail time, depending on such factors as the location of the offense and whether it was the first offense. For example, if an illegal drug was sold in a DRUG-FREE ZONE (often a school, playground, or similar area where children primarily congregate), the penalties attached to this offense are usually far more severe than if the drug was sold elsewhere. If the person has committed many crimes before, he or she may be seen as a habitual offender and one in need of INCARCERATION, in contrast to a person who has never committed a crime before and toward whom the justice system may take a more lenient view. State laws vary on sentencing guidelines.

Addictive Behaviors and Criminal Acts

Individuals addicted to alcohol or drugs are not the only ones with addictive behaviors who may turn to crime. Many different types of addictive behaviors may lead individuals to performing criminal acts because of the desperation of the individual and the fact that he or she may have no further financial resources to obtain what is needed in order to carry out the addiction. Compulsive gamblers may resort to crime because they nearly always need money to continue to gamble when they have exhausted their own finances. Individuals who are sex addicts may commit crimes such as engaging in illegal sexual acts with children.

In many cases, however, illegal acts are tied to drug or alcohol abuse. Sometimes the person may have sufficient funds, but the route to the desired substance is blocked by other means. For example, the desired item may be illegal or may be legal under some conditions (such as a SCHEDULED DRUG) but a physician has decided that it should not be given to the addicted person. For example, if a person is addicted to a prescription drug and a physician has refused to prescribe the drug, some patients will resort to stealing prescription pads and forging the doctor's order to obtain a prescription. (Most pharmacists are well aware of the ways that prescriptions can be faked and will not hesitate to alert law enforcement authorities when someone exhibits any of these behaviors.)

Other patients will perform less direct acts but with the same intent of obtaining the addicted item. Consequently, they may steal money or items of value to others in order to obtain money to purchase prescribed or illegal drugs. This situation is particularly painful for family members who are aware of the drug problem but do not wish to turn their relative over to the police. They may be fearful that jail would be worse than the individual's current unhappy situation.

Criminals Have High Rates of Alcohol and Drug Abuse

Studies of incarcerated individuals, under the Arrestee Drug Abuse Monitoring Program (ADAM), managed by the National Institute of Justice, has revealed that many inmates have a very high rate of substance abuse. Although it cannot be concluded that drug abuse and alcoholism inevitably lead to criminal behavior since many people with drug and alcohol problems are not incarcerated and do not appear to commit crimes, it does seem significant that large proportions of those who do commit crimes are also individuals with serious drug and alcohol problems.

Some patterns of behavior are also seen among the inmates that are instructive. For example, the ADAM data for 2000 looked at patterns of alcohol abuse as well as drug abuse. The data showed that compared with adult male arrestees who had their first alcoholic drink after age 21, those individuals who drank for the first time at or before age 13 were twice as likely to be at risk for alcoholism. In addition, the younger drinkers were also twice as likely to be at risk for drug addiction as an adult. This fact alone seems to underline the importance of denying alcohol to teenagers.

The arrestees were interviewed and were also drug tested for 10 drugs. Four drugs consistently showed up most often: COCAINE (CRACK COCAINE and powder), MARIJUANA, METHAMPHETAMINE, and OPIATES. Of these, marijuana was the most commonly used drug, followed by cocaine, opiates, and methamphetamine.

In half the sites where arrestees were tested, at least 40 percent of adult males tested positive for marijuana. In half the sites, at least 31 percent of the arrestees tested positive for cocaine. Opiate use varied considerably depending on the site. For example, the range was 2 percent of arrestees in Fort Lauderdale, Florida; Omaha, Nebraska; and Charlotte-Metro, North Carolina, but was a high, of 27 percent, in Chicago.

Methamphetamine abuse among the arrestees was the highest in the western United States. The top rate was seen in Honolulu, Hawaii, (36 percent), followed by Sacramento, California, (29 percent),

San Diego, California, (26 percent), San Jose, Puerto Rico, (22 percent), Portland, Oregon, (21 percent), and Spokane, Washington, (20 percent).

See also DRUG COURTS; DRUG ENFORCEMENT ADMINISTRATION; DRUG TESTING; IMPULSE CONTROL DISORDER; MENTAL ILLNESS/PSYCHIATRIC PROBLEMS; PROSTITUTION; VIOLENCE.

National Institute of Justice, Office of Justice Programs. *2000 Arrestee Drug Abuse Monitoring: Annual Report.* NCJ 193013. Washington, D.C.: U.S. Department of Justice, April 2003.

cross-tolerance   When the regular use of one drug results in the need for a higher-than-expected dosage level of another related drug in order to achieve the desired effect in a patient, whether the hoped-for effect of the second drug is pain control, sedation, or something else. Some drugs are similar enough in their effect on the brain that a tolerance and addiction to one drug will lead to an equivalent tolerance to another related or sometimes an unrelated drug. Such a cross-tolerance is found with alcohol and benzodiazepines, with methadone and heroin, and with oxycodone and hydrocodone. HEROIN abusers can become extremely tolerant and resistant to all opiate pain medication, and alcoholics can become very tolerant to BENZODIAZEPINES and related drugs.

Patients who have been taking opiate medications, whether legally or illegally, should be sure to advise their physician, and particularly the anesthesiologist, about their drug use before any procedure requiring anesthesia and/or PAIN MANAGEMENT. Sometimes a higher dose than usual of the anesthesia drug will be required in patients with a cross-tolerance.

See also TOLERANCE.

crystal meth   See METHAMPHETAMINE.

Darvon   See PROPOXYPHENE.

date/acquaintance rape   Forcible sexual intercourse with a person who is known to the victim. A date implies a potentially romantic relationship, while a reference to an acquaintance implies a more distant relationship. However, many experts use the terms date rape and acquaintance rape interchangeably.

Perpetrators

The rapist may be a person the victim has just met. It may be their first date, or they may have had an ongoing relationship. The rapist may be someone the victim knows casually and is not dating. In most cases of date rape, the rapist and/or the victim are intoxicated with alcohol and/or illegal drugs. BINGE DRINKING is a major factor in many cases of date rape. College campuses that are known for high rates of binge drinking have a higher risk of women being raped than other colleges, according to a 2004 study in the *Journal of Studies on Alcohol.*

In some cases, the victim unknowingly ingests drugs that have been administered by the assailant, often placed in an alcoholic drink or even a can of soda. These are called DATE RAPE DRUGS. More often, alcohol or drugs are consumed willingly by the victim.

Adolescent Victims

Most cases of date rape are perpetrated against adolescent and young adult females, although adolescent males, too, are date raped, usually (in 90 percent of cases) by other males. According to a 2001 statement from the Committee on Adolescence of the American Academy of Pediatrics (AAP) on adolescent sexual assault victims, adolescents suffer the highest rates of rapes and other sexual assaults compared with all other age groups, with female victims predominating in a ratio of 13.5 to 1.

About two-thirds to three-fourths of these adolescent rapes are perpetrated by an acquaintance or a relative. In the case of younger adolescents, the perpetrator may be someone in the extended family. In the case of older adolescents, the rape is more likely to occur on a date. Said the report, "Adolescents with developmental disabilities, especially those in the mildly retarded range, are at particular risk for acquaintance and date rape."

According to the statement from the AAP, adolescent rape victims are more likely to have used drugs or alcohol than adult rape victims. Some reports indicate that alcohol or drugs are a factor in at least 40 percent of sexual assaults. Adolescent victims often delay seeking medical attention and are also often reluctant to press charges with the police against their assailants. However, females are more likely to report sexual assaults than are male victims.

Many rape victims suffer from POSTTRAUMATIC STRESS DISORDER. Victims of date rape may wonder if their behavior before the act somehow led to the rape. According to the statement from the Committee on Adolescence, "Adolescent victims may feel that their actions contributed to the act of rape and have confusion as to whether the incident was forced or consensual." In addition, say the authors of the statement, "Self-blame, humiliation, and naivete may prevent the adolescent from seeking medical care." Adolescents need to be reassured that they were not to blame for acts of violence against them, such as rape.

College Student Victims

In one study that included date rape as well as other acts of sexual violence, researchers surveyed over 4,000 college women at two- and four-year colleges in the United States in 1997. They described their findings in *The Sexual Victimization of College Women,* a report for the National Institute of Justice, which is a division of the U.S. Department of Justice. According to this report, some of the women (23 percent of those who were raped) were raped more than once. The researchers found a rate of 19.3 completed rapes per 1,000 female students and 16.0 attempted rapes per 1,000 female students.

According to the researchers, in 90 percent of the cases, the victims knew the person who raped them. In most cases of completed rapes, the rapist was a classmate (35.5 percent), a friend (34.2 percent), or a boyfriend or ex-boyfriend (23.7 percent). Most rapes occurred at night, and only about 12 percent occurred between the hours of 6 A.M. and 6 P.M. The majority of the completed rapes (almost 60 percent) occurred in the victim's own residence, while 31 percent occurred in living quarters off the campus and about 10 percent occurred in a fraternity house.

Very few women reported the rapes to the police. Less than 5 percent of the women who suffered either completed or attempted rapes reported the incidents to the police, although about two-thirds of them told someone else, usually a friend.

The women said that they did not report a completed rape for several key reasons, and some women gave more than one reason for failing to report the incident to the police. These reasons included that they did not want other people to know about the rape (46.9 percent), they did not want their family to know about it (44.4 percent), they felt that there was a lack of proof that the incident had happened (42.0 percent), they were not sure that what had occurred was a crime or that harm had been intended (44.4 percent), they feared reprisals from the assailant or from others (39.5 percent), they feared the police would not think that their complaint was serious enough (27.2 percent), they did not know how to report a rape (13.6 percent), and they feared being treated hostilely by the police (24.7 percent).

The reason given most frequently for not reporting a completed rape was that the women did not think it was serious enough to report to police (65.4 percent). As of this writing, improved education regarding date rape is being evaluated by many college campuses.

The researchers found four risk key factors among the women who were most at risk for sexual victimization, including date rape. These included frequent drunkenness among the victims, being unmarried, a prior sexual assault before the school year began, and living on the campus.

Another study of rapes on college campuses used data from 119 schools and involved a sample of over 8,000 women in each year in 1997 and 1999 and about 7,000 in 2001. The findings were published in the *Journal of Studies on Alcohol* in 2004. The researchers found that 4.7 percent of women reported being raped. Most of the rapes (72 percent) had occurred when the victims were too intoxicated either to consent or to refuse to have sex.

Said the study authors, "College prevention programs must give increased attention to educating the male college student that one of the first questions he must ask himself before initiating sex with a woman is whether she is capable of giving consent. College men must be educated for their own protection that intoxication is a stop sign for sex. College women need to be warned not only about the loss of control through heavy drinking but also about the extra dangers imposed in situations where many people are drinking heavily."

Other risk factors that the researchers found for rape occurring in college were being under age 21, being white, living in a sorority house, using illicit drugs, having a past history of heavy drinking during high school, and attending a college that had a high rate of binge drinking. Although date rape drugs are still a cause for concern for students, the authors contend that the substance that women should be the most concerned about is the one that is still the most commonly abused in colleges and in the United States: alcohol.

Committee on Adolescence, American Academy of Pediatrics. "Care of the Adolescent Sexual Assault Victim," *Pediatrics* 107, no. 6 (June 2001): 1,476–1,479.

Fisher, Bonnie S., Francis T. Cullen, and Michael G. Turner. *The Sexual Victimization of College Women.* National Institute of Justice Research Report, MCJ 182369. Washington, D.C.: U.S. Department of Justice, December 2000.

Mohler-Juo, Meichun, et al. "Correlates of Rape While Intoxicated in a National Sample of College Women," *Journal of Studies on Alcohol* 65, no. 1 (2004): 37–45.

date rape drugs   Drugs that sexual assailants use to induce unconsciousness in others, including drugs such as flunitrazepam (ROHYPNOL, a sedating drug that is not legal in the United States), KETAMINE (generally used as an anesthetic), clonazepam (Klonopin, an antianxiety drug), fentanyl (a drug that is usually used by veterinarians to sedate animals), or gamma-hydroxybutyrate (GHB), another drug of abuse.

The assailant may be an acquaintance or someone met at a party, hence the term DATE/ACQUAINTANCE RAPE. The drugs are colorless and odorless and must be specifically sought for by toxicologists within about 72 hours after their unknowing ingestion.

Because of concern about this illegal use of drugs, in 1997, the manufacturer of Rohypnol reformulated the drug so that if it is mixed with a liquid, the fluid will become blue. However, some sexual predators place the drug in blue drinks or dark containers to hide the warning blue color.

The drugs work rapidly, usually within about 15 minutes after being consumed from a drink or food. In most cases, after the drug is administered to the unknowing victim (usually a woman, but sometimes a man) and its effects are apparent, the victimizer removes the drugged person to another place where the unconscious person is then sexually assaulted.

The drugs have an amnesiac effect, so the victim has no memory of the actual assault, although she may awaken without any clothes on or with her clothes in disarray and in a place that she has no memory of going to. Victims may be told that they consented to sex, and they may also be told (and may believe) that they were intoxicated when they agreed to have sex. Others around the person at the time of the drug's effects may have assumed that the victim was intoxicated. Often the assailant had easily convinced others that the victim needed to leave and required assistance, which the assailant would seemingly provide.

Because of concern for date rape drug victims, the federal Drug-Induced Rape Prevention and Punishment Act was passed in 1996, which provides for punishments of up to 20 years when controlled drugs are used without the victims' knowledge in order to rape or act violently against them.

See also CLUB DRUGS; ECSTASY; GHB.

dealers, drug   People who sell drugs to others illegally. Such substances may include COCAINE, HEROIN, MARIJUANA, or medications that can be prescribed by a doctor but are sold on the street to others without a prescription, such as OXYCONTIN, METHADONE, or other narcotics. In general, state and federal laws, as well as law enforcement officials and the courts, take a much harsher position against drug dealers than against individuals who are drug addicts but are not dealers themselves, and thus, drug dealers are usually given longer sentences.

See also COCAINE; CRACK COCAINE; CRACK HOUSES; DRUG COURTS; ZERO-TOLERANCE LAWS.

death   Cessation of life. Some addictive behaviors can lead to death, such as chronic ALCOHOLISM, ALCOHOL POISONING, DRUG ABUSE, and some eating disorders, such as ANOREXIA NERVOSA, BINGE EATING DISORDER, and BULIMIA NERVOSA. Years of smoking can lead to the development of diseases that cause death, such as LUNG CANCER and EMPHYSEMA. Participation in extreme sports or exercising to the point of addiction can lead to death. SEX ADDICTION can lead to death. If the individual participates in unprotected sex, exposure to the human immunodeficiency virus can lead to acquired immune deficiency syndrome, which is fatal.

In many cases, addicted individuals have been warned by their physicians, family members, and others that the addiction is killing them. In the case of some drugs, death may be caused the first time the substance is used, such as when a person takes ECSTASY. This may occur because of other underlying illnesses that the individual has (such as a respiratory or heart problem) or because of the extreme potency of the drug, the contaminants of a drug that was ingested, or a combination of factors.

Cocaine and Death

In some studies, COCAINE has been found to be a major cause of death. For example, researchers studied fatal injuries among nearly 15,000 residents of New York City over the period of 1990–92 and reported on their findings in a 1995 issue of the *New England Journal of Medicine*. Among the nearly 10,000 deceased persons who were ages 15–44 years old, benzoylecgonine, a metabolite of cocaine, was found in nearly 36 percent of the cases. In addition, ETHANOL (alcohol) was found in about 34 percent of the people who died, and free cocaine (cocaine that is not bound to serum protein and has not been metabolized) was present in about 25 percent.

About one-third of the deaths were directly linked to cocaine intoxication, but two-thirds of the deaths were caused by SUICIDES, HOMICIDES, traffic accidents, and falls. Said the researchers, "If fatal injury after cocaine use was considered as a separate cause of death, it would rank among the five leading causes of death among those 15 to 44 years of age in New York City." As of this writing, cocaine abuse continues to be a major problem in New York and many other cities in the United States.

See also ANABOLIC STEROIDS; CRACK COCAINE; HOMICIDE; METHAMPHETAMINE; VIOLENCE.

Marzuk, Peter M., M.D., et al. "Fatal Injuries After Cocaine Use as a Leading Cause of Death Among Young Adults in New York City," *New England Journal of Medicine* 332, no. 26 (June 29, 1995): 1,753–1,757.

delirium tremens (DTs)   Refers to a severe reaction of an alcoholic to the complete withdrawal from alcohol. Most alcoholics should undergo alcohol withdrawal only under the careful supervision of a physician, preferably in a treatment facility or hospital with specific programs for alcoholism. If an individual who is a long-term alcoholic undergoes withdrawal on his or her own, with no medical assistance, he or she may become severely ill, could become psychotic, and could also die.

Delirium tremens may cause the following symptoms:

- Confusion
- Hallucinations
- Extreme sweating
- Seizures
- Nausea and vomiting
- Insomnia
- Fever
- Emotional lability or mania

These symptoms may last for days or even for weeks. To help the patient tolerate the withdrawal and to prevent delirium tremens, physicians may prescribe antianxiety medications, sedatives, or even antipsychotic drugs.

See also ALCOHOLIC HEALTH PROBLEMS; ALCOHOLISM; DETOXIFICATION; HALLUCINATIONS.

depression   The common name to describe depressive illnesses, which cause chronically severely negative moods and a risk for suicidal behavior in some individuals. The presence of depression is very different from a passing sadness or a bad day. People with depression cannot cheer themselves up or pull themselves together. They need treatment. According to the National Institute of Mental Health (NIMH), in any given year in the United States, about 19 million people suffer from a depressive illness, and nearly two-thirds of them do not obtain the help that they need. Yet treatment can alleviate symptoms in an estimated 80 percent of all cases.

Many individuals with addictive behaviors such as the abuse of alcohol or drugs may have problems with an underlying clinical depression that may have been untreated for years. Some people may unconsciously seek to treat their depression with alcohol and/or illegal drugs. Doctors usually cannot determine which problem came first, the abuse/addiction or the depression. However, they can attempt to treat both problems or treat one problem and refer the patient for treatment of the other problem. For example, the physician may treat depression and refer the patient to a clinic for treatment of drug abuse.

Types of Depression

According to the NIMH, three types of depressive disorders are most common. The first is major depressive disorder (sometimes referred to as unipolar depression or clinical depression). It is often manifested by persistently sad or empty feelings and feelings of hopelessness, worthlessness, and guilt that make it difficult or impossible for the individual to carry on a normal life. Other symptoms that may occur are as follows:

- Fatigue
- Difficulty concentrating and making decisions
- Sleep problems, such as insomnia or oversleeping
- Weight problems, such as an unintended weight loss or gain
- Thoughts of death or SUICIDE or actual suicide attempts

Dysthymia is a second and less severe form of depression, with the same symptoms as already discussed but less intense. It is generally a longer-term and more chronic problem than major depressive disorder.

BIPOLAR DISORDER is another form of depression. It includes periods of depression that are alternated with periods of mania (severe highs). Mania can lead to a PSYCHOTIC BREAK if untreated. Individuals who are manic may engage in compulsive GAMBLING, promiscuous sexual behavior, excessive drug and alcohol use, and other addictive behaviors.

Some symptoms of mania are as follows:

- Racing thoughts
- Increased sexual desire
- Excessive elation
- Decreased need for sleep
- Grandiose ideas
- Rapid talking
- Increased energy level
- Inappropriate social behavior

Women and Depression

In general, women are about twice as likely to suffer from depression as men. This may be due to hormonal factors, such as menstrual cycle changes and menopause. It may also be due to the additional life stressors that they face, such as single parenthood or the need to care for aging parents. Some women develop a short-term depression after the birth of a child, which is called postpartum depression.

Men and Depression

Although fewer men experience depression than women, they have four times the rate of suicide. Men may mask their depression with ALCOHOLISM and drug use or by working very long hours. Many men are resistant to seeking help for their depressive symptoms.

Elderly and Depression

Many people believe that it is "normal" for senior citizens to feel depressed, but this is not true. According to the American Association for Geriatric Psychiatry, 15 percent of adults older than 65 suffer from depression, and the rate is higher if the individual is in a hospital or a nursing home. Some illnesses may trigger depression, such as cancer, diabetes, heart disease, or stroke. The loss of a loved one may also lead to depression. The loss of a loved pet may trigger depression in some elderly individuals.

Although they may have medical problems that are painful and difficult to cope with, if elderly individuals are depressed as well, the depression can and should be treated. Yet many elderly people are resistant to discussing their mood problems with doctors and, instead, may present with numerous minor physical complaints. It is also true that some medications that older people take, such as medications for hypertension, Parkinson's disease, and other illnesses, may induce depressive symptoms as a side effect.

Older people who are depressed may have worsening symptoms of their other health problems. This may be a cause or an effect of an increasing depression. (Depression can generate physical symptoms, causing patients to worry more about health problems that would not normally trouble them.) In the worst case, very depressed patients may choose suicide. The elderly population is at an increased risk for suicide, often because of depression rather than physical pain or suffering. Although they comprised about 13 percent of the population, they represented about 18 percent of all suicide deaths in 2000. The highest suicide rates were for white males age 85 and older, or 59 deaths per 100,000 persons in 2000. This rate was more than five times the national rate of 10.6 per 100,000.

Elderly people who are depressed are also likely to increase their SUBSTANCE ABUSE, particularly of alcohol.

Medications and short-term psychotherapy have been shown to be effective treatments for elderly people with late-life depression. Some studies have shown that combination therapy (both medication and psychotherapy) provides the best results to a large majority of patients with depression.

Depression in Children and Adolescents

Most experts accept that children and adolescents can and do suffer from depressive disorders. What they often disagree about, however, is the form of the appropriate treatment. Some experts support the use of antidepressants in youths, while others are very opposed to such use and strongly favor limiting treatment to psychotherapy alone. Others believe in a combination of medication and psychotherapy. Children and adolescents who are depressed may turn to substance abuse for relief from their symptoms.

Gender differences In general, high school girls tend to suffer more from depression than high school boys. According to data from *The Formative Years: Pathways to Substance Abuse Among Girls and Young Women Ages 9–22* from the National Center on Addiction and Substance Abuse (CASA) at Columbia University, 34.5 percent of high school girls say they feel sad or hopeless, compared with 21.6 percent of boys. In addition, teenage girls who smoke are almost twice as likely to be depressed (47 percent) than girls who have never smoked (25.3 percent). This higher rate of depression is also true for girls who drink (38.7 percent) and are depressed, versus those who do not drink and are depressed (20 percent).

High school girls have a greater risk of attempting suicide than boys, or about 11.2 percent versus 6.2 percent. Girls who use marijuana are twice as likely to have considered or attempted suicide (34.5 percent) compared with those who never used marijuana (19.5 percent).

Summarized the report, "This CASA report demonstrates that certain key risk factors for substance abuse are unique to girls and young women and pose a greater threat to them than to boys and young men. For example, girls are likelier than boys to experience eating disorders, depression and

sexual abuse, each of which propels a girl farther down the pathway to substance abuse."

Alcohol abuse According to data from *The Formative Years: Pathways to Substance Abuse Among Girls and Young Women Ages 9–22*, the researchers found that females, particularly eighth-grade girls, who reported ever drinking alcohol were also more likely to be depressed six months later than nondrinkers. In addition, the greater the quantity of alcohol consumed, the higher the probability of depression. It is commonly known that many people with alcoholism have severe underlying problems with depression.

Depression and Family Members of Substance Abusers

Depression may also be a problem for the family members of substance abusers, even if the depressed person does not abuse alcohol or drugs. For example, according to authors Linda J. Roberts and Barbara S. McCrady in their guide for marriage and family therapists, "Spouses with an actively drinking partner experience significant levels of anxiety, depression and psychophysiological complaints."

Drug Abuse and Addiction

Abuse of some drugs, such as ANABOLIC STEROIDS or marijuana, can lead to depression. The depressive symptoms associated with abuse of anabolic steroids may persist for longer than a year or more after the user ends the abuse, according to the DRUG ENFORCEMENT ADMINISTRATION. MARIJUANA users are four times more likely to have depressive symptoms than those who are not users of the drug, and they are also more likely to suffer from suicidal thoughts.

In a study reported in a 2001 issue of the *American Journal of Psychiatry,* the researchers sought to estimate the degree to which cannabis (marijuana) abuse was a risk factor for depression as opposed to an effort to self-medicate already-existing depression.

They found that patients who were marijuana abusers who had no depressive symptoms prior to marijuana use were four times more likely to subsequently develop depression than subjects who were not marijuana abusers. Thus, marijuana abuse was predictive for depression. However, among participants who had not been diagnosed with depression but who had depressive symptoms prior to their use of marijuana, their depressive symptoms failed to predict further marijuana abuse at follow-up assessment. As a result, depression was not a predictor for further marijuana abuse in their case.

Said the researchers, "Obviously, causal associations or other mechanisms that explain the higher risk of depression in cannabis abusers cannot be determined by an epidemiological survey. However, a physiological mechanism underlying a causal association of cannabis use and suicide has been proposed, although it is somewhat limited to young male subjects. Cannabis increases levels of interferon-gamma, which inhibits the activity of aromatase, the enzyme that converts androgens to estrogen. This in turn creates a deficiency in estrogen, a hormone that augments the synthesis of serotonin, thereby creating a deficiency in serotonin characteristic of major depression and suicide."

Individuals who are addicted to COCAINE are also prone to developing depression. In addition, withdrawal from many drugs, such as METHAMPHETAMINE, leads to depression.

Smoking

SMOKING CESSATION is more difficult among people who have problems with depression. This may explain why bupropion (ZYBAN), which is also an antidepressant medication, is effective in helping many people stop smoking. It appears that nicotine may affect the same neurotransmitters associated with depression as does Zyban.

Eating Disorders

Depression is common among people with eating disorders, especially ANOREXIA NERVOSA, BULIMIA NERVOSA, and BINGE EATING DISORDER.

Risk Factors for Suicide

Note that either drug or alcohol abuse in conjunction with depression are risk factors for suicide. Other risk factors, according to Dr. Mary Whooley and Dr. Gregory Simon in their article in a 2000 issue of the *New England Journal of Medicine,* include unemployment, male sex, age older than 65, a history of admission to a psychiatric ward, a family or personal history of one or more suicide attempts, a severe physical illness, and a plan for suicide and/or access to firearms or other means of self-destruction.

Diagnosis and Treatment of Depression

Depression is a common and highly treatable illness. The physician will take a medical history to determine how severe the symptoms are, when they started, whether they ever occurred before, and if so, what treatment was tried then and if it helped the patient. The medical history, as well as laboratory tests and a physical examination, are all important because sometimes other illnesses may present as depression. For example, the patient may seem apathetic and/or sad, and have experienced a weight loss and yet be suffering from another medical problem altogether, such as hypothyroidism, diabetes, or cancer. A serum thyroid-stimulating hormone test can rule out hypothyroidism. (It is also possible for a patient to have hypothyroidism, diabetes, or cancer *and* depression.)

Medications for depressive disorders Most patients do very well with ANTIDEPRESSANTS, and there is a wide variety from which to choose. If the patient has bipolar disorder, he or she may be treated with lithium or another MOOD STABILIZER such as valproate, or with an anticonvulsant, such as carbamazepine (Tegretol), lamotrigine (Lamictal), or gabapentin (Neurontin). The herbal remedy known as St. John's wort (*Hypericum perforatum*) has not been proven to be any more efficacious than placebo (sugar pill) and is not recommended for patients with depression. This finding has been documented in several studies, such as in the *Journal of the American Medical Association* in 2001 and 2002.

One problem with medications for depression is that often patients stop taking them when they feel better, mistakenly thinking that they are "cured." This is a common problem with many other types of drugs. However, following the doctor's orders is important because stopping the medication can lead to a recurrence of the depression. Also, medications should not be stopped abruptly without consulting the doctor because to do so may cause an adverse reaction.

In 2004, the Food and Drug Administration (FDA) requested a warning label be placed on most antidepressants to encourage the close observation of pediatric and adult patients at risk for worsening depression or suicide. These drugs include fluoxetine (Prozac), sertraline (Zoloft), paroxetine (Paxil), fluoxamine (Luvox), citalopram (Celexa), escitalopram

(Lexapro), buproprion (Wellbutrin), venlafaxine (Effexor), nefazodone (Serzone), and mirtazapine (Remeron). According to the FDA, no suicides occurred in any clinical trials of the medications. Close monitoring is encouraged at the beginning of treatment or with any increases or decreases of dosages.

Never assume that patients who are taking antidepressants are automatically "safe" and that families and others need not worry any longer about them. The medication may not be effective, or an alternate medication may be preferable. In addition, even if effective, many medications take time to take effect and may take weeks or longer to help the person recover from depression. As a result, the early stages of treatment are still times when the patient should be closely monitored by the physician. Any suicidal symptoms, behaviors, or statements should be taken very seriously by family members and reported to the treating psychiatrist immediately. Keeping the patient alive is more important than worrying about whether he or she may be angry about the violation of his or her confidence.

Psychotherapy   When psychotherapy is used with depressed patients, generally mental health professionals rely upon cognitive-behavioral therapy. This teaches patients to challenge irrational and negative thoughts about themselves, replacing them with positive and empowering thoughts. Psychodynamic and insight-oriented psychotherapy may help the patient resolve conflicted feelings, cope with traumatic experiences, and understand repetitive dysfunctional patterns in relationships and behaviors.

Electroconvulsive therapy   In cases of severe life-threatening depression in which the patient needs to be hospitalized, doctors may use electroconvulsive therapy (ECT). Before the ECT treatment, the patient is given a muscle relaxant.

With ECT, the brain is stimulated at brief intervals of less than two seconds with electricity that causes a brief mild seizure that lasts for about 30 to 60 seconds. The patient is under anesthesia during the procedure, to prevent the patient from experiencing full body seizures, and the seizure is limited to brain activity. An electroencephalogram is used to monitor these brain seizures. Current ECT involves focused low-voltage stimulation on one side of the brain, which is thought to significantly decrease side effects such as memory loss or confusion. Measures of cumulative seizure time are taken, and several sessions of ECT may be required.

It is unknown how ECT works, but it appears to cause changes in brain chemistry. It is most effective in severe depression but is also used in some patients with bipolar disorder.

In the early years of ECT, in the 1930s, physicians did not use anesthesia or muscle relaxants, and they used a much higher voltage of electricity to both sides of the brain, which sometimes led to violent seizures that caused patients to suffer from broken bones. The procedure is far more benign in the 21st century.

ECT may cause side effects, including muscle aches, confusion, nausea, hypotension (low blood pressure), and headaches. Some patients have memory gaps for the period surrounding the treatment.

The procedure is usually performed in a hospital or other facility and is given under general anesthesia administered by an anesthesiologist.

See also ANXIETY DISORDERS; DUAL DIAGNOSIS; MENTAL ILLNESS/PSYCHIATRIC PROBLEMS; OBSESSIVE-COMPULSIVE DISORDER; PSYCHIATRIC MEDICATIONS; PSYCHIATRISTS.

For further information on depression, contact the following organizations:

American Association for Geriatric Psychiatry
7910 Woodmont Avenue
Suite 1050
Bethesda, MD 20814
(301) 654-7850
http://www.aagponline.org

Depression and Bipolar Support Alliance
730 N. Franklin
Suite 501
Chicago, IL 60610
(312) 642-0049
http://www.DBSAlliance.og

National Alliance for the Mentally Ill
Colonial Place Three
2107 Wilson Boulevard
Suite 300
Arlington, VA 22201
(703) 524-7600
http://www.nami.org

National Foundation for Depressive Illness, Inc.
P.O. Box 2257
New York, NY 10116
(212) 268-4260
http://www.depression.org

National Institute of Mental Health
6001 Executive Boulevard
Room 8184, MSC 9663
Bethesda, MD 20892
(301) 443-4513
http://www.nimh.nih.gov

National Mental Health Association
2001 N. Beauregard Street
12th Floor
Alexandria, VA 22311
(703) 684-7722
http://www.nmha.org

Bovasso, Gregory B. "Cannabis Abuse as a Risk Factor for Depressive Symptoms," *American Journal of Psychiatry* 158, no. 12 (December 2001): 2,033–2,037.

Hypericum Depression Trial Study Group. "Effect of *Hypericum perforatum* (St. John's Wort) in Major Depressive Disorder: A Randomized Controlled Trial," *Journal of the American Medical Association* 287, no. 14 (April 10, 2002): 1,807–1,814.

Roberts, Linda J., and Barbara S. McCrady. *Alcohol Problems in Intimate Relationships: Indentification and Intervention: A Guide for Marriage and Family Therapists.* Washington, D.C.: National Institute on Alcohol Abuse and Alcoholism, February 2003.

The National Center on Addiction and Substance Abuse at Columbia University. *The Formative Years: Pathways to Substance Abuse Among Girls and Young Women Ages 8–22.* New York: February 2003.

Whooley, Mary A., M.D., and Gregory E. Simon, M.D. "Managing Depression in Medical Outpatients," *New England Journal of Medicine* 343, no. 26 (December 28, 2000): 1,942–1,950.

designer drugs See CLUB DRUGS.

detoxification A medically supervised WITH-DRAWAL and the process of tapering an addicted individual off drugs or alcohol. According to data from the Treatment Episode Data Set (TEDS), an annual nationwide compilation on admissions to publicly funded SUBSTANCE ABUSE treatment facilities, 436,000 patient admissions were for detoxification for alcohol and drugs in the United States in 2001. Alcohol was the primary substance of abuse in half (50 percent) of these cases. (See table below.)

In some cases, if the addiction is mild to moderate, patients can be detoxified on an outpatient basis. If the addiction is severe, however, the detoxification needs to occur in an inpatient treatment facility.

Some patients should always receive treatment in a facility, such as elderly patients, pregnant women, people with psychiatric illnesses, and patients who have experienced withdrawal seizures or DELIRIUM TREMENS in the past. This is true even if the addictive symptoms are mild. Those who have recently consumed a large quantity of alcohol and people who do not have family members or friends on whom they can depend upon at home should also be detoxified on an inpatient basis. Some groups, such as pregnant women, can have great difficulty finding facilities that will provide them with detoxification treatment until after the delivery. Individuals who are mentally ill may also have difficulty finding a facility that will treat a person with both a mental illness and a severe substance abuse problem, otherwise known as a DUAL DIAGNOSIS.

Individuals Admitted for Detoxification

According to data from TEDS, most patients who were admitted for detoxification in the United States in 2001 were male (75 percent) and white (55 percent), 24 percent were African American,

PRIMARY SUBSTANCES OF ABUSE IN DETOXIFICATION ADMISSIONS IN THE UNITED STATES, 2001, BY PERCENT

Alcohol	50 percent
Opiates	33 percent
Cocaine	10 percent
Other drugs	3 percent
Marijuana	2 percent
Stimulants	2 percent

Source: Office of Applied Studies, Substance Abuse and Mental Health Services Administration. "Admissions for Detoxification: 2001," *The DASIS Report.* (March 26, 2004). Available online. URL: http://www.oas.samhsa.gov/2k4/detox/detox.pdf. Accessed on April 15, 2004.

and 17 percent were Hispanic. The average age of patients admitted for detoxification was 38 years. About a third of patients admitted for detoxification were admitted for the first time. In about 26 percent of the cases, it is the fifth or greater time that patients were admitted for detoxification.

In an analysis of patients who underwent detoxification programs in the United States in 2000, reported in a 2004 issue of *The DASIS Report*, researchers found that patients whose primary substance of abuse was alcohol had the highest rate of detoxification completion (54 percent), and patients with marijuana abuse had the lowest rates (39 percent). The patients who left the facility against professional medical advice totaled 29 percent, while 9 percent were terminated by the facility. A small number, 8 percent were transferred to another facility. What happened to the other 2 percent of patients is unknown. (See table below.)

Health Risks

Depending on the level of addiction and the general health of the patient, detoxification can cause severe short-term health problems, such as HALLUCINATIONS, seizures, severe diarrhea and vomiting, and in the most extreme cases, death. This is why most patients who are detoxifying are appropriately treated in an inpatient treatment facility.

Alcohol Detoxification

Some patients who are detoxifying from alcohol dependence receive NALTREXONE, although studies are mixed on whether the drug is effective in treating these patients. Those undergoing alcohol detoxification generally also receive treatment with BENZODIAZEPINE medications for seven to 10 days, primarily in order to ease their symptoms of withdrawal. Many patients who are undergoing detoxification will also be malnourished and need vitamin supplementation, particularly of B vitamins and folate or folic acid.

Some patients with long-term alcoholism who undergo detoxification may suffer from delirium tremens. For this reason, they should be under the care of a physician in a medical facility. This is particularly true of elderly alcoholic individuals, who are also at risk of fatal heart attacks or seizures.

According to Dr. Max Bayard and colleagues in their article on alcohol withdrawal syndrome in a 2004 issue for *American Family Physician*, alcoholic patients who are being detoxified and treated on an outpatient basis should be evaluated each day. Say the authors, "The patient and support person(s) should be instructed about how to take the withdrawal medication, the side effects of the medication, the expected withdrawal symptoms, and what to do if symptoms worsen."

Detoxification treatment may be followed by referral to outpatient treatment, 12-step groups such as offered by ALCOHOLICS ANONYMOUS, and follow-up treatment with mental health therapists to help the person avoid a RELAPSE.

Opioid Detoxification

The primary opioid to which most Americans are addicted is HEROIN. According to Dr. Mori Krantz

DISCHARGES FROM DETOXIFICATION, BY REASON FOR DISCHARGE AND PRIMARY SUBSTANCE AT ADMISSION, 2000, UNITED STATES						
		Reason for Discharge				
Primary Substance at Admission	Total	Treatment Completed	Transferred to Further Treatment	Left Against Professional Advice	Terminated by Facility	Other
Alcohol	34,346	18,670	3,312	8,492	3,024	848
Opiates	25,643	12,634	541	10,273	1,898	297
Cocaine	8,632	4,335	817	1,927	1,466	87
Marijuana/hashish	1,936	732	493	369	284	58
Stimulants	1,841	902	362	374	164	39
Other/unknown	1,166	487	293	241	100	45
Total	73,564	37,760	5,818	21,676	6,936	1,374

and Dr. Philip Mehler in their 2004 article for *Archives of Internal Medicine,* about 3 million Americans have abused this drug.

When opioid-dependent patients receive detoxification treatment, the process must be done slowly and carefully. Dr. Krantz and Dr. Mehler said, "Although untreated alcohol withdrawal is potentially more dangerous, opioid withdrawal causes intensely disturbing symptoms." Withdrawal symptoms may include extreme anxiety and distress, insomnia, diarrhea, nausea, vomiting, and flu-like symptoms.

METHADONE is usually given to detoxify patients. It is tapered down steadily over the course of weeks to months. Some physicians have used BUPRENORPHINE to taper patients off opioids. Clonidine has also been used along with benzodiazepines to help combat anxiety symptoms that may occur. Some physicians have combined clonidine with naltrexone.

Detoxification Versus Maintenance

Many patients addicted to heroin do not receive detoxification treatment and, instead, are maintained on other drugs. The treatment drugs approved for maintenance treatment of heroin abuse are METHADONE, levomethadyl, and buprenororphine, although levomethadyl is very rarely used. An estimated 200,000 patients in the United States receive opioid replacement therapy, and there are about 1,000 opioid treatment programs. According to Dr. Krantz and Dr. Mehler, opioid-dependent patients often have psychiatric problems that cause them to need higher-than-normal methadone doses.

In one study, researchers compared the outcomes of patients who received methadone maintenance therapy to patients who received six-month methadone-assisted detoxification. They reported on their findings in a 2000 issue of the *Journal of the American Medical Association.* The researchers randomized 91 patients to methadone maintenance and 88 patients to detoxification. Each group also received psychotherapy. Some subjects also received therapy for cocaine.

The researchers found that the methadone maintenance group had significantly lower subsequent heroin use rates than the detoxification group, which seems to favor methadone maintenance as a treatment. However, even though they used drugs less than the detoxification group, half the methadone maintenance participants were found to have also used an illegal opioid at least once a month while under treatment.

The researchers said, "That 50% of participants used an illicit opioid at least once a month is not encouraging. Given that methadone doses were adequate, failure may rest in the realm of psychosocial treatment. Neither program in this study provided extensive legal, employment, family, or psychiatric services. Participants showed little change in these areas."

As a result, further studies are needed before detoxification should be ruled out in favor of methadone maintenance.

Rapid and Ultrarapid Opioid Detoxification

Some physicians believe that it is possible and advisable to withdraw patients who are addicted to opioids very rapidly under medical supervision. A general review of rapid and ultrarapid opioid detoxification is offered in a 1998 issue of the *Journal of the American Medical Medical Association.* The goal of rapid and ultrarapid detoxification (within a few days or a week) is to avoid an expensive and both physically and psychologically painful withdrawal process that could last months. The patient is sedated while undergoing detoxification. Dissenters believe that if the underlying problems that led the person to become addicted to opioids are not resolved, then rapid detoxification is unlikely to be successful in preventing relapse.

Rapid detoxification is complex and difficult. According to Dr. Thomas Kosten and Dr. Patrick O'Connor in their 2003 article in the *New England Journal of Medicine,* this process "should only be undertaken by clinicians who have had substantial experience working with simpler approaches to withdrawal, such as using clonidine alone or tapering the dosage of methadone in an inpatient setting."

See also ALCOHOLISM; ANTABUSE; BETTY FORD CENTER; DRUG ADDICTION; TREATMENT FACILITIES.

Bayard, Max, et al. "Alcohol Withdrawal Syndrome," *American Family Physician* 69, no. 6 (March 15, 2004): 1,443–1,450.

Kosten, Thomas R., M.D., and Patrick G. O'Connor, M.D. "Management of Drug and Alcohol Withdrawal," *New England Journal of Medicine* 348, no. 18 (May 1, 2003): 1,786–1,795.

Krantz, Mori J., M.D. and Philip S. Mehler, M.D. "Treating Opioid Dependence: Growing Implications for Primary Care," *Archives of Internal Medicine* 164, no. 3 (February 9, 2004): 277–288.

O'Connor, Patrick G., M.D. and Thomas R. Kosten, M.D. "Rapid and Ultrarapid Opioid Detoxification Techniques," *Journal of the American Medical Association* 279, no. 3 (January 21, 1998): 229–234.

Office of Applied Studies. "Discharges from Detoxification: 2000," *The DASIS Report,* Substance Abuse and Mental Health Services Administration, July 9, 2004. Available online. URL: http://www.oas.samhsa.gov/2k4/detoxDischarges/detoxDischarges.pdf. Accessed on August 15, 2004.

Sees, Karen L., et al. "Methadone Maintenance vs. 180-Day Psychosocially Enriched Detoxification for Treatment of Opioid Dependence: A Randomized Controlled Trial," *Journal of the American Medical Association* 283, no. 10 (March 8, 2000): 1,303–1,310.

diet pills   Over-the-counter or prescribed medications that are taken to decrease appetite and enable individuals who are overweight or obese to lose weight. Sometimes individuals who are not overweight, such as individuals with ANOREXIA NERVOSA, take diet pills and/or laxatives to lose weight, and they may become severely underweight.

In the past, AMPHETAMINES (stimulant drugs) were prescribed for weight loss. However, that treatment use is no longer medically approved because medical experts realized that some individuals were abusing the drugs or had become addicted to them. Prescribed diet pills that continue to be lawful to use for weight loss include sibutramine (Meridia), orlistat (Xenical), and phentermine (Fastin, Adipex-P).

In 2004, the Food and Drug Administration banned the use of ephedra, also known as ma huang, as a diet drug in the United States after several individuals died from using this herbal remedy.

See also BINGE EATING DISORDER; BULIMIA NERVOSA; OVEREATING/OBESITY.

diversion programs   Special rehabilitative programs that individuals may enter in order to avoid a serious consequence, such as losing an occupational license, entering jail, or losing the custody of a child. For example, if physicians or other healthcare professionals develop a SUBSTANCE ABUSE problem, many states have programs that enable them to enter a rehabilitation program specifically designed for the problems and pressures that they face.

See also PHYSICIANS AND HEALTHCARE PROFESSIONALS AND ADDICTION.

drinking games   Games in which the "loser" must drink alcohol. The purpose of such games is generally to get all the participants drunk. Drinking games should be avoided because they encourage BINGE DRINKING, which can be very dangerous, and at their most extreme, lead to ALCOHOL POISONING and death.

See also COLLEGE STUDENTS; TEENAGE AND YOUTH DRINKING.

driving, impaired   Operating a motor vehicle while under the influence of alcohol or drugs that impedes normal and alert driving. Impaired driving is defined by such factors as decreased reaction time, poor judgment, worsened night driving and peripheral vision, and decreased physical coordination. Alcohol and illegal drugs as well as some prescription drugs, over-the-counter medications, and some herbal supplements (such as valerian) have been shown to cause impairment in driving.

The National Center for Statistics and Analysis of the National Highway Traffic Safety Administration estimated that 17,419 alcohol-related traffic fatalities occurred in 2002, or 41 percent of all traffic fatalities. This is equivalent to an average of one alcohol-related fatality every 30 minutes. An estimated 258,000 people were injured in car crashes where alcohol was present in 2002, which is an average of one person injured about every two minutes. In addition, about 1.4 million drivers were arrested in 2001 for driving under the influence of alcohol or narcotics. The rate of alcohol involvement in car crashes increases by more than three times at night.

According to the National Highway Traffic Safety Administration (NHTSA), alcohol-related crashes cost the public more than $50 billion in 2000, and about 75 percent of these costs were incurred in crashes in which a driver or nonoccupant had a BLOOD ALCOHOL LEVEL of 0.10 or greater. The NHTSA says that impaired driving is the most frequently occurring violent crime in the United States.

If the individual is stopped by a police officer and found to be intoxicated, he or she may be charged with driving under the influence of alcohol. This is a serious crime that can lead to the loss of a driver's license, fines, and/or even jail time, depending on the circumstances of the situation, state law, and often on whether it is a first offense. However, not all state laws require drivers who are convicted of driving under the influence of alcohol or drugs to receive mandatory treatment despite the fact that untreated individuals are at high risk for further involvement in car crashes.

Some prescribed and over-the-counter medications can also impair driving and should be used only with caution or driving should be avoided altogether during their use. This is particularly true of sedating drugs and some cold remedies. Although states are primarily concerned with drivers who are impaired because of the use of alcohol and/or illegal drugs, impairment from any other drug can lead to charges of driving while intoxicated.

Police officers are trained to assess the signs of intoxication and are capable of evaluating and testing drivers. (It is true, however, that sometimes people with medical problems such as diabetes may appear intoxicated when they are not drunk.) However, beyond the ALCOHOL BREATH TESTS for alcohol, toxicologic screening for drugs such as COCAINE and MARIJUANA is often considered cumbersome and expensive. Consequently, it may not be used by the police unless evidence of the drug is present.

One study reported in a 1994 issue of the *New England Journal of Medicine* indicated that a significant number of subjects who were arrested for reckless driving but did not appear to be impaired were actually under the influence of cocaine and/or marijuana. In this study, the researchers used a rapid urine test to test the urine of 150 individuals who had been arrested for reckless driving. The results were disturbing. A majority, 59 percent, of the subjects tested positive for cocaine or marijuana or for both cocaine and marijuana. However, nearly half of the drivers who were intoxicated with cocaine were able to pass standard sobriety tests.

Driving Under the Influence of Drugs

An estimated 35 million people ages 12 and older used illegal drugs in 2002, according to the National Survey on Drug Use and Health (formerly known as the National Household Survey on Drug Abuse). Of these 35 million people, nearly 11 million drove vehicles when they were under the influence of illegal drugs. Most of those who drove while they were drugged were between the ages of 18 and 22 years, and 21 year olds had the greatest risk of driving with drugs (18 percent of all the 21-year-old individuals surveyed). (See figure on page 94.)

In looking at the differences between races and ethnicities, Native Indians and Alaskan Natives as a group had the greatest risk of driving while under the influence of illegal drugs. An estimated 6.2 percent of this population drove while drugged in 2002. They were followed by whites (5.0 percent of their population) and African Americans (4.5 percent).

Among individuals ages 18–22, individuals who were college undergraduates (18 percent) were more likely than their noncollege age peers (14 percent) to have driven under the influence of drugs. After graduation, however, college students were less likely to drive while under the influence of illegal drugs than their peers. For example, among adults ages 26–49 years old, about 4 percent of college graduates drove while drugged, compared with 6 percent of those with some college education and 5 percent who were high school graduates.

Another finding was that unemployed people have a significantly greater rate of driving while under the influence of illegal drugs. Among adults ages 26–49 years old, of those who were unemployed, 9.3 percent reported driving while under the influence of drugs. The percent of individuals driving under the influence of illegal drugs for people who were employed full-time was almost half that of unemployed individuals, or 5.1 percent. About 5 percent of part-time workers drove while under the influence of illegal drugs.

Driving Under the Influence of Alcohol

Alcohol continues to be a major contributor to car crashes and to many traffic deaths. For example, the NHTSA data show that alcohol was a factor in 9 percent of the cases of people injured in car crashes, or 225,000 out of 2,926,000 crashes in 2002.

When looking at all traffic deaths in 2002, in 41 percent of the cases in which alcohol was present

PERCENTAGES OF PERSONS AGES 12 AND OLDER REPORTING DRIVING UNDER THE INFLUENCE OF ILLEGAL DRUGS IN THE PAST YEAR, BY DETAILED AGE CATEGORIES: 2002

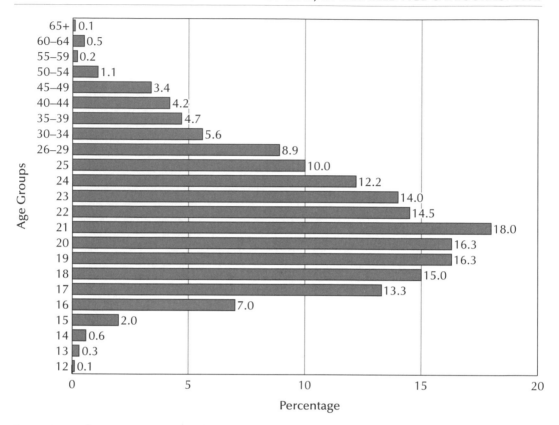

Source: National Survey on Drug Use and Health, "Drugged Driving: 2002 Update," *The NSDUH Report,* Rockville, Md.: Office of Applied Studies, Substance Abuse and Mental Health Services, September 16, 2003.

at all, whether in drivers or pedestrians, alcohol was found to be a factor in traffic fatalities.

Information provided by the NHTSA reveals that the percentage of fatalities from car crashes when alcohol was a factor varied by age of the person who died. This information was analyzed in an article in a 2003 issue of *Alcohol Research & Health* by Ralph Hingson and Michael Winter.

For example, among several age groups, traffic fatalities related to the use of alcohol by drivers and pedestrians represent the majority of all fatalities. This is true for people between the ages of 21 and 45 years. Fatalities linked to alcohol represent a significant percentage for other age groups. For example, they represent 37 percent of the deaths for individuals ages 16–20 years old. (See table at top of page 95.)

In addition, the higher the level of blood alcohol, the greater the risk for involvement in traffic death. As can be seen from the table at top of page 95, individuals who are between the ages of 16 and 20 years have a 7 percent risk of a traffic fatality if their blood alcohol level is between 0.01 and 0.07 percent. This risk increases to 13 percent for individuals whose blood alcohol is 0.08–0.14 percent and further to 17 percent for blood alcohol levels that are 0.15 percent or higher. This increased risk for death applies to every age level.

Men are more likely than women to die in an alcohol-related car crash. In 2002, 78 percent of the

TRAFFIC DEATHS BY AGE AND BLOOD ALCOHOL LEVEL, UNITED STATES, 2002

BAC *	Under Age 16	Ages 16–20	Ages 21–29	Ages 30–45	Ages 46–64	Ages 65+
0.0%	77%	63%	43%	47%	62%	85%
0.01–0.07%	5%	7%	7%	6%	5%	3%
0.08–0.14%	7%	13%	16%	13%	9%	5%
0.15%+	11%	17%	34%	35%	24%	7%
All BACs	100%	100%	100%	100%	100%	100%
Percentage alcohol involved	23	37	57	53	38	15
Number alcohol involved	573	2,329	4,595	5,682	3,192	971
Total of all fatalities	2,542	6,277	8,022	10,707	8,487	6,622

* BAC = the highest blood alcohol concentration of a driver or pedestrian involved in the crash.
Source: Hingson, Ralph and Michael Winter. "Epidemiology and Consequences of Drinking and Driving," *Alcohol Research & Health* 27, no. 1 (2003): 64.

individuals killed in accidents involving alcohol (as either drivers, passengers, or pedestrians) were male.

Although racial and ethnicity data is not routinely collected in car crashes, from 1990–94, death certificate information was available on people who died in car crashes in the United States. Based on that information, researchers found that 72 percent of those killed in alcohol-related crashes were white, followed by Hispanics (12.7 percent, including Mexican Americans, Puerto Ricans, and Cubans). Next were African Americans (12.1 percent), Native Americans (2.4 percent), and Asian Americans/Pacific Islanders (1.2 percent).

Based on this data and the fact that more men die from car crashes than women, white males apparently have the greatest risk of dying from an alcohol-related car crash.

Failure to Wear Seat Belts

Another problem among individuals who drink and drive is that they often fail to wear their seat belts (because they forget to buckle up, they do not think it is important, or for another reason). The higher the blood alcohol content, the lower the probability that individuals will wear their seat belt. As a result, these drivers have an increased risk of death. (See Table III.)

As can be seen from table at right, the lowest percentage of individuals involved in car crashes and using seat belts (20 percent) was also the group who had blood alcohol levels at or above 0.15 percent. Even with that high level of blood

alcohol level, of those who survived the car crash, 43 percent were belted. It should also be noted that although their seat belts may have protected them, which is important, among this group, the majority (57 percent) died.

Children and Impaired Drivers

Car crashes are the main cause of fatal injuries to children between the ages of four and 14 years. Impaired drivers are more likely to be involved with car crashes. If the impaired driver is a parent, he or she is less likely to use seat belts or child

SEAT BELT USE BY DRIVERS IN FATAL CRASHES, BY DRIVER'S BLOOD ALCOHOL LEVEL, 2002

Driver's BAC *	0.00%	0.01–0.07%	0.08–0.14%	0.15%+
Drivers in fatal car crashes who survived the crash, percent belted	79	56	51	43
Fatally injured drivers, percent belted	48	33	24	20

* BAC = the highest blood alcohol concentration of a driver or pedestrian involved in the crash.
Source: Hingson, Ralph and Michael Winter. "Epidemiology and Consequences of Drinking and Driving," *Alcohol Research & Health* 27, no. 1 (2003): 64.

CHILD ALCOHOL-RELATED TRAFFIC FATALITIES, 1994–2000

Year	Ages 0–5	Ages 6–9	Ages 10–14	Total Deaths
1994	682	441	693	1,816
1995	620	470	718	1,808
1996	656	454	707	1,817
1997	604	479	713	1,796
1998	575	518	683	1,776
1999	557	507	664	1,728
2000	539	484	645	1,668
Totals	4,233	3,353	4,823	12,409

Source: Fatality Analysis Reporting System (FARS), National Highway Safety Administration, U.S. Department of Transportation, 2002.

restraints. The more intoxicated the driver, the lower the probability his or her children will be safely buckled up. In 2000, more than 1,668 children died in alcohol-related traffic accidents. (See table above.) This is lower than in previous years but is still far too high.

See also ALCOHOL/ALCOHOL CONSUMPTION; ALCOHOLISM; COLLEGE STUDENTS; DRIVING WHILE INTOXICATED/DRIVING UNDER THE INFLUENCE; TEENAGE AND YOUTH DRINKING.

Brookoff, Daniel, et al. "Testing Reckless Drivers for Cocaine and Marijuana," *New England Journal of Medicine* 331, no. 8 (August 25, 1994): 518–522.

Hingson, Ralph and Michael Winter. "Epidemiology and Consequences of Drinking and Driving," *Alcohol Research & Health* 27, no. 1 (2003): 63–70.

National Center for Statistics and Analysis, National Highway Traffic Safety Administration. "Traffic Safety Facts 2002: Alcohol," Department of Transportation, DOT HS 809 606, 2003.

National Survey on Drug Use and Health. "Drugged Driving: 2002 Update," *The NSDUH Report.* Rockville, Md.: Office of Applied Studies, Substance Abuse and Mental Health Services, September 16, 2003.

driving while intoxicated/driving under the influence   Legal terms that refer to individuals operating motor vehicles while under the influence of intoxicants, including drugs or alcohol. According to the National Highway Traffic Safety Administration (NHTSA), about 1.5 million arrests are made nationwide each year for driving while intoxicated.

This is second only to the 1.6 million arrests per year for SUBSTANCE ABUSE–related crimes. Some experts have estimated that a person can drive drunk from 300–2,000 times before being detected and arrested, based on roadside breath test surveys.

All states have laws on blood alcohol levels, and drivers who test positive for exceeding these levels are considered impaired. Testing for drugs varies from state to state, but most states can readily test for common drugs of abuse, such as MARIJUANA, COCAINE, and HEROIN.

According to the NHTSA, 17,000 people were killed in 2002, and 258,000 people were injured in car crashes in which ALCOHOL was a contributing factor.

For many age groups, the majority of traffic fatalities are related to high blood alcohol levels of either the driver or a pedestrian. For example, among people ages 21–29 years old, 57 percent of traffic fatalities are alcohol-related, according to the NHTSA.

Some states have provisions to remove the driver's license if a person has a certain number of driving-while-intoxicated convictions. State laws vary in their severity of punishment. Lobbying organizations such as Mothers Against Drunk Driving have been successful at increasing the penalties for drunken driving in many states.

Driving While Intoxicated (DWI) Courts

According to the NHTSA in their 2003 report, there were 68 DWI courts nationwide, modeled after DRUG COURTS. DWI courts can provide supervision and monitoring to DWI offenders. Some studies on DWI courts in Wisconsin and Georgia have found the recidivism rate (repeat offense rate) dropped by more than 40 percent. The NHTSA plans to collaborate with the Department of Justice to encourage increased use of DWI courts.

Repeat Offenders

About a third of all drivers who are arrested or convicted of driving while intoxicated or driving under the influence are repeat offenders. To help cope with this problem, Section 164 of title 23, United States Code requires that states have laws for repeat intoxicated drivers or lose a portion of federal highway funds. To date, many states have met this requirement, including Alabama, Arizona,

Arkansas, Colorado, Delaware, Florida, Georgia, Hawaii, Illinois, Indiana, Idaho, Iowa, Kansas, Kentucky, Maine, Maryland, Michigan, Mississippi, Missouri, Nebraska, Nevada, New Hampshire, New Jersey, North Carolina, Oklahoma, Pennsylvania, Tennessee, Texas, Utah, Virginia, Washington, and Wisconsin.

According to the NHTSA, compliance with Section 164 requires that for a second and subsequent offense of driving while intoxicated or driving under the influence of alcohol, states will:

- Require a minimum one-year driver's license suspension for repeat intoxicated drivers

- Require that all motor vehicles of repeat intoxicated drivers be impounded or immobilized for a specified period when the license is suspended or require the installation of an ignition interlock system on the motor vehicles of these drivers for a specified period after the suspension

- Require mandatory assessment of repeat intoxicated drivers' level of alcohol abuse and referral to treatment as needed

- Establish a mandatory minimum sentence for repeat intoxicated drivers of no fewer than five days imprisonment or 30 days of community service for the second offense and no fewer than 10 days imprisonment or 60 days of community service for the third or subsequent offense

See also ALCOHOL BREATH TESTS; BLOOD ALCOHOL LEVELS; DRIVING, IMPAIRED; TEENAGE AND YOUTH DRINKING.

National Highway Traffic Safety Administration. *Initiatives to Address Impaired Driving,* December 2003. Available online. URL: http://www.nhtsa.dot.gov/people/injury/alcohol/IPTReport/FinalAlcoholIPT-03.pdf. Accessed on April 16, 2004.

National Highway Traffic Safety Administration. *"Traffic Safety Facts:* Repeat Intoxicated Driver Laws," 1, no. 1 (May 2003).

Voas, Robert B. and Deborah A. Fisher. "Court Procedures for Handling Intoxicated Drivers," *Alcohol Research & Health* 25, no. 1 (2001): 32–42.

drug abuse   Use of drugs that is excessive, illegal, and dangerous for the body but that does not rise to the level of DRUG ADDICTION. A drug abuser may eventually become a drug addict, although not all drug abusers become addicted. Some individuals are able to use an illicit substance, such as COCAINE, MARIJUANA, or other drugs, once, twice, or intermittently. In contrast, others use the drug once or twice and then are drawn to a repeated and chronic abuse and sometimes to addiction. Some individuals abuse drugs that are prescribed to themselves or others.

Determining which individuals are more prone to drug abuse or addiction than others is difficult.

Drug abuse can be very harmful to the body and cause many serious health effects, up to and including death.

See also DRUG ABUSE/ADDICTION AND HEALTH PROBLEMS; SUBSTANCE ABUSE; TEENAGE AND YOUTH DRUG ABUSE.

drug abuse/addiction and health problems
Acute or chronic health problems that are caused by the abuse of or addiction to illegal, prescribed, or some over-the-counter drugs. Although many medications can greatly enhance lives, some illegal drugs and some prescribed drugs can cause short-term or long-term severe health problems, up to and including death. Some over-the-counter drugs, when abused, can also cause serious health consequences. In addition, pregnant women who abuse illegal drugs or prescribed drugs can harm the development of the fetus and may cause life-long problems in the child after birth.

According to the National Center for Health Statistics, 2,718 people died of ACCIDENTAL OVERDOSES from the use of opiates and related narcotics in the United States in 1998.

Note that an addiction to a drug is not necessary for harmful effects to occur. Abuse of illegal, prescribed, or some over-the-counter drugs can be harmful on the first use, depending on the type of drug and the dosage taken.

Health Problems Caused by Illegal Drugs
Drug abuse can cause a wide variety of health problems, depending on the particular drug, the extent of the abuse, and other issues, such as the use of alcohol along with drugs. In the most severe cases, death may result. The abuse of some drugs, such as AMPHETAMINES or COCAINE, may lead to or apparently trigger a PSYCHOTIC BREAK, similar to the

symptoms seen with SCHIZOPHRENIA. Some individuals do not recover from this psychotic break.

Individuals who abuse ANABOLIC STEROIDS may suffer long-term effects. Men may develop shrunken testicles and gynecomastia (abnormal breast development). They may lose their sexual drive and develop diminished sperm production because of their decreased levels of testosterone.

Women who abuse anabolic steroids may develop increased facial hair growth and decreased breast size as well as irregular or stopped menstruation. They may develop a permanently deepened voice.

Anabolic steroid abuse may impair fertility in men and women. Users may also develop problems with hypertension and high blood cholesterol, putting them at risk for stroke and heart attack. Psychiatric effects may also occur. Anabolic steroids may cause mood swings and mania. Users may suffer from DEPRESSION.

Individuals who abuse cocaine face many health risks, in part because many users inject the drug. Many health risks are associated with using contaminated needles, such as the transmission of the human immunodeficiency virus (HIV) or forms of HEPATITIS. Other health risks associated with cocaine abuse and addiction include heart attack, stroke, respiratory failure, seizures, and the loss of the sense of smell.

The abuse of 3-4 methylenedioxymethamphetamine (MDMA), known as ECSTASY, also has many serious health risks. MDMA abuse can cause a very rapid sudden rise in the body temperature. If not treated in time, this hyperthermia can cause death. Other health risks with MDMA are heart attack, kidney failure, and brain damage. In addition, the abuse of MDMA can induce severe psychiatric symptoms, such as anxiety, depression, confusion, panic attacks, and paranoia.

The abuse of gamma-hydroxybutyrate (GHB) can induce a comalike sleep, as well as delusions, HALLUCINATIONS, seizures, a slowed heart rate, respiratory distress, and lowered blood pressure.

HEROIN abuse can lead to addiction as well as to serious health effects, such as pneumonia, tuberculosis, and liver and kidney disease. Pregnant women who use heroin may have a miscarriage or a premature delivery. There is also an increased risk

of sudden infant death syndrome (SIDS) in the newborn that survives the delivery to a woman addicted to heroin.

The abuse of illegal inhalants incurs many health risks. Some inhalant abusers die the first time they use an inhalant, often because of erratic heart rhythms (arrhythmias) that have been triggered, which lead to heart failure. Inhalant abuse may also cause permanent memory loss and learning problems caused by brain damage. It may also damage major organs, such as the lungs, kidneys, liver, and heart.

Hallucinogens such as lysergic acid diethylamide (LSD) may cause permanent health effects, such as a psychotic break, and serious psychiatric problems, such as depression.

Chronic abuse of MARIJUANA, often considered to be relatively benign by many people, also has serious health consequences. This may be in part because the marijuana available in the 21st century is about twice as powerful as the drug that was used by some people in the 1960s. Marijuana abuse may lead to deficits in short-term thinking and memory. Regular users may also develop an increased heart rate. They may experience problems with depression and panic attacks.

METHAMPHETAMINE abuse, too, has many serious consequences to the health of the user. Chronic use of methamphetamine can lead to auditory and visual hallucinations. Paranoia and extreme rages may also occur, precipitating VIOLENCE. Some chronic users of methamphetamine suffer from the terrifying delusion that insects are crawling underneath their skin. Users of crystal methamphetamine risk the development of psychotic symptoms that may persist for months or years.

Regular methamphetamine users may develop pneumonia, tuberculosis, and diseases of the kidneys and the liver. Withdrawal symptoms from the drug may include depression, paranoia, aggression, and fatigue as well as an intense CRAVING for more methamphetamine.

Abuse of phencyclidine (PCP) can cause serious health problems, such as hyperthermia and severe muscle contractions. High doses of PCP may cause convulsions, coma, and death. PCP also causes psychiatric symptoms that can be permanent. It induces auditory and visual hallucinations in users and may cause a psychotic break. PCP users may experience paranoia and symptoms that are difficult to distinguish from schizophrenia. They may not recover.

Health Problems Caused by Abuse and Addiction of Prescribed Drugs

Prescribed drugs can be misused by failing to follow the physician's instructions and taking too many (or not enough) drugs, or by taking other drugs (or alcohol) with the drug, risking a serious interaction. Some people abuse prescribed drugs, such as BENZODIAZEPINES or OPIATES. It is also abusive and illegal for a patient to give or sell his or her own drugs to any other person. Some addicted individuals steal prescribed drugs or forge prescriptions.

Individuals who abuse the prescribed analgesic OXYCONTIN will become addicted and need higher doses to achieve the same euphoric result. New or inexperienced users of the drug who take a large dose can cause a severe respiratory depression that causes death. OxyContin abusers who illegally inject the drug risk contracting diseases such as the human immunodeficiency virus, hepatitis B and C, and other bloodborne viruses.

Health Problems Caused by Abuse of Over-the-Counter Medications

Most over-the-counter medications are not used as drugs of abuse; however, a few drugs are. One example of such a drug is COUGH SYRUP that contains dextromethorphan. Some adolescents and young adults buy large quantities of cough syrup to induce euphoria and subsequently become addicted to the drug.

Large quantities of dextromethorphan may induce hallucinations and dissociative effects (a feeling of not really being present). Other serious health consequences that may occur are hyperthermia, irregular heartbeat, high blood pressure, loss of consciousness, brain damage, and death.

The abuse of high doses of PROPOXYPHENE (Darvon) can lead to coma, seizures, and accidental death. Long-term use can cause stomach bleeding and may damage the kidneys and the liver.

See also ALCOHOLIC HEALTH PROBLEMS; AMPHETAMINE PSYCHOSIS; CRACK COCAINE; DRUG ABUSE; DRUG ADDICTION; INHALANTS, ABUSE OF; KETAMINE; METHADONE; SMOKING AND HEALTH PROBLEMS.

drug addiction   A physical, emotional, and psychological compulsion to take a specific drug illicitly. Without this drug, the individual becomes ill as well as suffers from other physical and psychological symptoms. Some experts refer to drug addiction as drug dependence.

The symptoms of drug addiction vary depending on the drug. The drug addict has developed a TOLERANCE to the drug such that increasingly larger doses are needed to achieve the same effect. The addict eventually needs to take the drug not to achieve any EUPHORIA but because the body needs the substance in order to feel normal again. Individuals can become addicted to some prescription drugs as well as to illegal drugs.

In general, individuals addicted to drugs should undergo WITHDRAWAL from drugs only under the supervision of trained medical professionals, preferably in a treatment facility that is set up to assist drug addicts.

Amphetamine Addiction

Some individuals become addicted to amphetamines that they have used illegally. Some adolescents in high school abuse amphetamines, sometimes to the point of dependency/addiction. In the past, amphetamines were used as DIET PILLS. Today, amphetamines are sometimes used to treat ATTENTION DEFICIT HYPERACTIVITY DISORDER.

In patients with ADHD, stimulants do actually stimulate the brain. Individuals with this disorder are better able to focus and feel calmer when the electrical activity of the brain is increased, as happens when they take stimulants. This has been described as a paradoxical effect. Patients with ADHD are carefully monitored by physicians.

Individuals who are addicted to amphetamines should withdraw from the drug under medical supervision. Groups such as NARCOTICS ANONYMOUS may help individuals who are dependent on amphetamines to overcome the problems that led to their addiction.

Benzodiazepine Addiction

Some people become addicted to antianxiety medications known as benzodiazepines. For example, alprazolam (Xanax) has a high risk of causing addiction and even more so when an individual is taking a high dose of the drug. If the person stops taking the drug, withdrawal symptoms, such as increased blood pressure, increased heart rate, and tremor, will quickly occur. A sudden stopping of the medication may also cause the patient to experience HALLUCINATIONS, grand mal seizures, and DELIRIUM TREMENS. For these reasons, withdrawal should occur only under medical supervision.

Cocaine Addiction

Addiction to COCAINE is a serious and growing problem in the United States today. According to the *2002 National Survey on Drug Use and Health,* an estimated 2 million people in the United States were current cocaine users in 2002. Of these, 567,000 were CRACK COCAINE users. Most cocaine users are male and over age 18. About 800,000 people received treatment for cocaine addiction in the United States in 2002.

Drugs such as NALTREXONE are used to treat cocaine addiction. During withdrawal from cocaine, many patients benefit by taking ANTIDEPRESSANTS. Some doctors have found that bromocriptine has decreased the craving for cocaine in some patients.

Heroin

According to the *2002 National Survey on Drug Use and Health,* there were about 166,000 HEROIN users in the United States in 2002. Most were male and over age 18.

Many patients addicted to heroin are treated with METHADONE maintenance therapy. According to Dr. Mori Krantz and Dr. Philip Mehler in their article on treating opioid dependence in a 2004 issue of the *Archives of Internal Medicine,* opioid replacement therapy serves heroin patients in the United States in more than 1,000 treatment programs nationwide.

According to Dr. Krantz and Dr. Mehler, before methadone maintenance therapy was introduced into the United States, 21 of every 1,000 heroin patients died. After methadone was introduced, the death rate dropped significantly to 13 heroin addicts per 1,000 patients.

Methadone is a legally authorized SCHEDULED DRUG under the CONTROLLED SUBSTANCES ACT. It is also a drug given to treat some patients with severe chronic pain who are not addicted to heroin or other drugs. As a result, it should not be assumed that patients taking methadone are heroin addicts

or that they are addicted to any other drugs. If they are under a doctor's care and are healthy, that is all most people need to know.

The two other medications given to heroin addicts as part of opioid maintenance therapy are levomethadyl and BUPRENORPHINE. Buprenophine is a Schedule III drug, in contrast to levomethadyl and methadone, which are both Schedule II drugs; thus, buprenorphine is considered a safer medication. The Drug Addiction Treatment Act authorizes approved physicians to treat patients who are addicted to heroin in their offices with buprenorphine.

Heroin addicts can also be treated with DETOXIFICATION from the drug. This is usually performed in an inpatient treatment facility. However, it is very difficult for most heroin addicts to maintain ABSTINENCE from the drug.

Marijuana

Experts disagree on whether MARIJUANA is addictive. Certainly, though, some users become heavily dependent on the drug, using it for 20 or more days per month. For example, according to the *2002 National Survey on Drug Use and Health,* 4.8 million marijuana users (about a third of all users) take the drug this frequently. Many patients who are heavily dependent on marijuana use can recover, based on treatment statistics.

About two-thirds of all new marijuana users are under the age of 18 years, and about half of all new users are females. About 974,000 people ages 12 years old and older received treatment for marijuana abuse or dependence in 2002.

Methamphetamine

Some individuals become addicted to METHAMPHETAMINE, for which there are no simple treatments. Physicians may use antidepressants for the depression that usually occurs with withdrawal from this drug. If patients have possible methamphetamine toxicity, they require urgent treatment in a hospital emergency room. They may also need antipsychotic medications to treat their hyperactivity or agitation. Sometimes benzodiazepines are used for these symptoms. Other medications are used to treat the symptoms of hypertension, hypotension, hyperthermia, and the metabolic and electrolyte abnormalities that may occur with the use of this drug.

Prescription Drugs Used Nonmedically

According to the *2002 National Survey on Drug Use and Health,* about 6.2 million people abused prescription-type drugs nonmedically, including 4.4 million people who abused pain relievers, 1.8 million who abused tranquilizers, 1.2 million who abused stimulants, and 0.4 million who abused sedatives. Not all of these individuals could be classified as addicts, and many people abuse a drug once or several times. However, they are all illicit drug users, and the drugs they are abusing have addictive potential.

Substance Abuse or Dependence

The *2002 National Survey on Drug Use and Health* included questions to assess dependence (addiction) and abuse of illicit drugs and alcohol. The responses to these questions provided valuable information for educators, researchers, policy makers, and others. For example, the rate of substance dependence or abuse by age was 8.9 percent for youths ages 12–17 years old. The rate increased to 21.7 percent for adults ages 18–25 years old. The rate dropped to 7.3 percent for those ages 26 years old and older. Based on this information, it can be concluded that SUBSTANCE ABUSE and dependence peak sometime before the age of 26 years for most people.

In considering race and ethnicity, the rate of dependence or abuse was highest among Native Americans/Alaska Natives (14.1 percent), followed by persons reporting two or more races (13.0 percent). Asians had the lowest rate (4.2 percent). Rates for other races and ethnicities were 10.4 percent for Hispanics, 9.5 percent for African Americans, and 9.3 percent for whites.

More than a third (36.2 percent) of adults over age 18 who were paroled or on a supervised release from jail during the past year were classified with dependence or abuse of a substance, compared with 9.2 percent of other adults. This is significant for those who are involved in any way in the criminal justice system and who are hopeful that people released from prison will not reoffend. The more likely they are to use drugs again, the higher the probability that individuals will commit crimes and return to jail. Thus, the goal is to keep ex-offenders from using drugs again for their own sakes as well as for the sake of society at large.

Mandated Treatment Can Work

Some experts believe that effective treatment cannot be mandated, but others do not agree. According to *Principles of Drug Addiction Treatment: A Research-Based Guide,* a manual published by the National Institute on Drug Abuse (NIDA) in 1999 and that covers the basic principles of effective treatment for drug addiction, "Treatment does not need to be voluntary to be effective. Strong motivation can facilitate the treatment process. Sanctions or enticements in the family, employment setting, or criminal justice system can increase significantly both treatment entry and retention rates and the success of drug treatment interventions."

Drug treatment must be monitored with regular DRUG TESTING, according to NIDA. In fact, just knowing that drug testing is part of a program can help individuals to resist the lure of drugs in many cases.

Coexisting Psychiatric Problems Need to Be Identified and Treated

Many drug addicts have coexisting psychiatric problems, such as DEPRESSION, ANXIETY DISORDERS, BIPOLAR DISORDER, and/or antisocial personality disorder. (This is also called a DUAL DIAGNOSIS.) Both the drug addiction and psychiatric disorders must be treated, otherwise the cycle is likely to be repeated and the recovered addict will quickly relapse and begin using drugs again. Finding a facility that is willing to treat a patient with both an addictive disorder and a psychiatric problem may be difficult since each problem alone is difficult to treat and the problems taken together are extremely challenging.

Inpatient Versus Outpatient Treatment

Some patients addicted to drugs can be treated on an outpatient basis. Examples include heroin addicts who enter a methadone maintenance program or some heavy marijuana smokers who wish to enter a day program in their community. Others may need to be removed from their environment and experience a radical change, such as in a residential treatment setting.

There are more than 11,000 specialized drug treatment facilities in the United States. Some specialize in treating youths, while others specialize in other types of populations. Many facilities receive funding from the federal government and state governments as well as from private insurance companies.

To locate a drug or alcohol treatment facility on the Internet, go to the Substance Abuse and Mental Health Services Administration at http://findtreatment.samhsa.gov/facilitylacatordoc.htm.

Patients may need to receive treatment more than once, and relapses commonly occur. Drug addiction is not an easy problem to overcome nor is it easy to treat. However, with work, it can be overcome.

See also AMPHETAMINES; BENZODIAZEPINES; DRUG ABUSE; DRUG ABUSE/ADDICTION AND HEALTH PROBLEMS; DRUG ENFORCEMENT ADMINISTRATION; MORPHINE; OPIATES; OXYCONTIN; PHYSICIANS AND HEALTH CARE PROFESSIONALS AND ADDICTION; TEENAGERS AND YOUTH DRUG ABUSE.

Krantz, Mori J., M.D. and Philip S. Mehler, M.D. "Treating Opioid Dependence: Growing Implications for Primary Care," *Archives of Internal Medicine* 164, no. 3 (February 9, 2004): 277–288.

National Institute on Drug Abuse. *Drug Addiction Treatment: A Research-Based Guide.* National Institutes of Health, NIH Publication 99–4180, Washington, D.C.: National Institutes of Health, October 1999.

Substance Abuse and Mental Health Services Administration (SAMHSA). *Results from the 2003 National Survey on Drug Use and Health: National Findings.* Office of Applied Studies, NHSDA Series H-22, DHHS Publication Number SMA 03-3836. Rockville, Md. SAMHSA, 2003.

drug courts   Judicial systems that are specifically set up to deal with offenders who have been accused of using drugs illegally or committing crimes while under the influence of drugs. The first drug court was established in Miami, Florida, in 1989. As of 2003, there were more than 940 drug courts in 49 states nationwide in the United States, up from only about six drug courts in 1991. In addition, 441 more drug courts were in the planning stages. There are many different types of drug courts in the United States because states have chosen different models to follow.

One of the key provisions of the Violent Crime Control and Law Enforcement Act, passed by the United States Congress in 1994, was to set up a grant system to encourage states and local areas to set up drug courts that would provide supervision and services for offenders. Subsequent to that date, drug courts began to proliferate throughout the country.

The basic idea behind such courts is that drug offenders chosen for the program will be given a treatment plan to follow and will agree to submit to regular monitoring, including DRUG TESTING. If they comply with the plan and refrain from using drugs or alcohol, then former drug offenders will not go to jail. Conversely, if their urine tests positive for drugs or they violate their program in some other way, they will be incarcerated immediately.

The Initial Impetus for Drug Courts: Crack Cocaine

A key reason for the nationwide spread of drug courts was the prevalent abuse of CRACK COCAINE by many individuals in the 1980s, which became a severe problem that strained the judicial system to the breaking point. Many people were arrested and incarcerated. After they served their terms and were then released, very often they were quickly rearrested for the same offenses.

Experts decided that rather than concentrating on using solely punitive measures such as INCARCERATION, which obviously were not working with this population, a more therapeutic model might be effective. As a result, the idea of separating some offenders into a drug court system developed. The idea was based on the premise that offenders would be given a chance to receive therapy and rehabilitative services. Experts determined that the best candidates for drug courts would be individuals who were nonviolent offenders that local experts considered possible to rehabilitate.

Repeat Offenses Are Down with Drug Courts

The concept of drug courts seems to be working well. According to a report funded by the U.S. Department of Justice, *Recidivism Rates for Drug Court Graduates: Nationally-Based Estimates, Final Report,* statistics from the study have shown that recidivism (repetition of crimes) is lower among drug court graduates than among individuals who go through the regular court system.

Researchers John Roman et al. studied about 2,000 individuals who were involved in a drug court system, and they found that their recidivism rate was 16.4 percent after one year and 27.5 percent after two years. This compares favorably to the rate of drug offenders who go through the regular courts, who have a rearrest rate of 43.5 percent after one year and 58.6 percent after two years.

In another study on drug courts, performed by the Washington State Institute for Public Policy and released in 2003, the researchers studied the results from six adult drug courts in Washington. The researchers found that two-thirds of the drug court participants were males, with an average age of 34 years.

They also found that the drug courts initially cost more than criminal courts on average. However, the ultimate financial return was better because recidivism dropped by 13.3 percent in five out of six of the drug courts. For these courts, the researchers found that the benefits per drug court participant in terms of cost were $6,779 each, including $3,759 in criminal justice costs avoided and $3,020 in crime victim costs avoided. The actual drug court cost per participant was $3,891. As a result, there was a net gain of $2,888 per participant.

Considering Juvenile Drug Courts

Because the adult drug courts have worked effectively for many adult offenders as well as for the court system itself, some experts also decided that the model of the drug court would work well in the juvenile justice system. As a result, between 1995 and 2001, about 140 juvenile drug courts were created and 125 more were in the planning stages.

The juvenile drug court model creates a team with a judge as one member. Other members often include social services workers, school officials, law enforcement personnel, probation officers, and others. In contrast to the adult drug courts, the juvenile drug court team works not only with children who have broken the drug laws but also with their immediate family members.

See also DIVERSION PROGRAMS; ZERO-TOLERANCE LAWS.

Barnoski, Robert and Steve Aos. *Washington State's Drug Courts for Adult Defendants: Outcome Evaluation and Cost-Benefit Analysis.* Olympia, Wash.: Washington State Institute for Public Policy, March 2003.

Bureau of Justice Assistance. *Juvenile Drug Courts: Strategies in Practice.* Washington, D.C.: U.S. Department of Justice, March 2003.

Roman, John, Wendy Townsend, and Avinash Bati Singh. *Recidivism Rates for Drug Court Graduates: Nationally Based Estimates, Final Report.* New York: The Urban Institute, July 2003.

The White House. *National Drug Control Strategy Update,* Washington, D.C.: Office of National Drug Control Policy, February 2003.

Drug Enforcement Administration (DEA) A federal organization in the United States that was formed in 1973, the DEA is responsible for the enforcement of the laws on the illegal use of narcotics and other SCHEDULED DRUGS, such as COCAINE, HEROIN, MARIJUANA, as well as some prescribed medications that are sometimes abused, such as OXYCONTIN and other narcotic analgesics (painkillers) such as METHADONE.

The DEA is the primary federal agency that is responsible for enforcing the CONTROLLED SUBSTANCES ACT. There are five schedules of drugs, and drugs that are classified as Schedule I are illegal drugs.

The DEA investigates and prosecutes criminals who are engaged in drug trafficking. It also manages a national drug intelligence program that cooperates with federal, state, local, and foreign law enforcement officials. In addition, it seizes and retains assets that are related to illicit drug trafficking.

In 2002, the DEA made 27,635 arrests in the United States. The agency also seized 61,594 kg of cocaine, 705 kg of heroin, 195,644 kg of marijuana, 118,049,279 dosage units of methamphetamine, and 11,532,704 dosage units of hallucinogens.

DEA regulations for Schedule II prescription drugs, unlike those for other prescription medications, require that the doctor write and sign each prescription. Prescriptions are not permitted to be telephoned in to the pharmacy unless the situation is an emergency. In addition, they are not to be refilled, and a new prescription is required each time a patient needs more medication. The DEA also sets limits on the quantity of Schedule II drugs that may be produced every year.

See also NARCOTICS; OPIATES.

For further information, contact the DEA at:

2401 Jefferson Davis Highway
Alexandria, VA 22301
(202) 307-1000
http://www.usdoj.gov/dea

drug-free zones Areas where, according to law, the use or sale of illegal drugs is punished more severely than it is outside these areas. Drug-free zones are generally places where children are likely to be found, such as elementary and secondary schools and playgrounds, although some states, such as Virginia, have extended the provisions of the law to colleges. States vary in the severity of their punishments for violations as well as in enforcement of the law.

The concept of drug-free zones became popular after the passage of the federal Drug-Free School Zones Act of 1984. Most states passed laws describing drug-free zones. In 1994, the Violent Crime Control and Law Enforcement Act created or enhanced penalties for individuals trafficking in drugs in drug-free zones as well as for drug trafficking near public housing, in prisons, and in other situations.

See also DRUG COURTS; ZERO-TOLERANCE LAWS.

David Teasley. "95025: Drug Supply Control: 104th Congress," CRS Issue Brief, Available online. URL: http://www.fas.org/irp/crs/95-025-htm. Accessed on March 15, 2004.

drug testing Refers to laboratory tests that are taken to determine if a person has illegal drugs and/or alcohol within the body, which often (but not always) indicate that he or she has used these substances. These tests do not provide evidence of every drug that the person may take, and instead, they only screen for the substances that are of concern to the tester. As a result, the tester will not receive a printout of all medications that a person takes but instead will receive either positive or negative results to the substances for which tests were performed.

Drug testing may be done in the form of tests of the blood, urine, hair, saliva, and even body perspiration. Many companies require such drug testing before they will hire an individual, and they may also require periodic testing on some current employees. Employees in safety-sensitive positions, such as airline pilots and commercial truck drivers, may be subjected to random drug tests for the purpose of public safety to ensure that employees are not impaired while on the job. The military services often use random drug screening. Some vocational schools do random drug testing.

Other populations are also routinely and/or randomly subjected to drug testing. Individuals who are referred to diversion programs for SUBSTANCE ABUSE are subjected to random drug tests. Recently released prisoners who were known to have had a prior drug problem may be subject to random drug tests as a condition of their release. In addition, public schools may legally require the drug testing of students who participate in extracurricular activities, based on a 2002 United States Supreme Court decision, *Board of Education of Independent School District No. 92 of Pottawatomie County v. Earls.*

Professional athletes may be tested for drug use, as are Olympic athletes.

In general, some employees who may be tested for drugs include:

- Known past drug users
- Those having an annual physical examination
- Those who have just had an accident
- People who have completed drug treatment
- People being considered for a promotion
- Those being considered for a new position involving money, security, or safety

Pros and Cons of Drug Testing

One key advantage of drug testing is that the public is better protected when people who are abusing drugs are prevented from driving large trucks, flying airplanes, or acting in other ways against the common good. The drug-testing policy also acts as a deterrent. When employees and students know that such a policy exists, they may be less likely to abuse drugs or alcohol. In addition, drug testing gives students an opportunity and an excuse to resist PEER PRESSURE toward trying drugs.

The disadvantages are that drug testing may seem invasive and annoying to those who are being tested, particularly when urine tests are used. Drug testing has grown into a small industry, and detractors feel employers overly depend on it.

If drugs are detected, then serious consequences are usually attached to this finding. For example, an employee who is found to have drugs in the blood or urine may be suspended from work and/or required to undergo immediate drug treatment. An athlete may be suspended or even forced off a team altogether, depending upon the circumstances. The consequences may seem very harsh and unreasonable to the person who suffers them and to his or her family. The person may suffer severe financial and emotional hardship. However, proponents of drug testing say that the benefits far outweigh the disadvantages.

Types of Drug Testing

The most common form of drug testing is the urine test, which can test for drugs or metabolites (drug residues) in the urine. It is the lowest-cost test, and the various assays used to perform the test can help to ascertain the largest number of illegal substances. According to the DRUG ENFORCEMENT ADMINISTRATION, urinalysis is the only methodology for drug testing approved by the U.S. Department of Health and Human Services.

A urine test can detect drug usage that has occurred within about one to five days (with some exceptions, such as marijuana, which can persist in the urine for weeks to months after the last use). The Federal Drug-Free Workplace program uses a urine test that detects the presence of MARIJUANA, OPIATES, COCAINE, AMPHETAMINES, and phencyclidine. Urine tests are also available that can detect the presence of alcohol, lysergic acid diethylamide, and other drugs.

The hair can be tested for drugs. Testing of the hair can determine drug use that has occurred within as long as the past 90 days, depending on the length of the hair. However, it cannot detect drug use within about one to seven days of the test. As a result, the hair test is a better way to check for long-term drug use.

Hair cannot be used to detect alcohol intake. Hair testing is usually limited to law enforcement agencies like the Federal Bureau of Investigation when testing for cocaine, heroin, or their metabolites, and has been used in criminal investigations.

For example, according to an article on the forensic application of testing hair for drugs of abuse, a child died of cocaine intoxication while in the care of her mother and father. The mother and the father both accused each other of drug abuse, but hair testing revealed that the father was a cocaine user and the mother was not. The father then confessed to having possessed the cocaine.

Saliva can also be used to test for drugs. This test can be taken under direct observation, in contrast with the urine test, which can be substituted or adulterated by the subject. (However, most organizations have procedures in place to protect against deception so that it is very difficult for subjects to substitute someone else's urine for their own.) Usually the saliva sample is taken by swabbing the inside of the cheek. The disadvantage of this test is that it is less efficient than the urine or hair test. The oral fluids test detects drug use within the past 10–24 hours.

The sweat patch is another means of drug testing, although some studies have found it to be unreliable. This is a skin patch that is placed on the subject for a time frame ranging from one to seven days, depending on the type of patch used. The disadvantage is that not many laboratories process the sweat patch results. Also, subjects with any cuts, abrasions, or excessive hair cannot wear the sweat patch. The patch detects drug use within the past seven days.

False-Positive Drug Test Results

A positive urine test does not necessarily mean that the person has just used a particular drug. However, it does usually mean that he or she used the drug within the past few days. Occasional FALSE POSITIVE results occur with tests. For example, if subjects take cough syrup with dextromethorphan, they may test positive for opiates even if they have not used opiates.

Eating foods rich in poppy seeds can also sometimes cause false positive opiate tests. In addition, patients taking common antibiotics, particularly quinolones, such as levofloxacin (Levaquin) and ofloxacin (Floxin) that are used for patients with urinary tract infections, prostate infections, or bronchitis, may test positive for opiates with some tests used to detect substance abuse.

This false-positive issue was proven in a study reported in a 2001 issue of the *Journal of the American Medical Association.* For example, one dose of 500 mg of levofloxacin caused a false-positive test result within two hours that lasted for 22 or more hours in three healthy non-substance-abusing volunteers. The same pattern was observed with a single dose of 400 mg of ofloxacin.

Any person who receives a false positive on a drug test should point out to authorities that false positives do exist, because many officials are unaware that this is true. More sophisticated screening may need to be done. If the person who was screened was taking an antibiotic, a retest could be performed when he or she is no longer taking the medication. Specific tests are also available to assess further whether the positive opiate finding was related to the recent consumption of poppy seeds, dextromethorphan, and so forth.

Patients Taking Legitimate Medications That May Show Up in Drug Screens

Patients with chronic pain who are taking prescribed opiates for PAIN MANAGEMENT or patients with ATTENTION DEFICIT HYPERACTIVITY DISORDER who are taking prescribed amphetamines will test positive for these drugs, even though they are taking them legally. Such patients must tell their employers or their school beforehand about their medication use to avoid drug-screening results that cause officials to mistakenly assume illicit drug use. The employer or school may require a note from the prescribing physician verifying that the individual does have a medical need to take the specific drug and that the drug could cause a positive result in some drug screens.

Attempts to Hide the Use of Drugs

Some students and employees purchase products on the Internet to try to mask their drug use. However, these products are usually costly, and often they do not work. Sometimes the products mask the drug use, but the product use itself shows up in a drug test because employers are aware that such products exist. When these problems are detected, they automatically signal employers or schools to be concerned about the person's likely drug use, even if no drugs are found.

See also ALCOHOL BREATH TESTS; EMPLOYEE ASSISTANCE PROGRAMS; INTERNET; LSD; PCP; WORK.

Baden, Lindsey R., M.D. et al. "Quinolones and False-Positive Urine Screening for Opiates by Immunoassay Technology," *Journal of the American Medical Association* 286, no. 24 (December 26, 2001): 3,115–3,119.

Miller, Mark L., Brian Donnelly, and Roger M. Martz. "The Forensic Application of Testing Hair for Drugs of Abuse," in *The Validity of Self-Reported Drug Use: Improving the Accuracy of Survey Estimates,* Edited by Lana Harrison and Arthur Hughes. NIDA Research Monograph 167, NIH Publication No. 97-4147. Washington, D.C.: National Institute of Health, 1997, pages 146–160.

Office of National Drug Control Policy. *What You Need to Know About Drug Testing in Schools.* Office of the President, NCJ 195522. Available online. URL: http://www.whitehousedrugpolicy.gov/pdf/drug_testing.pdf. Accessed on May 15, 2004.

dual diagnosis   The presence of one or more psychiatric problems as well as problems with alcohol and/or drug addiction. Many people who abuse or are addicted to alcohol and/or to drugs also have psychiatric problems, such as ANXIETY DISORDERS, BIPOLAR DISORDER, or DEPRESSION. An estimated 5 million people with a serious mental illness in the United States used an illegal drug in 2002. (See table on page 109.) Individuals with depressive episodic generalized anxiety disorder, panic attacks, and agoraphobia are especially likely to abuse legal and illegal substances. (See table at top of page 108.) According to the 2002 National Survey on Drug Use and Health, 17.5 million adults had a serious mental illness in the United States (8.3 percent of all adults in the United States). Of these individuals, an estimated 4 million adults met the criteria for both a serious mental illness and a problem with SUBSTANCE ABUSE or dependence (addiction) in the past year. The prevalence of a mental illness was greater than twice as likely among individuals who used illicit drugs in the past year (17.9 percent) than among those who did not (6.9 percent).

It should be emphasized that although many mentally ill people use drugs illegally and/or abuse alcohol, the problems of alcoholism and drug abuse should not be generalized to all mentally ill people, further stigmatizing them. In addition, neither should it be assumed that all or most drug abusers, addicts, or alcoholics are mentally ill. Only a mental health professional should make a determination of a serious mental illness.

Treatment of Both Problems Is Essential

A dual diagnosis makes it difficult for experts to treat the patient. Many treatment facilities concentrate on treating either the substance abuse or the psychiatric illness and not treating both problems concurrently. However, if the person with a dual diagnosis is not treated for both problems, then it will be difficult or impossible for the patient to recover. Often the psychiatric problem and the substance abuse are inextricably linked, and treating only one problem will eventually cause the person to relapse. For example, if a patient with alcoholism has an underlying problem with depression and only the alcoholism is treated, eventually the untreated depression is likely to cause the patient to wish to drink again, and he or she will resume drinking. Treatment of the depression as well as treatment of the alcoholism can help the patient to resist the urge to drink.

The psychiatrist may not be able to determine which is the cause and which is the effect (if there is, in fact a cause and effect relationship between the psychiatric problem and the substance abuse). However, treatment may facilitate a recovery and break the link between the psychiatric problem and the substance abuse. In addition, self-help organizations, such as ALCOHOLICS ANONYMOUS, may be effective in helping patients to continue to resist the lure of drugs or alcohol.

According to the 2002 National Survey on Drug Use and Health, about half of adults with a serious mental illness and a drug abuse or alcoholism problem received mental health treatment.

High-Risk Patients

According to a 2004 pamphlet from the National Drug Intelligence Center, patients with some mental illnesses have particularly high risks of developing a problem of drug abuse. For example, patients who are diagnosed with antisocial personality disorder have a 15.5 percent risk of developing a drug abuse problem, followed closely in risk by patients with a manic episode (14.5 percent) and then by patients with SCHIZOPHRENIA (10.1 percent). Note that other experts indicate that the risk for sub-stance abuse in patients with schizophrenia is about 50 percent, although most of this risk appears to be for alcohol abuse.

Antisocial personality disorder is a personality type that tends toward criminal behavior. Schizophrenia is a psychotic disorder characterized by irrational thinking, paranoid delusions, and auditory and visual hallucinations. Patients with schizophrenia may use drugs to try to dampen their symptoms as well as to alleviate some of the side effects of some of their antipsychotic medications.

Other patients with psychiatric problems who are at risk for developing drug abuse problems are those with panic disorder (4.3 percent), major depressive disorder (4.1 percent), OBSESSIVE-COMPULSIVE DISORDER (3.4 percent), and phobias (2.1 percent). Other disorders associated with an increased risk of drug abuse are POSTTRAUMATIC STRESS DISORDER and ATTENTION DEFICIT HYPERACTIVITY DISORDER (ADHD)—although some physicians argue that patients with ADHD are not receiving the appropriate psychiatric medication if they are taking illegal drugs.

Alcohol Abuse and Mental Illness Treatment

An analysis of data from the admissions of patients with both a substance abuse problem and a psychiatric disorder as reported to the Treatment Episode Data Set, an annual compilation of data, provided valuable data. This data was summarized in a 2004 issue of the *DASIS Report*. According to this data, the number of patients who were admitted for co-occurring substance abuse and psychiatric disorders increased from 12 percent in 1995 to 16 percent in 2001.

This population of patients was more likely than other patients who were admitted to report alcohol as the primary substance of abuse. They were also more likely to be females than among admitted patients who were not diagnosed with psychiatric problems. In 2001, 56 percent of the patients with both substance abuse and psychiatric disorders were female, compared with only 29 percent of females for all other admissions.

Alcoholism and Psychiatric Problems

A 2002 issue of *Alcohol Research & Health*, based on the National Comorbidity Survey in 1996 and the Epidemiologic Catchment Study in 1990, showed that in a one-year period, nearly a third (29.6

PAST-YEAR SUBSTANCE USE (PERCENT) BY MENTAL SYNDROME, U.S. POPULATION, AGE 18 AND OLDER, 1996

Substance	Total Adult Population	Major Depressive Episode	Generalized Anxiety Disorder	Agoraphobia	Panic Attack
Cigarettes	33.2	50.4	55.5	47.0	49.2
Alcohol (heavy use) *	18.9	23.6	23.0	14.3	20.1
Any illicit drug	10.1	20.6	14.4	15.7	19.9
Psychotherapeutics **	2.9	7.8	4.9	7.7	8.6
Cocaine	1.9	5.0	4.4	2.0	4.0

* Heavy alcohol use is defined as being "drunk" or "very high" on three or more days in the past year.
** Psychotherapeutics refer to the nonmedical use of any prescription-type stimulant, sedative, tranquilizer, or analgesic. It does not include over-the-counter medications.
Source: Beatrice A. Rouse, editor, Web mounted version prepared by Rick Albright, *Substance Abuse and Mental Health Services Administration (SAMHSA) Statistics Source Book, 1998.*

percent) of patients with alcoholism suffered from mood disorders. Most of the risk of a mood disorder lay with major depressive disorder (depression), or 27.9 percent of the 29.2 percent, and the balance of the patients had bipolar disorder. The researchers also calculated that an alcoholic was 3.6 times more likely to suffer from a mood disorder than a person who was not an alcoholic. (See table below.)

The researchers also found that over one year, 36.9 percent of alcoholic patients had a risk of suffering from ANXIETY DISORDERS, and the calculated risk ratio was 2.6. The anxiety disorders were further divided into generalized anxiety disorder,

PREVALENCE OF PSYCHIATRIC DISORDERS IN PEOPLE WITH ALCOHOL DEPENDENCE (ALCOHOLISM)

Comorbid Disorder	1-Year Rate (Percent)	Odds Ratio
Mood disorders	29.2	3.6
Major depressive disorder	27.9	3.9
Bipolar disorder	1.9	6.3
Anxiety disorders	36.9	2.6
Generalized anxiety disorder (GAD)	11.6	4.6
Panic disorder	3.9	1.7
Posttraumatic stress disorder	7.7	2.2
Schizophrenia	24	3.8

Source: Petrakis, Ismene L., M.D., et al. "Comorbidity of Alcoholism and Psychiatric Disorders," *Alcohol Research & Health* 26, no. 2 (2002): 81–89.

panic disorder, and posttraumatic stress disorder. The researchers found alcoholics had nearly five times the risk of the nonalcoholic person of developing generalized anxiety disorder.

In addition, the researchers found that psychiatric problems were significantly greater for people with alcoholism than for people with alcohol abuse. For example, 29.2 percent of the alcoholics had a problem with mood disorders, but the rate of mood disorders among those with alcohol abuse was 12.3 percent. That is about the same rate as that found in the general population.

Drug Addiction and Psychiatric Problems

As mentioned, many people who are addicted to drugs also suffer from psychiatric problems. As with alcoholism, these psychiatric problems need to be treated along with the addiction so that the person can attain a recovery.

Sometimes drug abuse or addiction can cause psychiatric problems. For example, methylenedioxymethamphetamine (ECSTASY) can cause symptoms such as anxiety, depression, confusion, panic attacks, and paranoia, and these symptoms may continue. Drugs such as COCAINE and METHAMPHETAMINE may induce a psychotic break in some individuals. In others, they may create a rage that leads the user to uncharacteristic VIOLENCE and even to HOMICIDE.

Some psychiatric problems can be resolved with DETOXIFICATION from the drug under medical supervision, while others may be lifelong. For example, some hallucinogens such as lysergic acid

PERSONS AGES 18 OR OLDER WITH SERIOUS MENTAL ILLNESS IN THE UNITED STATES IN THE PAST YEAR, BY PAST YEAR USE OF ANY ILLICIT DRUG AND DEMOGRAPHIC CHARACTERISTICS: NUMBERS IN THOUSANDS, 2002

Demographic Characteristic	Any Illicit Drug Use[1]		
	Total	Yes	No
Total	17,483	5,061	12,423
Age			
18–25	4,085	1,965	2,120
26–49	9,534	2,730	6,804
50 or older	3,865	366	3,499
Gender			
Male	6,041	2,282	3,759
Female	11,442	2,779	8,663
Race			
White	12,639	3,751	8,888
Black or African American	2,032	547	1,485
American Indian or Alaska Native	161	39	122
Native Hawaiian or Other Pacific Islander	40	16	23
Asian	600	53	546
Two or More Races	289	86	203
Hispanic	1,724	569	1,155
Education			
Less than High School	3,591	1,115	2,476
High School Graduate	5,839	1,516	4,323
Some College	4,991	1,724	3,267
College Graduate	3,062	705	2,357
Current Employment			
Full-Time	8,453	2,562	5,891
Part-Time	2,664	829	1,834
Unemployed	1,078	548	530
Other[2]	5,289	1,122	4,167

[1] Any illicit drug includes marijuana/hashish, cocaine (including crack cocaine), heroin, hallucinogens, inhalants, or any prescription-type psychotherapeutic drug used nonmedically.
[2] Retired person, disabled person, homemaker, student, or other person not in the labor force.
Source: Epstein, J., et al. *Serious Mental Illness and Its Co-occurrence with Substance Use Disorders, 2002*. Substance Abuse and Mental Health Services Administration, Office of Applied Studies, Department of Health and Human Services Publication No. SMA 04-3905, Analytic Series A-24. Washington, D.C.: Department of Health and Human Services, June 2004.

diethylamide may induce hallucinations or flashbacks that can be terrifying to the individual. These may occur months or even years after the individual has ceased to use the drug.

The Homeless and Dual Diagnosis

Many homeless people have both psychiatric problems and substance abuse problems. In a study on the prevalence of substance use disorders and mental illness among 216 homeless women, published in a 1998 issue of the *American Journal of Psychiatry,* the researchers found greater than two-thirds of the homeless women were given at least one lifetime diagnosis of a serious psychiatric disorder. About one-third of the women had been diagnosed with three or more disorders.

Note that the prevalence of both depression and substance abuse was significantly higher among two groups of women, homeless women and low-income women, than among all women in the National Comorbidity Survey, according to the authors. Thus, dual diagnosis may occur more frequently among poor women than among women in the general population, although further research is needed before that determination can be made.

See also ANTIDEPRESSANTS; BENZODIAZEPINES; HOMELESSNESS; IMPULSE CONTROL DISORDER; LSD; MENTAL ILLNESS/PSYCHIATRIC PROBLEMS; MOOD STABILIZERS; PSYCHIATRIC MEDICATIONS; PSYCHIATRISTS; PSYCHOTIC BREAK; RECOVERY; TREATMENT FACILITIES.

Bassuk, Ellen L., M.D., et al. "Prevalence of Mental Health and Substance Use Disorders Among Homeless and Low-Income Housed Mothers," *American Journal of Psychiatry* 155, no. 11 (November 1998): 1,561–1,564.

Epstein, J., et al. *Serious Mental Illness and Its Co-occurrence with Substance Use Disorders, 2002.* Substance Abuse and Mental Health Services Administration (SAMHSA), Office of Applied Studies, Department of Health and Human Services Publication No. SMA 04-3905. Rockville, Md.: SAMHSA, June 2004. Available online. URL: http://www.drugabusestatistics.samhsa.gov/CoD/Cod.pdf. Accessed on July 15, 2004.

National Drug Intelligence Center. *Drug Abuse and Mental Illness Fast Facts.* NDIC Product No. 2004-L0559-005. Washington, D.C.: U.S. Department of Justice, 2004. Available online. URL: http://www.usdoj.gov/ndic/pubs7/7343/7343p.pdf. Accessed on June 1, 2004.

Petrakis, Ismene L., M.D., et al. "Comorbidity of Alcoholism and Psychiatric Disorders," *Alcohol Research & Health* 26, no. 2 (2002): 81–89.

Ecstasy Common nickname for 3–4 methylene-dioxymethamphetamine (MDMA), a very dangerous illegal drug that is popular among some adolescents and young adults. It has also been called a CLUB DRUG because Ecstasy is often sold or given away at clubs and parties for young people as well as being distributed in college dormitories, shopping malls, and other sites. The drug has also often been available at all-night dance parties called *raves*. Areas with the highest use and distribution of MDMA have included such cities as Los Angeles, California; Miami, Florida; and New York City, New York.

An estimated 8 million people ages 12 and older have used Ecstasy at least once, according to the National Household Survey on Drug Abuse. About 676,000 people used Ecstasy in 2002, according to the National Survey on Drug Use and Health published in 2003. Among young people ages 18–25 years old who had ever used drugs, the use of hallucinogens increased from 14.3 percent in 1992 to 24.2 percent in 2002, largely due to increases in the use of MDMA.

Most of the MDMA used by people in the United States was produced in other countries. According to the Office of National Drug Control Policy, in 2002, most MDMA (about 80 percent) was produced illegally in western Europe, primarily in Belgium and the Netherlands, with some production also occurring in Poland.

The drug was first developed in Germany in 1912 as a possible appetite suppressant, although it was never marketed for this purpose. Some therapists later used MDMA in psychotherapy prior to 1988, when the drug was classified as a Schedule I substance under the CONTROLLED SUBSTANCES ACT.

Because of increasing concern over the use of MDMA, the Ecstasy Anti-Proliferation Act was passed in 2000, authorizing increased federal guideline sentences for drug dealers who sold MDMA to others. In 2001, the recommended sentence for selling 800 Ecstasy pills was five years, up from the earlier sentence of 15 months.

MDMA Primary Users

Most Ecstasy users are under age 25 years, and many are ages 12–17 years, according to federal studies of drug use. They also are significantly more likely than other age groups to use other drugs, particularly hallucinogenic drugs such as LSD or PCP as well as MARIJUANA. In addition, Ecstasy users who are ages 18–25 years old are more likely than nonusers to have also used COCAINE.

When considering geographic regions, Ecstasy users in 2001 ages 18–25 were more concentrated in the Northeast (9.4 percent were users), compared with other regions, such as the West (7.0 percent), the South (7.1 percent), and the Midwest (4.8 percent). However, little regional difference of Ecstasy use occurred among young people ages 12–17, where usage was 2.7 percent for the Northeast, 2.7 percent for the West, 2.4 percent for the South, and 1.8 percent for the Midwest.

When considering gender, females ages 12–17 were more likely to use Ecstasy in 2001. Conversely, in the age group of 18–25, males were more dominant users of the drug than females.

Usage statistics by race alone show that Asians ages 12–25 years were most likely to use Ecstasy (3.5 percent) in 2001, followed by whites (2.8 percent), Hispanics (1.7 percent), and African American (1.0 percent).

Effects of Ecstasy

MDMA is generally taken in a pill form, and its effect lasts between four to six hours. Some individuals believe that MDMA can provide a sexual high; however, there is no evidence that this is true.

MDMA is taken for its stimulant and psychedelic effects. However, the drug can also cause such psychiatric symptoms as anxiety, depression, confusion, panic attacks, and paranoia. Some physical effects may include nausea, tremors, sweating, or chills, involuntary teeth clenching, sleeplessness, and other effects.

Some individuals risk dehydration from hyperthermia (very high fevers) because MDMA can cause a very rapid sudden rise in the body temperature. If not treated in time, this hyperthermia can cause death. Other risks of taking this drug are heart attack, kidney failure, and brain damage. Emergency department visits that involved MDMA increased in the United States from 253 visits in 1994 to 4,511 in 2000, according to data from the Drug Abuse Warning Network (DAWN). As of this writing, the most recent data from DAWN are 2002 data, and MDMA emergency visits were down to 4,026, still a high level.

There are also long-term effects caused by the use of MDMA. Researchers at the National Institute of Mental Health demonstrated in 2001 that MDMA can damage the nerve cells that use serotonin, an important brain chemical. In addition, MDMA affects dopamine and acetylcholine, other key brain chemicals needed by the body for normal functioning.

Other Unknown Substances May Be Included with Ecstasy

Another risk that individuals take by buying or accepting what they think is MDMA from others is that they may be receiving another drug altogether or the drug may include MDMA and other substances as well. As a result, HEROIN, ephedrine, KETAMINE, PCP, caffeine, and other substances may be unknowingly ingested by the MDMA user. Because selling MDMA is illegal, no Food and Drug Administration oversight or purity in packaging rules and regulations apply, as with legal medications. Consequently, the buyer or Ecstasy user must trust that the drug dealer is providing a pure and unadulterated product, which is hardly a safe risk to take.

Some users who think that they have received MDMA have actually been given paramethoxyamphetamine (PMA) instead of MDMA. Because the effects of PMA take somewhat longer to appear, some individuals become impatient and then take even more of the drug, which is very dangerous and can lead to death when the drug takes effect.

See also DATE RAPE DRUGS; TEENAGE AND YOUTH DRUG ABUSE.

National Drug Intelligence Center. *National Drug Treatment Assessment 2003.* U.S. Department of Justice, Product Number 2003-Q0317-001. Washington, D.C.: U.S. Department of Justice, January 2003.

Office of National Drug Control Policy (ONDCP). *MDMA (Ecstasy).* ONDCP Clearinghouse Fact Sheet, NCJ-188745. April 2002. Available online. URL: http://www.expomed.com/drugtest/files/mdmafacts.pdf. Accessed on February 2004.

U.S. Department of Justice (DOJ). *PCP Tablets Sold as MDMA.* Information Bulletin Number 2001-L0424-003. Washington, D.C.: DOJ, April 2001.

education Providing instruction and information on a topic. Public policy experts and social scientists hope that by educating children and adolescents about various addictions, young people can better understand the risks involved and subsequently make better life choices. Nearly every study shows that addictive behaviors, particularly of alcohol, drugs, and tobacco, are most common among low-income and less-educated individuals, despite the fact that some high-income and highly educated individuals also engage in these behaviors.

Educating adults about issues surrounding addictive behaviors that they or other family members may suffer from is also important. Many government and nonprofit organizations seek to provide information to the public on these issues.

See also TEENAGE AND YOUTH DRINKING; TEENAGE AND YOUTH DRUG ABUSE; TEENAGE AND YOUTH GAMBLING; TEENAGE AND YOUTH SMOKING.

Office of Applied Studies, Substance Abuse and Mental Health Services Administration. "Substance Use Among School Dropouts," *The NSDUH Report,* November 28, 2003. Available online. URL: http://www.oas.samhsa.gov/2k3/dropouts/dropouts.htm. Accessed on January 15, 2004.

elderly/older adults Older individuals, usually older than age 65, although some sources define older adults as those who are 55 years and older.

Older individuals may have or develop problems with a wide array of addictive behaviors, such as ALCOHOLISM, DRUG ABUSE, GAMBLING, and other forms of addictions.

Alcoholism and Older Individuals

How many seniors are alcoholics is unknown. However, experts estimate that 2–4 percent of the population in the United States may have this problem, and this estimate may be low. In general, alcoholism is a greater problem among males, although often it is also a hidden problem among older women. Older drinkers are more likely to be unmarried or widowed and to use alcohol to avoid their problems. Studies indicate that elderly individuals who start drinking late in life have a much better prognosis for recovery than those who have been drinking their entire lives.

Alcoholism causes many serious health problems, including CIRRHOSIS, alcoholic HEPATITIS, diseases of the kidneys and heart, and PANCREATITIS. These diseases may not present until the individual is older than age 65, after many years of chronic drinking. Alcoholics are also at risk for osteoporosis (bone loss). Seniors already have an increased risk for bone loss by virtue of their age. The added disadvantage incurred by alcoholism greatly increases their risk of developing fractures when they fall, whether from intoxication or from falls that occur when they are sober.

Seniors are more prone to developing most forms of cancer. Alcoholism further exacerbates the risk of developing cancers, especially esophageal cancer, cancers in the head, neck cancer, and liver cancer. If the alcoholic person also smokes, the risk for LUNG CANCER is increased.

Many alcoholics suffer from vitamin and mineral deficiencies, especially of vitamin B_{12}. This deficiency may present with symptoms, such as mental confusion, that are similar to those seen with Alzheimer's disease. Tragically, the older person with alcoholism and a vitamin deficiency may sometimes be misdiagnosed with Alzheimer's disease if appropriate laboratory work is not performed.

Many elderly people already have hypertension, and alcoholism can exacerbate it further. If not already present, hypertension can be created by excessive drinking. Excessive drinking can also damage the immune system, causing seniors to become more susceptible to illnesses such as pneumonia or influenza. Many seniors fail to obtain their flu or pneumonia shots, and this can be a fatal mistake.

Older individuals who are alcoholic can respond well to sessions with ALCOHOLICS ANONYMOUS. However, the older person who decides to stop drinking should also seek medical help because sudden ABSTINENCE could trigger DELIRIUM TREMENS, which could be very dangerous and even fatal. Instead, DETOXIFICATION from alcohol should occur under medical care in a hospital or rehabilitation facility with experience in treating elderly alcoholics.

Smoking and Seniors

About 3.7 million older individuals in the United States continue to smoke when age 65 and older, or about 10 percent of older men and 9 percent of older women. Many older people wrongly believe that there would be no benefit to quitting smoking and that the damage to their bodies is "already done." This is dangerously incorrect, with the one exception of patients who have terminal illnesses. Instead, for most older people, the risk of lung cancer declines among those who stop smoking, as does the risk of other forms of cancer and heart disease. For example, three months after stopping smoking, lung function improves by as much as one-third. In one to nine months, chronic coughing and shortness of breath abates.

Some older people quit smoking with the help of NICOTINE REPLACEMENT THERAPY, while others use bupropion (ZYBAN) to end their smoking habit. Some studies have shown that a combination approach of both nicotine replacement therapy and bupropion is most effective, although those studies were not performed on older individuals. Hypnosis is effective for some individuals.

Drug Abuse and the Elderly

Most elderly individuals are not addicted to HEROIN, METHAMPHETAMINE, or other drugs typically associated with drugs of abuse. However, they may take analgesic or antianxiety medications largely because the elderly are more likely to have more health problems than younger individuals and may build up a tolerance to them. Although people over age 65 comprise about 13 percent of the population, they receive about 30 percent of all prescription medications. The abuse of these drugs is usually accidental. Often older individuals may forget whether they have taken their medications and they may take double doses of drugs. This may result in an ACCIDENTAL OVERDOSE.

Another accidental problem that seniors sometimes create is that they receive their prescriptions from different physicians and they also fill them at different pharmacies. Because medications can interact with each other, this is a very dangerous practice. It is best to tell all doctors about all drugs that are taken (and to bring a list of medications to each doctor's visit or to bring the actual drugs) and to obtain all medications from one pharmacy so that the pharmacist can act as an additional safeguard against any potential medication interactions.

Sometimes seniors may share their medications with others, and this is another form of drug abuse. It is also illegal. A drug that helps treat one patient with diabetes, pain, or hypertension can harm another person with the same illness because of different weight, blood pressure, and other issues that their physician has taken into consideration.

ALL ADMISSIONS: BY AGE GROUP, GENDER, AND RACE/ETHNICITY: 2001

	Percent	
Age:	Under 55	55 and Older
Gender		
Male	70	80
Female	30	20
Race/ethnicity		
White	59	61
African American	24	23
Hispanic	12	11
American Indian/Alaska Native	2	3
Asian/Pacific Islander	1	1
Other	2	1

Source: Office of Applied Studies, Drug and Alcohol Services Information System. "Older Adults in Substance Abuse Treatment: 2001," *The DASIS Report,* (May 11, 2004). Available online. URL: http://www.oas.samhsa.gov/2k4/olderAdultsTX/olderAdultsTX.htm. Accessed July 15, 2004.

Older Adults Admitted to Treatment Facilities

According to a report released by the Office of Applied Studies in 2004 on 2001 admissions, there were 58,000 admissions for treatment of people ages 55 years and older for SUBSTANCE ABUSE problems in the United States of the 1.7 million total admissions (about 3 percent of all admissions). Among older adults who were admitted for treatment, alcohol was the primary substance of abuse in most cases (74 percent) compared with 44 percent of the cases of individuals younger than age 55.

As can be seen from the table at bottom left, a greater percentage of the older admissions (80 percent) were male than the younger admissions (70 percent).

Gambling and Seniors

Some older people engage in playing bingo, buying lottery tickets, or playing cards or games of chance. Others develop compulsive gambling habits. They may develop a problem with gambling because they are lonely or bored. Some seniors seek to make a major win in the face of their dwindling retiring income. It is unknown how prevalent a problem compulsive gambling is among senior citizens.

See also ALCOHOLIC HEALTH PROBLEMS; CANCER; CARISOPRODOL; EMPHYSEMA; ORAL CANCER; PRESCRIPTION DRUG ABUSE; SMOKING AND HEALTH PROBLEMS.

Kandel, Joseph, M.D. and Christine Adamec. *The Encyclopedia of Senior Health and Well-Being.* New York: Facts On File, Inc., 2003.
Office of Applied Studies, Drug and Alcohol Services Information System. "Older Adults in Substance Abuse Treatment: 2001," *The DASIS Report,* (May 11, 2004). Available online. URL:http://www.oas.samhsa.gov/2k4/olderAdultsTX/olderAdultsTX.htm. Accessed on July 15, 2004.

emergency treatment   Care received on an urgent basis, often in the emergency department/emergency room of a hospital. Individuals who abuse alcohol and/or drugs may need immediate attention in order to save their lives, and may need emergency treatment for one or more of the following reasons:

• They may react to contaminants in illegal drugs.

• They may take a dosage higher than their bodies can tolerate.

- They may have underlying medical problems that they do not know about, such as undiagnosed heart disease, and the drug may trigger a heart attack.

- The drug may induce severe unanticipated side effects, such as hyperthermia, convulsions, or a psychotic reaction.

- Individuals may seek to commit SUICIDE by overdose (others may discover them after they have overdosed on drugs, or they may seek medical attention on their own behalf).

The emergency room staff can often save lives, stabilize patients, and relieve severe pain and symptoms such as seizures. However, they cannot provide the continuing treatment or long-term care needed by people with SUBSTANCE ABUSE problems. The emergency department may refer patients back to their own physicians as well as to rehabilitative facilities and to self-help organizations such as ALCOHOLICS ANONYMOUS or NARCOTICS ANONYMOUS. Even with emergency care, some individuals will not survive, regardless of their previous health status.

The Drug Abuse Warning Network

The Drug Abuse Warning Network (DAWN) is a database system of the federal government that relies upon nationwide data from hospital emergency departments that operate 24-hour emergency rooms in the coterminous United States (all states except Alaska and Hawaii, and including Washington, D.C.). DAWN obtains information from these units on the number of emergencies that doctors found were drug related. This information is useful because it is derived from individuals who have suffered from the extremes of substance abuse. It does not provide the entire picture of drug and alcohol abuse and dependence in the United States, however, since many substance abusers do not end up in hospital emergency rooms.

The data reported by DAWN is on children and adults with a presenting problem that was induced by or related to drug use. It does not include the following types of cases:

- An accidental ingestion or an inhalation of a substance with no intent to abuse the drug

- Adverse reactions or side effects to prescribed or over-the-counter medications that were taken as directed

- Ill effects from drugs taken against a victim's knowledge or will, as in DATE/ACQUAINTANCE RAPE cases

Up to four different substances may be reported for each emergency department episode. In 2002, the majority of the cases (54 percent) that were reported involved more than one drug. As a result, determining which drug is the cause of the problem requiring emergency medical attention can often be hard.

According to the most recent report available as of this writing, derived from *Emergency Department Trends from the Drug Abuse Warning Network, Final Estimates 1995–2002,* there were 681,957 incidents of patients requiring emergency services because of major substances of abuse in 2002 in the United States. This was a 49 percent increase since 1995, due to increased emergencies caused by use of MDMA, marijuana, inhalants, cocaine, and alcohol in combination with other drugs possibly due to increased abuse of methamphetamine). (See table at top of page 116.) Of the substances that were abused, alcohol-in-combination, which means alcohol and at least one other drug, was the most dominant problem, followed by COCAINE abuse and then MARIJUANA abuse.

As can be seen from the table at top of page 116, in the case of some drugs, there were much lower rates of abuse than in past years. For example, in 2002, there were 891 visits for LSD, compared with 2,821 in 2001. Ketamine usage was significantly down as well. Increases occurred in other areas, such as with methamphetamine, methylene dioxymethamphetamine (Ecstasy), and inhalant abuse, all of which required emergency treatment in 2002. Inhalant abuse was also sharply up, although why is not clear. Despite this fact, the numbers are still low, although any increase is still cause for concern.

According to the DAWN data for 2002, the most common reason that was cited for patients' visits to the emergency room was an overdose (39 percent), followed by an unexpected reaction (20 percent) to a substance. These two reasons taken

**TOTAL EMERGENCY DEPARTMENT VISITS FOR MAJOR SUBSTANCES OF ABUSE,
ESTIMATES FOR THE CONTERMINOUS UNITED STATES
(48 STATES AND WASHINGTON, D.C., EXCLUDING ALASKA AND HAWAII) BY YEAR, 1995–2002**

Drug Category	Total 1995	Total 1996	Total 1997	Total 1998	Total 1999	Total 2000	Total 2001	Total 2002
All major substances	457,773	478,387	510,284	548,582	575,163	623,999	669,340	681,957
Alcohol-in-combination	166,897	166,166	171,894	184,989	196,178	204,500	217,940	207,395
Cocaine	135,711	152,420	161,083	172,011	168,751	174,881	193,034	199,198
Heroin	69,556	72,980	70,712	75,688	82,192	94,804	93,064	93,519
Marijuana	45,259	53,770	64,720	76,842	87,068	96,426	110,512	119,472
Amphetamines	9,581	9,772	10,496	12,183	12,496	17,134	18,555	21,644
Methamphetamine	15,933	11,002	17,154	11,486	10,447	13,505	14,923	17,696
MDMA (Ecstasy)	421	319	637	1,143	2,850	4,511	5,542	4,026
Ketamine	—	81	—	209	396	263	679	260
LSD	5,682	4,569	5,219	4,982	5,126	4,016	2,821	891
PCP	5,963	3,441	3,626	3,436	3,663	5,404	6,102	7,648
Miscellaneous hallucinogens	1,463	1,600	1,629	1,849	1,533	1,849	1,788	1,428
GHB	145	638	762	1,282	3,178	4,969	3,340	3,330
Inhalants	736	1,030	1,539	1,735	650	1,141	522	1,496
Not tabulated	163	383	201	125	34	127	298	—

Source: Substance Abuse and Mental Health Services Administration (SAMHSA), Office of Applied Studies. *Emergency Department Trends from the Drug Abuse Warning Network, Final Estimates 1995–2002.* Rockville, Md.: SAMHSA, DAWN Series: D-24, DHHS Publication No. (SMA) 03-3780, July 2003.

**UNEXPECTED REACTIONS AND
OVERDOSES AS PREDOMINANT REASONS FOR
EMERGENCY DEPARTMENT CONTACT IN 2002
IN THE UNITED STATES BY PERCENT AND
TYPE OF DRUG**

Type of Drug	Percent of Cases
GHB	88
Miscellaneous hallucinogens	78
PCP	63
Inhalants	78 (62 percent for overdose alone)
MDMA (Ecstasy)	69
Amphetamines	63
Ketamine	59
Marijuana	57
LSD	56
Alcohol-in-combination	54

Source: Substance Abuse and Mental Health Services Administration, Office of Applied Studies. *Emergency Department Trends from the Drug Abuse Warning Network, Final Estimates 1995–2002.* Rockville, Md.: DAWN Series: D-24, DHHS Publication No. (SMA) 03-3780, July 2003.

together (overdose and unexpected reaction) were the predominant reasons for emergency room contact in 88 percent of the cases involving the drug GHB. (See table at left.) Interestingly, seeking DETOXIFICATION was a reason for emergency room contact in 37 percent of the cases involving heroin and 28 percent involving cocaine.

See also ACCIDENTAL OVERDOSE; AMPHETAMINES; CLUB DRUGS; DEATH; DRIVING IMPAIRED; DRIVING WHILE INTOXICATED/DRIVING UNDER THE INFLUENCE; HEALTH PROBLEMS; ECSTASY; GHB; HEROIN; INHALANTS, ABUSE OF; KETAMINE; METHAMPHETAMINE; TEENAGE AND YOUTH DRUG ABUSE.

Substance Abuse and Mental Health Services Administration (SAMHSA), Office of Applied Studies. *Emergency Department Trends from the Drug Abuse Warning Network, Final Estimates 1995–2002.* DAWN Series: D-24, DHHS Publication No. (SMA) 03-3780, Rockville, Md.: SAMHSA, July 2003.

emphysema   A serious and incurable lung disease usually caused by years of smoking cigarettes as well as cigars or pipes. An estimated 90 percent of all cases of emphysema are caused by smoking. A small number—about 50,000–100,000—of patients in the United States with emphysema have a deficiency of alpha 1-antitrypsin, which may develop into a hereditary form of emphysema.

Emphysema is a form of chronic obstructive pulmonary disease (COPD). The other diseases also diagnosed as forms of COPD are chronic asthma and bronchitis.

Emphysema destroys the lung sacs, causing large holes in them and making it difficult for patients to breathe. As a result, shortness of breath (dyspnea) is a common symptom for patients with emphysema. However, the disease may destroy 50–70 percent of a person's lung tissue before any symptoms are actually noticeable to the patient. When symptoms do occur, shortness of breath after physical exertion is often the earliest sign of emphysema.

Who Gets Emphysema

About 2.8 million people in the United States have been diagnosed with emphysema, including 1.6 million men and 1.2 million women. Approximately 16,000 Americans die from emphysema annually. Some patients with emphysema die from heart failure, while others die from their inability to breathe.

Most people diagnosed with emphysema are older than 44 years. (See table at right.) The disease heavily predominates among whites, and about 2.6 million of all emphysema victims are Caucasians. Emphysema transcends socioeconomic status, and it is not a disease of the poor only. However, as can be seen from the table, the percent of the poor (2.2 percent) and near-poor (2.4 percent) who have emphysema is more than double the rate found among those who are not poor (1.0 percent). The largest number of emphysema patients reside in the South, or nearly 1.2 million people, while the fewest number of emphysema patients are in the western United States, or about 349,000 people.

Interestingly, some research has shown that postmenopausal women with emphysema are more prone to panic attacks than other same-age patients, although the reason for this is unknown.

Diagnosis and Treatment

Spirometry is a diagnostic tool that may be used to detect emphysema in its earliest stages. The patient

PERCENTS OF PERSONS 18 YEARS OF AGE AND OLDER WITH EMPHYSEMA, UNITED STATES, 1999

Total	1.4
Sex	
Male	1.7
Female	1.1
Age	
18–44 years	0.2
45–64 years	1.6
65–74 years	4.9
75 years and older	5.2
Race	
White	1.6
African American	0.5
American Indian or Alaska Native	1.6
Asian	0.4
Hispanic or Latino	0.4
Poverty status	
Poor	2.2
Near poor	2.4
Not poor	1.0
Region	
Northeast	1.5
Midwest	1.4
South	1.6
West	0.9

Source: Centers for Disease Control and Prevention, National Center for Health Statistics. "Summary Health Statistics for U.S. Adults: National Health Interview Survey, 1999," Series 10, number 212, August 2003.

takes a deep breath and exhales as quickly as possible into a tube that is connected to a machine. This machine measures how much air the patient's lungs can hold as well as how much air the patient expels in one second. This technique is an effective way to determine whether a patient's airway is obstructed.

Arterial blood gas, which includes the levels of oxygen and carbon dioxide in the blood leaving the lungs, can be measured to help with a diagnosis of emphysema. It is measured by blood that is drawn from an artery and is primarily used to evaluate whether supplemental oxygen is needed by a patient with emphysema.

In the middle to late stages, emphysema is often easy for doctors to spot. Patients have a characteristic severe shortness of breath and extreme coughing, and nearly all patients eventually (or immediately) will require supplemental oxygen in order to breathe adequately. Suspected cases of emphysema can be confirmed with imaging tests, such as X-rays.

Medication Treatment

No cure is available for advanced emphysema, although people in the early stages of the disease can improve their condition by immediately stopping smoking. Some patients with moderate emphysema can use bronchodilators to improve their breathing, while others with more serious illness require oxygen intermittently or continuously in order to breathe. Inhaled steroids may help some patients. Pulmonary specialists and their staff may also instruct patients in breathing exercises than can help some patients.

Surgical Treatment

In severe cases, some doctors recommend lung-volume-reduction surgery. This procedure is covered by Medicare for high-risk patients. In a study of 1,218 patients with severe emphysema, reported in a 2003 issue of the *New England Journal of Medicine*, researchers studied whether this procedure could increase survival for patients. The patients were randomized, and 608 patients had surgery while 610 had medical therapy.

The researchers found that if patients had predominantly upper-lobe emphysema with low exercise capacity (as measured by the patients' performance pedaling on a stationary bicycle), the surgery did provide a survival advantage. However, for other patients, the death rate was higher among those who received surgery than among those who received medical therapy.

The most extreme form of treatment for emphysema is a lung transplantation. It is reserved for patients who would otherwise die and who are healthy enough to survive the procedure.

Preventive Recommendations

Patients with emphysema are strongly encouraged to receive annual shots for both influenza (flu) and pneumonia since if they contracted such illnesses, they would become extremely ill and could die. They should also avoid air pollution and smog, and stay indoors whenever the pollution levels are high.

See also LUNG CANCER; ORAL CANCER; SMOKING AND HEALTH PROBLEMS.

For further information on emphysema, contact the following organizations:

The American Lung Association (ALA)
1740 Broadway
New York, NY 10019
(212) 315-8700
http://www.lungusa.org

National Heart, Lung, and Blood Institute
NHLBI Health Information Center
P.O. Box 30105
Bethesda, MD 20824
(301) 592-8573
http://www.nhlbi.nih.gov

National Center for Health Statistics, Summary Health Statistics for U.S. Adults: National Health Interview Survey, 1999. Centers for Disease Control and Prevention, Series 10, number 212, August 2003.
National Emphysema Treatment Trial Research Group. "A Randomized Trial Comparing Lung-Volume-Reduction Surgery with Medical Therapy for Severe Emphysema," *New England Journal of Medicine* 348, no. 21 (May 22, 2003): 2,059–2,073.
Smoller, Jordan W., M.D. "Prevalence and Correlates of Panic Attacks in Postmenopausal Women," *Archives of Internal Medicine* 163, no. 17 (September 22, 2003): 2,041–2,050.

employee assistance programs (EAPs) Company programs designed to help individual employees with serious personal problems, including addictions as well as underlying emotional or psychiatric problems that may be present and impeding workers from adequately performing their jobs. These programs were largely encouraged in the 1970s by the then newly created NATIONAL INSTITUTE ON ALCOHOL ABUSE AND ALCOHOLISM. The majority of corporations in the United States offer some form of employee assistance program, although companies with fewer than 100 employees are unlikely to have such a program.

Initially formed to cope with employee ALCOHOLISM, EAPs today are charged with dealing with a broad array of issues, including employee financial problems, work problems, and mental health issues. Some experts have become concerned that too little attention is given to addictive behaviors that may persist even after individuals are employed (or that may develop after employment).

Some EAPs are managed within the company itself, but many corporations have contracted out the responsibility for their EAP to other organizations. Most employees who come to EAPs are self-referrals, although research indicates that they often report feeling pressured by others, such as coworkers or supervisors. In other cases, employers order employees referred to the program because of their poor job performance if it is believed to be related to a problem that can be resolved through EAP assistance, such as alcoholism or DRUG ABUSE.

Some researchers believe that the current corporate emphasis on "wellness" programs could also encompass alcohol screening and could be used successfully in EAPs. Said Paul Roman in his article on EAPs, "Wellness programs can best address early alcohol programs if they adopt a 'back door' approach by incorporating specific information about alcohol's negative effects on other health conditions rather than focusing exclusively on drinking. For example, a woman who doesn't see any need to reduce her alcohol consumption, even though she is drinking excessively in an attempt to reduce stress, might very well enroll in a stress reduction program in which she would learn that having more than one drink a day elevates her risk for breast cancer."

See also DRUG TESTING; WORK.

Paul M. Roman. "Employee Assistance Programs: Workplace Opportunities for Intervening in Alcohol Problems," Available online. URL: http://www.ensuring solutions.org/images.primers/prim5.pdf Downloaded on June 18, 2004.
Roman, Paul M. and Terry C. Blum. "The Workplace and Alcohol Problem Prevention," *Alcohol Research & Health* 26, no. 1 (2002): 49–57.

emotions   Moods that may be extreme, moderate, or calm. All healthy people have emotions, and how they cope with these emotions is important. Individuals who are impaired by alcohol, ille-

gal drugs, and even some prescribed medications may experience mood disorders as a result of the effect of the ingested substance. In addition, some individuals have emotional or psychiatric disorders, such as ANXIETY DISORDERS, BIPOLAR DISORDER, DEPRESSION, and SCHIZOPHRENIA, that can be further exacerbated by consuming alcohol or drugs. Many people with psychiatric disorders are at risk for a problem with either SUBSTANCE ABUSE or substance dependence (addiction).

Some drugs, such as AMPHETAMINES and COCAINE, are particularly dangerous for highly emotional individuals to use because they may cause patients to lose control over their emotions. In some cases, the patient may experience a psychotic break, as with AMPHETAMINE PSYCHOSIS.

See also DUAL DIAGNOSIS; PSYCHIATRISTS.

enablers   Individuals who act in such a way that an addicted person does not have to face the consequences of the addiction. For example, the enabler of an alcoholic may hide empty liquor bottles, call in sick to the employer for the alcoholic when the person is hung over, and take other actions to cover up evidence of the alcoholism. A person who enables a compulsive shopper may complain about the bills but will still pay them and continue to allow the compulsive shopper to maintain credit card accounts. Nonaddicts can enable any type of addictive behavior.

Often the intentions are meant in a loving way because the enabler (usually a spouse or a family member) does not want the addicted person to suffer harmful consequences. Unfortunately, the effect is to allow the addiction to continue. Sometimes the enabler acts out of a sense of shame or embarrassment, not wishing others to know about the addicted person's behavior.

Taking the car keys away from a drunk or drugged person is *not* an example of enabling behavior. Instead it is commonsense behavior that prevents the intoxicated person from harming himself, herself or others.

Most enablers usually have great difficulty understanding that some of their actions are helping to perpetuate the addiction. They often instead believe that they are protecting the addict and/or their family. Sometimes individuals are completely unaware that they are enabling addictive behaviors to continue by their actions, and others need to point this out to them.

Organizations such as AL-ANON and ALATEEN teach the relatives and friends of alcoholics that they need to stop helping the alcoholic continue his or her drinking and that they should stop lying for the individual. Other organizations provide similar advice to the friends and families of addicted individuals.

See also CODEPENDENCY; TWELVE STEPS.

ethanol A substance present in all forms of alcohol consumed by individuals, such as beer, wine, and distilled spirits. The ethanol is what causes the intoxicating effect.

See also ALCOHOL/ALCOHOL CONSUMPTION; ALCOHOL POISONING; BEER; BLOOD ALCOHOL LEVELS.

euphoria An advanced state of giddy elation and happiness and one of the key reasons why many people exhibit some addictive behaviors: they wish to attain and then stay in this euphoric state. Nicotine can provide a transient and virtually unnoticeable euphoric rush. Some legal and illegal drugs induce a state of euphoria in users. Compulsive gamblers report that they are euphoric when they are on a winning streak. Sex addicts also experience euphoria, much as compulsive gamblers do. Hallucinogenic drugs may produce a heightened happy mood in users, as may drugs such as MARIJUANA. Unfortunately, just as addictive behaviors can produce an artificial high, they can also often produce the opposite effect: a severe depressive reaction.

See also BIPOLAR DISORDER; CRAVING; MOODS.

exercise addiction/dependence An excessive participation in sports, calisthenics, or other activities that exercise the body to the point that it begins to be overstressed, otherwise harmed, or at risk for experiencing harm. If individuals who are overly dependent on exercise cannot exercise for some reason, they usually become extremely anxious and distressed. Although not recognized as a clinical disorder by the AMERICAN PSYCHIATRIC ASSOCIATION as of this writing, exercise dependence has been anecdotally recognized by physicians and other experts as an addictive behavior.

Many people in the United States are either overweight or obese and actively need to exercise in order to reduce their weight. In comparison, relatively few people are addicted to exercise, so the issue of exercise dependence is rarely discussed. Instead physicians and others emphasize the value of exercise for most people. Obviously, in most cases, exercise is an important component of a healthy lifestyle. However, even positive actions can be taken to extremes, and this is also true for exercise.

In their article for the *Psychology of Sport and Exercise*, researchers Heather Hausenblas and Danielle Symons Downs recommended that exercise dependence be defined in terms of a manifestation of three or more of the following items, including as follows:

1. Development of tolerance, or a need for increased amounts of exercise each day to achieve the same effect
2. Withdrawal symptoms, such as anxiety or fatigue if the individual does not exercise; exercising may also be done in order to avoid withdrawal symptoms
3. Intention effects, such as when the person regularly exercises over a longer period than planned
4. Loss of control or the inability to cut back on exercising
5. Time spent on exercising is excessive; for example, vacations are devoted to exercising
6. Conflict: Exercising is causing the individual to give up other important work or social activities
7. Continuance: Exercising continues even though the individual is aware that he or she has a physical problem that would be worsened by further exercising, such as when a person continues to run even though the person knows that he or she has shin splints

Those at Risk for Exercise Dependence

Both men and women can become addicted to exercise. Some ATHLETES are at risk for developing an exercise dependence, particularly those for whom weight is most important, such as dancers or jockeys. People in the public eye, such as actors, may also become addicted to exercise. Individuals with an exercise addiction also often have an eating disorder, such as ANOREXIA NERVOSA or BULIMIA NERVOSA. Individuals who are compulsive about exercising may sometimes also have an underlying ANXIETY DISORDER.

Pathology and Exercise

A study in a 2000 issue of the *British Journal of Sports Medicine* reported on 291 women in the United Kingdom who were recruited from aerobic dance classes, from running clubs, and through various other means. The researchers administered instruments including an exercise dependence questionnaire, an eating disorder examination self-report questionnaire, and a general health questionnaire.

Based on their responses to the exercise dependence and eating disorder questionnaires, the participants were assigned to one of four different groups. For example, women who met the exercise dependence criteria but had no evidence of an eating disorder were assigned to the exercise dependence group. Women who met the criteria for a possible eating disorder but not for exercise dependence were assigned to another group. Women who fulfilled the criteria for both exercise dependence and eating disorders were assigned to the both group. The control group was made up of women with no evidence of either eating disorders or exercise dependence.

As a result, 43 women were assigned to the exercise dependence group, 14 to the eating disorders group, 27 to the both group, and 110 to the control group. In considering various traits based on the responses to the Eysenck personality questionnaire (revised), a measure of personality dimensions, the researchers found that, on the addictiveness subscale, the control group scored lowest in terms of average addictiveness (9.3), while the both group scored highest (15.9). The exercise addicts only group scored an average of 11.8 in addictiveness, and the eating disorders group scored an average of 13.2. The control group also scored lowest in neuroticism and impulsiveness and highest in empathy. As a result, slavish devotion or dependence to exercise is apparently related to other pathological traits.

College Students and Studies on Exercise Dependence

Some studies have indicated that college students may be particularly prone to excessive exercising.

A study of 257 students at the school of physical education and dance at the Kutztown University of Pennsylvania, published in a 2004 issue of the *Journal of American College Health,* revealed that about 22 percent of the students exercised 36 or more hours per week and that they also exhibited atypical exercise patterns. The researchers stated, "Although clinicians and educators should promote the many advantages of regular participation in physical activity, they should acknowledge that, for some, it may have undesirable consequences that occur at a frequency parallel to other age-related negative behaviors."

In a study at the University of Florida, the researchers found that men were more likely than women to become obsessed with or dependent on exercising. The study showed that men had twice the risk of women of exercising excessively. They were also more likely to exhibit behaviors of tenseness and irritability if they were compelled to miss an exercise session. The researchers found that men who primarily exercised in order to feel better (both physically and mentally) rather than to improve their appearance were also more likely to become dependent on exercising. In contrast, women who wanted to change their physical appearance were more likely to become exercise dependent.

Of the 408 exercise participants, about 3 percent (2 percent of the college age men and 1 percent of the women) were at risk for excessive exercising based on their high scores on a scale that measured exercise dependency tendencies. The men were more likely to be irritable and tense if they missed scheduled workouts.

In another article about this study, in the *Psychology of Addictive Behaviors*, the researchers looked at the impact of imagery on exercise dependence in men and women, using exercise dependence scales and exercise imagery subscales. Exercise imagery would include, for example, "When I think about exercising, I imagine my form and body position," and "To get me energized, I imagine exercising." The researchers also used an exercise dependence scale on the subjects.

The researchers found that exercise imagery was predictive of exercise dependence; however, male subjects usually had more exercise dependence symptoms. The exceptions were in cases of withdrawal effects or individuals who were exercising to avoid feeling anxious or irritable, in which case women scored about the same.

The researchers also stated, "Primary exercise dependence can be differentiated from secondary dependence by clarifying the ultimate objective of the exerciser. In *primary* exercise dependence the physical activity is an end in itself. In contrast, for *secondary* exercise dependence the compelling motivation for physical activity is the control and manipulation of body composition and, therefore, exercise is secondary to an eating disorder."

Perfectionism may be another problem among people who become addicted to exercise. In a study published in a 2003 issue of the *American Journal of Health Studies,* the authors studied 79 college students who completed self-reports on their exercise behavior and their perfectionistic and exercise dependence symptoms. Based on the results, the researchers split the groups into high exercise dependency (40 subjects) and low (39 subjects). They found that the high-exercise-dependent group not only exercised more but they also exercised more intensely. In addition, the high-exercise-dependent group was more perfectionistic.

See also COLLEGE STUDENTS; COSMETIC SURGERY, ADDICTION TO.

Bamber, Diane, Ian M. Cockerill, and Douglas Carroll. "The Pathological Status of Exercise Dependence," *British Journal of Sports Medicine* 34, no. 2 (2000): 125–132.

Garman, J. G., et al. "Occurrence of Exercise Dependence in a College-Aged Population," *Journal of American College Health* 52, no. 5 (March/April 2004): 221–228.

Hagan, Amy L. and Heather Hausenblas. "The Relationship Between Exercise Dependence Symptoms and Perfectionism," *American Journal of Health Studies* 18, no 2/3 (Spring/Summer 2003): 133–137.

Hausenblas, Heather and Danielle Symons Downs. "Exercise Dependence: A Systematic Review," *Psychology of Sport and Exercise* 3 (2002): 89–123.

Hausenblas, Heather and Danielle Symons Downs. "Relationship Among Sex, Imagery, and Exercise Dependence Symptoms," *Psychology of Addictive Behaviors* 16, no. 2 (2002): 169–172.

extreme sports, addiction to   Compulsion to participate in dangerous and even life-threatening sports activities. Although it is not a common addictive behavior, some individuals are clearly compelled to repeat life-threatening activities, such as race car driving, mountain climbing in extremely dangerous conditions, and other actions. It is not known if such individuals have a "death wish," have low impulse control, or have a strong desire to repeat actions that provide them with an adrenaline rush.

As with other addictive behaviors, such individuals feel irresistibly drawn to repeating dangerous actions. They feel this way despite any adverse consequences that may have occurred in the past to themselves (such as serious injuries) or to their friends or others they care about (such as injuries or deaths).

See also ATHLETES; ATTENTION DEFICIT HYPERACTIVITY DISORDER; IMPULSE CONTROL DISORDER.

false positives Refers to a test result that indicates that drugs or alcohol is or was recently present in the body when in fact, the individual does not or has not used the substance that was tested for. For example, the individual may have taken common medications such as antibiotics that may present as opiates in the test. False positives may lead to an assumption of guilt. The individual may be faced with serious consequences, such as the loss of a job or failure to be promoted. False-positive test results are a disadvantage of drug testing.

See also DRUG TESTING.

Baden, Lindsey R., M.D., et al. "Quinolones and False-Positive Urine Screening for Opiates by Immunoassay Technology," *Journal of the American Medical Association* 286, no. 24 (December 26, 2001): 3,115–3,119.

fatty liver disease/steatosis An enlargement of the liver, which may be a consequence of chronic alcoholism. There is also a nonalcoholic form of fatty liver disease that is often induced by diabetes or by chronic use of medications such as aspirin, calcium channel blockers, glucocorticoids, methotrexate, tetracycline, and other drugs. Sometimes fatty liver disease is exacerbated by a combination of prescribed medications and alcohol.

The early stages of alcoholic fatty liver disease may be reversible if the person stops drinking altogether. With total abstinence from alcohol, and assuming that the damage has not progressed to ALCOHOLIC HEPATITIS or CIRRHOSIS, the liver can show signs of dramatic improvement within two to four weeks.

Fatty liver disease is usually not life threatening. Most patients do not have symptoms from this disease, and their condition may be discovered in a routine physical examination or laboratory screening. However, if it is caused by alcoholism and the

individual continues to drink, the liver will usually become damaged further. The risk for developing liver cancer will also be increased.

Fatty liver disease is the first stage of alcoholic liver disease and is the stage that occurs before alcoholic hepatitis, a serious condition in which the liver is severely damaged by chronic drinking. Alcoholic hepatitis itself is the stage of alcoholic liver disease that occurs before cirrhosis, or the scarring and damage of the liver, which is the third and final stage of alcoholic liver disease. About 40–50 percent of patients with alcoholic hepatitis will develop cirrhosis of the liver.

Risk Factors

People who are heavy drinkers are at high risk for developing fatty liver disease, as are individuals who are obese. For example, according to the American College of Gastroenterology in their consumer health guide on alcoholic liver disease, a woman who drinks a pint of wine per day or three 12-ounce beers or four ounces of distilled spirits is consuming 20–40 grams of alcohol and risking liver damage. Some studies indicate that patients with HEPATITIS C are at risk for developing fatty liver disease.

Women who drink alcohol develop a more severe alcoholic disease faster and at lower doses of alcohol than men, possibly because of gender differences in how the body metabolizes alcohol and other factors. For example, according to the American College of Gastroenterology, women have lower levels of alcohol dehydrogenase, an enzyme that breaks down alcohol in the stomach. As a result, this may be the reason why lower amounts of alcohol cause more severe damage in women than in men.

Signs and Symptoms

Often patients with fatty liver disease have no signs or symptoms; however, indicators may occur. An enlarged liver (hepatomegaly) is the most common indicator of fatty liver disease in hospitalized patients. Patients may also present to their doctors with abdominal pain, nausea, and lack of appetite. Jaundice (yellowing of the skin) may also be a sign of fatty liver disease, especially in hospitalized patients.

Diagnosis and Treatment

A physician who suspects fatty liver disease will take a complete medical history and perform a physical examination. The doctor needs to know about all drugs that have been taken by the patient, whether legal or not, in order to arrive at an appropriate diagnosis. Ordinary toxicology screens that doctors may order do not show all possible drugs that may have been taken, so the cooperation of the patient or family members is necessary.

The doctor also needs honest information about alcohol consumption. Many patients are hesitant to provide such information, fearing the doctor's disapproval.

Generally, abnormal findings on routinely ordered liver function tests in an annual physical examination will lead doctors to be concerned and to order further testing for liver disease. Patients with liver disease may have elevated blood levels of both bilirubin and aminotransferases.

Diagnostic tests may include a computerized tomography scan or a magnetic resonance imaging scan of the liver. Sometimes a liver biopsy is performed. However, experts report that a biopsy is usually not necessary with fatty liver disease unless the doctor feels that the liver disease may have advanced further to alcoholic hepatitis or cirrhosis.

The key form of treatment is for the patient with fatty liver disease to stop drinking altogether. No medications are available to treat fatty liver disease. A low, steady weight loss is also recommended among obese patients, although alcohol abstinence is far more important.

Patients with fatty liver disease may also be deficient in vitamins and minerals, and such deficiencies should be identified and corrected. Patients also need to be evaluated for malnutrition and infections. Alcohol abuse can weaken the immune system and increase the risk for developing pneumonia and other serious infections.

See also ALCOHOLIC HEALTH PROBLEMS; ALCOHOLISM; LIVER.

American College of Gastroenterology. "Common Gastrointestinal Problems: A Consumer Health Guide. Alcoholic Liver Disease," Available online. URL: http://www.acg.gi.org/patientinfo/cgp/pdf/alcoho~1.pdf. Accessed on July 1, 2004.

Mohammad K. Ismail, M.D. and Caroline Riely, M.D. "Alcoholic Fatty Liver," Available online. URL: http://www.emedicine.com/med/topic99.htm. Accessed on June 4, 2004.

Narayanan Menon, K. V., M.D., Gregory J. Gores, M.D., and Vijay H. Shah, M.D. "Pathogenesis, Diagnosis, and Treatment of Alcoholic Liver Disease," *Mayo Clinic Proceedings* 76, no. 10 (2001): 1,021–1,029.

Tilg, Herbert, M.D. and Anna Mae Diehl, M.D. "Cytokines in Alcoholic and Nonalcoholic Steatohepatitis," *New England Journal of Medicine* 343, no. 20 (November 16, 2000): 1,467–1,476.

fetal alcohol syndrome (FAS)   A lifelong condition of developmental disabilities caused by the excessive consumption of alcohol during the mother's pregnancy. The mother may be an alcoholic or may not meet the criteria for alcoholism but has engaged in episodes of BINGE DRINKING or heavy drinking during pregnancy.

Individuals with FAS have an increased risk for alcohol or drug problems later in life. However, a study reported in a 2004 issue of the *Journal of Developmental and Behavioral Pediatrics* indicated that both an early diagnosis and a stable environment significantly decreased the risks of these and other adverse life experiences.

According to the Centers for Disease Control and Prevention (CDC), FAS is one of the leading known preventable causes of mental retardation and birth defects. The condition was first identified by Dr. Kenneth Jones and Dr. David Smith in their 1973 article in *Lancet*. In 1981, the Surgeon General of the United States first issued a public health advisory warning that alcohol consumption during pregnancy could cause birth defects. In 1989, mandated public labeling of alcohol products provided warnings that alcohol was not recommended for pregnant women. Yet the CDC estimates that 13 percent of pregnant women in the United States continue to drink during pregnancy.

According to the CDC, rates of FAS in the United States range from 0.2–1.5 per 1,000 live births per year. This means that about 1,000–6,000 infants are born each year with FAS.

How much alcohol is required to cause FAS is not known. Some studies, though, have shown that a pregnant woman drinking an amount as small as 0.5 ounces of alcohol per day can lead to fetal development problems. Binge drinking is particularly dangerous to the developing fetus, and it can lead to serious problems in brain development. Because physicians cannot determine any safe level of drinking, doctors recommend that all pregnant women abstain from drinking alcohol altogether during their pregnancy to avoid any risk of FAS.

However, it should also be noted that even if pregnant women who drink stop drinking at a later point during their pregnancies, it is possible that some damage to the developing fetus may be avoided. Thus women who have been drinking during their pregnancy should not assume that there is no point in giving up alcohol. For example, one of the problems caused by heavy drinking is microcephaly, a condition in which the baby has an unusually small head. According to Wei-Jung A. Chen and colleagues in their article in *Alcohol Research & Health,* some studies have shown that if pregnant women stop drinking before the end of their second trimester, their infants had larger head circumferences than the babies of women who had kept drinking throughout their pregnancies.

Possible Effects of Alcohol on a Developing Fetus

Physicians have done autopsies on the deceased infants of mothers who were binge drinkers during pregnancy to determine the possible effects of maternal alcohol consumption during fetal development. In one case, Chen and colleagues described a two-month-old baby who was born to a mother who binged heavily, mostly during the first trimester of her pregnancy. The infant was described as having "absent olfactory bulbs and tracts (which the brain uses to sense odors); poorly developed optic tracts; fused anterior brain structures such as the septum, thalamus, and the head of the caudate nucleus; fewer cells in the dentate gyrus, which is part of the hippocampus (an area crucial for memory); and fewer nerve cells in the cerebellum (which regulates balance, posture, movement, and muscle coordination) known as Purkinje cells, and disorientation of these cells." This one case is considered illustrative of the potential damage that excessive drinking can cause to a developing fetus, although damage can be greater or less extensive, depending on the individual case.

Some Racial Groups Have Higher Rates of FAS

Some racial and ethnic groups have a higher rate of children with FAS, presumably because they have a greater rate of consuming alcohol (although it may be due to a greater sensitivity to the effects of alcohol among members of these groups). For example, according to Dr. Sokol and his colleagues, African-American children have a five times greater risk of having FAS than white children, and American Indian/Alaskan Native children have a 16 times greater risk than white children.

Alcohol-Related Neurodevelopmental Disorder and Alcohol-Related Birth Defects

The terms alcohol-related neurodevelopmental disorder (ARND) and alcohol-related birth defects (ARBD) describe children who have the diagnostic features of FAS but in whom the symptoms present at a less severe level than with FAS. Fetal alcohol effect (FAE) was the former term used to describe these children. However, many experts continue to use the term FAE. Others use another term, fetal alcohol spectrum disorders (FASD), to encompass the range of effects that can occur in an individual whose mother drank alcohol during her pregnancy.

According to the CDC, ARND and ARBD are believed to occur at about three times the rate of FAS in the United States.

Signs and Symptoms of FAS

In the most extreme case, FAS causes death. Children with FAS are characterized by abnormal facial features, growth problems, central nervous system problems, and psychiatric problems. Both children with FAS and children with ARND may have the following characteristics:

- Small stature
- Small head
- Thin upper lip

- Facial abnormalities, such as small eyes that seem excessively widely spaced
- Poor coordination
- Developmental disabilities, such as language and speech delays
- Mental retardation or low intelligence
- Hyperactivity
- Epilepsy
- Learning disabilities
- Cerebral palsy
- Attention difficulties

In addition, children with FAS are at risk for developing psychiatric problems later in life, particularly mood disorders. They are also at risk for experiencing problems with law enforcement and the criminal justice system, primarily as adolescents and adults.

Diagnosing FAS by appearance (unless it is very severe) is often difficult until a child is age two or older. Diagnosing FAS after children have reached adolescence is also difficult. Once diagnosed, children with FAS will need special attention in school for their learning disabilities, memory problems, IMPULSIVITY, hyperactivity, distractibility, and mood disorders.

Diagnosis of FAS

In 2004, the CDC published new diagnostic guidelines for FAS as a result of a prior mandate from Congress: *Fetal Alcohol Syndrome Guidelines for Referral and Diagnosis.* It was believed that providing clear diagnostic markers for physicians would allow doctors to identify more infants and children with FAS, ARND, and ARBD.

According to the CDC, some doctors mistakenly believed that only alcoholics had babies with these illnesses. (As mentioned, binge drinking and heavy drinking can also cause these birth defects.) In addition, some physicians mistakenly believed that only minority women could have children with FAS, which is also untrue. Some minorities have an increased risk for having children with FAS but, for example, a white woman who binge drinks or drinks heavily during her pregnancy is also at risk for bearing a child with FAS. The primary risk factor for FAS is the alcohol consumption by the mother, not her ethnicity.

As a result, criteria were set for diagnosing FAS. These include the diagnostic need for the presence of facial dysmorphia (specific facial features different from the norm, as set by the guidelines, such as a smooth philtrum, the tiny groove between the nose and the upper lip), growth problems in the child's prenatal and/or postnatal height and weight (at or below the tenth percentile), and also the presence of central nervous system abnormalities, such as a head circumference that is at or below the tenth percentile for children of the same age and gender.

Ann P. Streissguth and her colleagues reported in 2004 in the *Journal of Developmental and Behavioral Pediatrics* that they had interviewed caregivers and other informants about the life span experiences of 415 patients with either FAS or FAE, including 236 males and 179 females. The patients had a median intelligence quotient (IQ) of 86. (An IQ of 100 is considered normal and below 100 is below normal. *Median* is a statistical term that means that half the population was below this number and half was above it. It is not the same as an average.) The racial mix included 60 percent white patients, 25 percent Native Americans, 7 percent African Americans, and 6 percent Hispanics.

Only about 20 percent of the patients were raised by their biological mothers, and most were raised by adoptive and foster families. Some studies indicate that children with FAS have a markedly greater risk of entering the foster care system, compared with other infants and children, not only because of the alcohol abuse of their mother but also because of child abuse and/or neglect.

The patients were diagnosed in the 1970s, 1980s, and the 1990s. They were enrolled in the Fetal Alcohol Follow-up Study of the University of Washington's Fetal Alcohol and Drug Unit. The respondents were adoptive mothers (33 percent), either foster mothers, biological fathers or stepmothers (25 percent), biological mothers (17 percent), other relatives or current or former caretakers (20 percent), and others. Most of the respondents (80 percent) had known the patients with FAS for half or more of the patient's lives.

When considering problematic behaviors among adolescents and adults with FAS or FAE, the researchers found that promiscuity (26 percent) and inappropriate sexual advances (18 percent) were the most frequently mentioned inappropriate sexual behaviors.

Many of the adolescents and adults with FAS had a disrupted school experience, with 53 percent of the FAS/FAE adolescents suspended from school, 29 percent expelled, and 25 percent dropped out of school. Learning problems were very common, especially attention problems (70 percent) and repeatedly incomplete schoolwork (58 percent).

The researchers found that many of the adolescents and adults had been in trouble with the law, including 14 percent of the children and 60 percent of the adolescents and adults. A large amount, 35 percent, of the adults had been incarcerated for a crime.

According to *Fetal Alcohol Syndrome Guidelines for Referral and Diagnosis,* individuals with FAS are at risk for entering the juvenile and criminal justice systems. The report says, "Their lack of executive functioning skills (i.e., poor judgment), fluid language skills and naïve social skills make them particularly vulnerable to participating in criminal activity. However, these same deficits demand that when they do encounter the justice system, their deficits should be taken into account during all aspects of justice proceedings (i.e., charges, process, punishment, and rehabilitation). As such the juvenile and criminal justice systems are major social systems in need of education regarding FAS."

Many of the FAS/FAE patients in the University of Washington study had also experienced problems with drugs and alcohol, and 29 percent of the adolescents and 46 percent of the adults had SUBSTANCE ABUSE problems. Alcohol abuse was a greater problem than drug abuse. Some of the adolescents and adults, 15 percent, had been hospitalized for alcohol or drug treatment.

Early Diagnosis and Stable Home Are Key Factors for Improved Outcomes

In Ann Streissguth and colleagues' study, some of the study individuals with FAS or FAE had a twofold to fourfold improvement in their odds of escaping the adverse life experiences typically predicted by FAS and FAE. These include confinement for criminal violations, inappropriate sexual behavior, and problems with drugs and alcohol. The researchers found that two key factors, including an early diagnosis of FAS/FAE and living in a stable and nurturing environment, were both conducive to an improved outcome.

Said the researchers, "In summary, this study documents the adverse postnatal environments and the corresponding risk of adverse life outcomes among many patients diagnosed FAS or FAE. These include major disruptions in schooling, trouble with the law, inappropriate sexual behaviors, extensive confinements, and alcohol and drug problems. Adverse life outcomes are not restricted to those with or without the classic facial features of FAS or to those with or without mental retardation. We find that good stable families, with enduring relationships with their children with FAS/FAE, appear to be a critical protective factor for helping children avoid adverse life outcomes.

"We also observed a significant reduction in the risk of adverse life outcomes with an earlier diagnosis."

See also ALCOHOLIC HEALTH PROBLEMS; CHILD ABUSE AND NEGLECT; PREGNANCY.

For further information on FAS, contact the following organization:

National Organization on Fetal Alcohol Syndrome (NOFAS)
900 17th Street NW
Suite 910
Washington, DC 20006
(202) 785-4585
http://www.nofas.org

Chen, Wei Jung A., et al. "Alcohol and the Developing Brain: Neuroanatomical Studies," *Alcohol Research & Health* 27, no. 2 (2003): 174–180.

National Center on Birth Defects and Developmental Disabilities, Centers for Disease Control and Prevention, Department of Health and Human Services, In Coordination with National Task Force on Fetal Alcohol Syndrome and Fetal Alcohol Effect. *Fetal Alcohol Syndrome: Guidelines for Referral and Diagnosis.* Atlanta, Ga.: Centers for Disease Control and Prevention, July 2004.

Sokol, Robert J., M.D., Virginia Delaney-Black, , M.D., and Beth Nordstrom. "Fetal Alcohol Spectrum Disorder,"

Journal of the American Medical Association 290, no. 22 (December 10, 2003): 2,996–2,999.

Streissguth, Ann P., et al. "Risk Factors for Adverse Life Outcomes in Fetal Alcohol Syndrome and Fetal Alcohol Effects," *Journal of Developmental and Behavioral Pediatrics* 25, no. 4 (2004): 228–238.

Warren, Kenneth R. and Laurie L. Foudin. "Alcohol-Related Birth Defects—The Past, Present, and Future," *Alcohol Research & Health* 25, no. 3 (2001): 153–158.

food addiction   See ANOREXIA NERVOSA; BINGE EATING DISORDER; BULIMIA NERVOSA; OVEREATING/OBESITY.

G

Gamblers Anonymous A self-help organization for pathological or compulsive gamblers, modeled on the abstinence and other principles of ALCOHOLICS ANONYMOUS. The organization was originally formed in 1957 by two men with serious gambling problems. The only membership requirement is that the individual give up all gambling activities. The purpose of the organization is to help compulsive gamblers to stop their gambling.

Gamblers Anonymous also offers 20 questions to people who may have a gambling problem in order to perform a self-evaluation. Most compulsive gamblers will answer "yes" to at least seven of these questions. The questions are as follows:

1. Did you ever lose time from work or school due to gambling?

2. Has gambling ever made your home life unhappy?

3. Did gambling affect your reputation?

4. Have you ever felt remorse after gambling?

5. Did you ever gamble to get money with which to pay debts or otherwise solve financial difficulties?

6. Did gambling cause a decrease in your ambition or efficiency?

7. After losing did you feel you must return as soon as possible and win back your losses?

8. After a win did you have a strong urge to return and win more?

9. Did you often gamble until your last dollar was gone?

10. Did you ever borrow to finance your gambling?

11. Have you ever sold anything to finance gambling?

12. Were you reluctant to use "gambling money" for normal expenditures?

13. Did gambling make you careless of the welfare of yourself or your family?

14. Did you ever gamble longer than you had planned?

15. Have you ever gambled to escape worry or trouble?

16. Have you ever committed, or considered committing, an illegal act to finance gambling?

17. Did gambling cause you to have difficulty in sleeping?

18. Do arguments, disappointments, or frustrations create within you an urge to gamble?

19. Did you ever have an urge to celebrate any good fortune by a few hours of gambling?

20. Have you ever considered self destruction or suicide as a result of your gambling?

Source: Gamblers Anonymous.

See also GAMBLING, PATHOLOGICAL; IMPULSE CONTROL DISORDER.

For further information on this organization and to find local chapters, contact Gamblers Anonymous at:

Gamblers Anonymous
International Service Office
P.O. Box 17173
Los Angeles, CA 90017
(213) 386-8789
http://www.gamblersanonymous.org

gambling, pathological Offering money or other items of value in exchange for a game of chance to the point of frequency at which it affects individuals and their families both financially and socially. Pathological/compulsive gamblers are often divorced because they cannot separate the needs of their family from their own need to gamble. Sometimes gambling begins as early as the teen years and continues into adulthood.

It is estimated that about 1–1.5 percent of the population in the United States are pathological gamblers. Some people go on gambling binges, similar to the way that others go on drinking binges.

Gambling can take many forms, including but not limited to casino gambling, purchasing lottery tickets, playing cards, betting on horse races, or playing slot machines. Gambling is legal in many states for most adults. Some people gamble on the INTERNET. Pathological gamblers can nearly always find something on which they can bet.

As with other forms of addictive behaviors, the gambler feels an intense CRAVING to gamble. If he or she resists, the emotional pain of withstanding the desire eventually becomes too great and the pathological gambler usually succumbs to the urge. Experts argue over whether gamblers truly believe that they will win. Some experts say that the rush or EUPHORIA that accompanies the risk entraps gamblers rather than actually winning. Others say that gamblers irrationally believe that they can and will win despite the unlikelihood of it happening time after time.

Pathological Gambling Versus Problem Gambling

Problem gambling is behavior that causes significant difficulty to a person's life but does not rise to the level of pathological gambling. It is estimated that about 3–4 percent of adults in the United States are problem gamblers. Problem gambling can develop into pathological gambling in the same way that alcohol abuse can become ALCOHOLISM.

Risk Factors for Pathological Gambling

In general, men have two to three times the risk for pathological gambling that women face. Studies have shown that individuals with either problem gambling or pathological gambling have higher rates of divorce, bankruptcy, arrest, incarceration, and mental health treatment. They may become involved in criminal activities as they become increasingly desperate for the money that they need to enable them to continue to gamble.

Pathological gamblers are more likely to lose their jobs than nongamblers. They also often lose their friends due to behaviors such as lying, borrowing money, and failing to pay back loans. They are at greater risk for legal problems and SUICIDE than nongamblers.

Some studies have shown that adults in SUBSTANCE ABUSE treatment centers and mental health centers have rates of pathological gambling that are four to 10 times greater than the rate found among the general adult population.

Causes of Pathological Gambling

Although what causes pathological gambling is not known for certain, there are several major theories. One key theory is that it may be an IMPULSE CONTROL DISORDER. Another theory is that people with this problem may have an abnormal serotonin function, while others believe there are problems with the neurotransmission of dopamine, another brain chemical. Some studies have implicated the limbic brain regions as a problem area causing pathological gambling.

Gambling and Alcohol Abuse

Alcohol and pathological gambling have many links. Many compulsive gamblers are also heavy drinkers. Alcohol also disinhibits people toward more reckless behavior in gambling, causing them to take more risks than they would normally take if they were sober. Gambling establishments realize this, and they often provide free drinks to their customers.

Illegal Drug Use

Pathological gambling is linked to an increased risk for illegal drug use. In a study of COCAINE-addicted outpatients, the researchers sought to determine the prevalence of pathological gambling among this population, reporting on their findings in a 2000 issue of the *American Journal of Psychiatry*.

The researchers found that of the 313 cocaine-dependent outpatients they studied (of whom 200 were also addicted to OPIATES), 3.8 percent had engaged in pathological gambling in the past month. They also found a lifetime prevalence of 8.0 percent for pathological gambling, which means that 8 percent of the patients had a past or current problem with pathological gambling. The authors concluded, "Pathological gambling is substantially more prevalent among cocaine-dependent outpatients than in the general population."

The researchers also found that the pathological gambling problem occurred before the cocaine addiction in 72.0 percent of the patients and that it came after opiate addiction in 44.4 percent of the patients.

Psychiatric Problems

Pathological gamblers are also at risk for other compulsive behaviors, such as COMPULSIVE SHOPPING. They may be at risk for SEXUAL ADDICTION. As mentioned, pathological gambling could be an underlying impulse control disorder. In addition, pathological gamblers are also at risk for many psychiatric problems, such as DEPRESSION and ANXIETY DISORDERS.

In a study of 30 subjects with a pathological gambling problem, reported in a 1998 issue of *Psychiatric Services*, the researchers found that half the subjects currently had major depressive disorder. In addition, 59 percent were OBSESSIVE-COMPULSIVE and 23 percent had generalized anxiety disorder, a form of anxiety disorder.

In another study of pathological gamblers and psychiatric problems, reported in a 2001 issue of the *American Journal of Psychiatry*, the researchers sought to determine what percent of the gamblers had psychiatric problems in addition to their pathological gambling. They found that 62 percent of the 43 gamblers they studied had psychiatric problems and 16 of the gamblers were alcohol abusers or alcoholics (which is considered a psychiatric problem). Other problems that the pathological gamblers had were adjustment disorders, mood disorders, personality disorders, antisocial personality disorders, and anxiety disorders.

The researchers said that with a greater number of psychiatric disorders came an increased risk for more severe gambling behavior. In addition, they said, "Because pathological gambling is frequently treated in specialized clinics, there is a risk that treatment may focus on gambling alone. Our findings underscore the need to conduct comprehensive evaluations of pathological gamblers and to devise treatment plans that appropriately address their comorbid [simultaneously existing] illnesses."

In another study, researchers evaluated gamblers in treatment for their gambling according to the psychiatric problems that they had, by gender. These findings were reported by Dr. Westphal in *Gambling Research*. In this study, male gamblers were much more likely to have alcohol use problems (20.5 percent) than female gamblers (7.7 percent). The females, though, were much more likely to have problems with compulsive shopping (19.5 percent) than the males (1.3 percent) and more likely to have OVEREATING problems (26.9 percent) than the males (12.8 percent).

The research revealed that two problems exacerbated gambling behavior: depression and problem drinking. Both males and females were equally likely to report that depression caused them to gamble more. However, for females, problem drinking escalated their gambling more than this behavior did for males.

Medication for Gambling

Some studies have shown that NALTREXONE, a drug used to treat alcoholism and sometimes used to treat eating disorders, has been effective in the short-term treatment of pathological gambling. The dosages that were needed were higher than those used with alcoholics (188 mg per day, on average, compared with 50 mg per day for alcohol dependence). More studies are needed over longer time periods to determine if medications can continue to help gamblers control their urge to gamble.

Other studies have shown that some ANTIDEPRESSANTS were effective at controlling the urge to gamble. For example, a small study of patients with pathological gambling indicated that fluvoxamine (Luvox) was effective in some patients. In this study, published in a 1998 issue of the *American Journal of Psychiatry*, seven of 10 patients who completed the study responded to the fluvoxamine and they stopped gambling. This may indicate that pathological gambling has links to obsessive-compulsive behaviors. Further studies are needed to determine if the drug has a long-term effect and also if it works on larger populations.

A study in a 2002 issue of the *Journal of Clinical Psychiatry* indicated that lithium and valproate (Depakote) were effective in treating patients with pathological gambling. Further studies on this medication and others should offer more information to help people with pathological gambling.

See also BINGE DRINKING; BIPOLAR DISORDER; GAMBLERS ANONYMOUS; TEENAGE AND YOUTH GAMBLING.

For further information on self-help in gambling, contact the following organizations:

Gam-Anon International Service Office, Inc.
P.O. Box 157
Whitestone, NY 11357
(718) 352-1671
http://www.gam-anon.org

Gamblers Anonymous
International Service Office
P.O. Box 17173
Los Angeles, CA 90017
(213) 386-8789
http://www.gamblersanonymous.org

Black, Donald W., M.D. and Trent Moyer. "Clinical Features and Psychiatric Comorbidity of Subjects with Pathological Gambling Behavior," *Psychiatric Services* 49, no. 11 (November 1998): 1,434–1,439.

Grant, Jon E., M.D., Matt G. Kushner, and Suck Won Kim, M.D. "Pathological Gambling and Alcohol Use Disorder," *Alcohol Research & Health* 26, no. 2 (2002): 143–150.

Hall, Gladys W., et al. "Pathological Gambling Among Cocaine-Dependent Outpatients," *American Journal of Psychiatry* 157, no. 7 (July 2000): 1,127–1,133.

Hollander, Eric, M.D., et al. "Short-Term Single-Blind Fluvoxamine Treatment of Pathological Gambling," *American Journal of Psychiatry* 155, no. 12 (December 1998): 1,781–1,783.

Ibanez, Angela, M.D., et al. "Psychiatric Comorbidity in Pathological Gamblers Seeking Treatment," *American Journal of Psychiatry* 158, no. 10 (October 2001): 1,733–1,735.

Pallanti, S., et al. "Lithium and Valproate Treatment of Pathological Gambling: A Randomized Single-Blind Study," *Journal of Clinical Psychiatry* 63, no. 7 (2002): 559–564.

Potenza, Marc N., M.D., Thomas R. Kosten, M.D., and Bruce J. Rounsaville, M.D. "Pathological Gambling," *Journal of the American Medical Association* 286, no. 2 (July 11, 2001): 141–144.

Wellford, Charles. "When It's No Longer a Game: Pathological Gambling in the United States," *National Institute of Justice Journal* 247 (April 2001): 15–18.

Westphal, James R., M.D., and Lera Joyce Johnson. "Gender Differences in Psychiatric Comorbidity and Treatment-Seeking among Gamblers in Treatment," Available online. URL: http://www.camh.net/egambling/issue8/research/westphal-johnson/index. Accessed on January 15, 2004.

genetic predispositions Refers to the propensities of individuals to inherit traits from their parents and ancestors. A predisposition means that an individual has an increased possibility of developing certain behaviors or traits, but it does not mean that the individual will definitely develop them. Thus, for example, if both biological parents have addictions to drugs or alcohol, this may mean that their children are more likely to abuse alcohol or drugs than the children of nonaddicted parents. However, the children may also grow up without problems with alcohol or drug abuse.

Some researchers argue that the problem is an underlying lack of impulse control or an attraction to novelty seeking that leads some individuals to problematic behaviors rather than a specific predilection to abusing drugs or alcohol or engaging in other addictive behaviors. Thus, the mountain climber may be driven by the same or a similar underlying thrill seeking as the individual who decides to try dangerous drugs, such as cocaine or heroin. If this goal is successfully channeled into a socially acceptable field, it may lead people to successful lives. If it is not, then individual lives may be destroyed. At this time, knowing whether these researchers are correct in this assumption is impossible.

Whether some individuals may have a particular genetic predisposition to an avoidance of alcohol or drugs is unclear. (This is the reverse of a predisposition toward a use of alcohol or drugs.)

Adoption and Twin Studies

Complicating the issue of genetic predispositions is the fact that most people are reared by and continue to live with their biological families until adulthood. Thus, they are also affected by environmental aspects, such as watching their parents drink heavily (or refrain from drinking) or use drugs (or not), and the children may model their own behaviors on those of their parents. To evaluate whether behavior is largely driven by environment or heredity, many researchers have performed studies comparing adopted children to their biological parents, primarily relying upon data from Sweden, Finland, and other countries. This data is extremely difficult to obtain or track in the United States because of laws on confidentiality and differing state laws on adoption.

Adoption studies have seemed to find a genetic link between alcoholism, drug use, and mental illness. A major problem with many adoption studies, however, is that most researchers fail to distinguish between children who were adopted as infants from children adopted at later ages after the child's removal from abusive and neglectful families.

When researchers have identified the populations of children in terms of when they were adopted, study after study has shown that children adopted as babies usually develop normally, with no greater risk of alcohol or drug abuse than that of the general population. However, children adopted as older children (older than three or four years of age) are much more likely to exhibit serious problems in adolescence and adulthood, such as addictive behaviors or mental illness.

Other researchers have performed studies of identical twins who were raised apart in different families, comparing the adult twins to each other and to their biological families. Both adoption and twin studies have shown some apparent genetic predispositions to some addictive behaviors, such as alcoholism. Some studies, though, have also shown that adopted children have a *lower* rate of alcoholism than their biological siblings who were raised by the birth parents. In such cases, the adoptive environment appeared to have a positive and mitigating effect, not eliminating the increased biological risk for alcoholism but reducing it.

Because of these contradictory results, scientists will likely continue to argue about the impact of heredity and environment on addictions and other behaviors for a very long time.

Adamec, Christine and William Pierce. *The Encyclopedia of Adoption,* 2nd ed. New York, N.Y.: Facts On File, Inc., 2000.

GHB (gamma-hydroxybutyrate)/GHB analogs

A laboratory-created drug that was first synthesized in the 1920s and was under development as an anesthetic in the 1960s. It was sold as a bodybuilding formula until the Food and Drug Administration (FDA) banned this use in 1990. GHB is categorized as a CLUB DRUG or designer drug.

GHB is a central nervous system depressant and was first listed as a Schedule I controlled substance in 2000. It has also sometimes been used as a DATE RAPE DRUG and may be used more frequently than other drugs used for this purpose, such as ROHYPNOL and KETAMINE. About 2 percent of high school seniors in the United States used GHB at least once in 2002.

In 2002, Xyrem, a drug with an active ingredient of GHB, was approved by the FDA to treat cataplexy in patients with narcolepsy, a very rare disease that causes individuals to fall asleep uncontrollably. Cataplexy is a condition of very weak or paralyzed muscles. When used for this purpose, Xyrem is a Schedule III controlled substance. This is the only legal medical use for any form of GHB in the United States. The illegal use of Xyrem is subject to the same penalties that apply to the abuse of a Schedule I drug.

GHB generally appears as a white powder or a clear fluid, and it may have a salty taste. GHB is taken orally and is often mixed with another beverage. If it is mixed with clear fluid, it will cause the liquid to become cloudy.

GHB may cause euphoria, induce amnesia, and increase the libido and passivity. It can induce a comalike sleep. When users awaken, they may be very aggressive and combative. Side effects of the use of GHB include nausea and vomiting, delusions, HALLUCINATIONS, seizures, a slowed heart rate, respiratory distress, and lowered blood pressure.

Continued use of GHB can lead to addiction and withdrawal symptoms, such as insomnia, tremors, agitation, and tachycardia (very fast heart rate). These symptoms will occur within one to six hours of the last dose that was taken.

It is very dangerous for a person under the influence of GHB to drive a motor vehicle. However, individuals on GHB could generally pass an ALCOHOL BREATH TEST unless they were also taking alcohol. According to the National Drug Intelligence Center, some police organizations began screening for GHB in 2002. Routine toxicological tests will not screen for GHB, and thus, police laboratories must order special blood or urine tests for screening. These blood tests must be taken within five hours of when the GHB or the analog was ingested by the individual. Urine tests can be performed within 12 hours of ingestion.

GHB Analogs

There are analogs to GHB that are very similar to GHB. These analogs are found as industrial solvents that are used to produce pesticides, pharmaceuticals, and other products. Some analogs metabolize to GHB within the body, while others metabolize into substances that produce the same effects caused by GHB. These illegal drugs are sold to bodybuilders. GHB analogs may be marketed as dietary supplements, diet pills, or sleep aids.

Some examples of GHB analogs are gamma-hydroxyvalerate methyl-GHB (GHV), gamma-valerolactone 4-pentanolide (GVL), gamma-butyrolactone furanone di-hydro dihydrofuranone (GBL), and 1,4-butanediol tetramethylene glycol sucol-B butylenes glycol (BD).

GHB analogs cause essentially the same effects as GHB causes in the body, such as euphoria and sedation. In addition, they may also cause side effects such as incontinence, kidney failure, and even death. As with GHB, GHB analogs are addicting.

Users may purchase GHB analogs at health clubs, nightclubs, raves (all-night dance parties), and on college campuses. GHB analogs may also be sold at some disreputable health food stores, and they may also be available on the Internet.

These analogs are considered controlled substances when they are used for human consumption. Their use and sale can be prosecuted in the same manner as GHB is prosecuted.

Office of National Drug Control Policy. *Gamma Hydroxybutyrate (GHB)*, ONDCP Clearinghouse Fact Sheet, NCJ-194881. November 2002.

National Drug Intelligence Center, "GHB Analogs: GBL, BD, GHV, and GVL," *Information Bulletin*, Product, No. 2002-L0424-003.

glue   A common household item normally used to make items adhere to each other. Examples include rubber cement, airplane glue, and household glue. Glue is also misused as an illegal inhalant and a means of attaining a chemical euphoria.

According to the data from the "Youth Risk Behavior Surveillance—United States, 2001," published in *Morbidity and Mortality Weekly Report* by the Centers for Disease Control and Prevention (CDC), 14.7 percent of all students in the United States had sniffed glue or inhaled paints or sprays in order to get high. Many states have passed laws making it illegal to use inhalants for the purpose of intoxication. In Massachusetts, minors may not purchase glue or other cements unless they show identification and provide information that is recorded in a book that is made available to law enforcement officials.

See also INHALANTS, ABUSE OF.

hallucinations Refers to sights, sounds, or even odors and skin sensations (such as the feeling of being touched) that are experienced by an individual and perceived as real events yet are not actually happening. Hallucinations may result from the use of some legal and illegal drugs, particularly lysergic acid diethylamide (LSD), PEYOTE, psilocybin, and phencyclidine.

Sometimes individuals who are going through WITHDRAWAL from drugs or alcohol experience hallucinations. Individuals who are mentally ill, such as those with SCHIZOPHRENIA or sometimes those with bipolar disorder, may experience hallucinations as part of their illness. Rarely, a side effect of a medication may be the inducement of hallucinations. For example, elderly cancer patients may hallucinate when given high doses of MORPHINE to cope with the pain.

Although not dangerous in themselves, hallucinations can be confusing or terrifying and may lead to dangerous behaviors. During withdrawal from drugs, hallucinations frequently represent a potentially life-threatening symptom because they usually occur at an advanced stage of withdrawal that is particularly difficult for physicians to treat.

In some cases, use of drugs such as LSD, METHAMPHETAMINE, or COCAINE may lead to permanent brain damage, with symptoms of hallucinations and other psychiatric illness that persist long after the drugs are stopped. This may be a permanent effect.

See also AMPHETAMINE PSYCHOSIS; DELIRIUM TREMENS; MUSHROOMS/PSILOCYBIN; PCP; PSYCHOTIC BREAK.

hashish Drug derived from the Indian hemp plant *Cannabis sativa*, the same plant from which MARIJUANA is also derived. Hashish is a compressed form of the resinous secretions of the flowering parts of the hemp plant, while marijuana is derived from the leaves, flowers, stems, and seeds. Hashish oil is made by repeatedly extracting the resin with alcohol and heat, which creates a concoction that ranges in color from light to very dark brown. Hashish is highly potent.

Hashish is a Schedule I drug under the CONTROLLED SUBSTANCES ACT and is illegal to use in the United States. It is smoked and sometimes is mixed with tobacco in cigarettes and pipe tobacco. It may also be smoked in a water pipe. The tetrahydrocannabinol (THC) content may range from 5–12 percent. Hashish oil has a much higher THC content of 20–80 percent.

The effects of hashish depend on the potency of the drug, and a greater potency brings more intense effects. Excessive use of hashish can lead to a psychotic intoxication that can last for 48 hours or more after ingesting the drug. Some individuals develop a psychological tolerance to hashish, while others develop a physical dependency (addiction).

It is unknown how many people use hashish in the United States because statistical data is reported as either marijuana or as marijuana/hashish when use of the drug is reported.

See also TEENAGE AND YOUTH DRUG ABUSE.

O'Brien, Robert, et al. *The Encyclopedia of Understanding Alcohol and Other Drugs,* vol. I. New York: Facts On File, Inc., 1999.

hepatitis Inflammation of the LIVER. The term *hepatitis* usually refers to the viral illness in the liver. HEROIN and COCAINE addicts and others who inject drugs intravenously and share needles are prone to contracting viral hepatitis. Chronic hepatitis B and

C can lead to CIRRHOSIS of the liver and may further lead to liver cancer.

ALCOHOLIC HEPATITIS refers to the severe liver condition that is caused by chronic ALCOHOLISM. In this case, it is a nonviral hepatitis. (However, a person can have both alcoholic hepatitis and viral hepatitis, which is a very dangerous combination of illnesses for the patient.)

Hepatitis A, B, and C

The most common forms of viral hepatitis in the United States are hepatitis A, B and C.

Hepatitis A, also known as HAV, can be communicated through household contact with an infected person, and it is the most common form of hepatitis among hepatitis A, B, and C. It may also be contracted in the course of international travel. HAV can be spread in food by food preparers who have not washed their hands after using the toilet. Men who have sex with other men may transmit hepatitis to them as may injecting drug users.

Males are more likely to contract HAV than females. According to the Centers for Disease Control and Prevention (CDC), in 2001 the rate of HAV in the United States among males was 5.4 per 100,000 people compared with 2.9 per 100,000 females. There were 10,615 people in the United States with acute viral hepatitis in 2001, down from 13,397 in 2000.

Hepatitis B, also known as HBV, can be transmitted through the sharing of intravenous needles for illegal drug use or through sexual contact with an infected person. Men who have sex with other men are at risk for contracting hepatitis B, as are individuals with multiple sex partners. As with HAV, males are at greater risk than females for contracting HBV. According to the CDC, the rate of acute HBV in males in 2001 was 3.4 per 100,000, compared with 1.9 per 100,000 females. There were 7,844 people with acute HBV in the United States in 2001, down from 8,036 in 2000.

Hepatitis C, also known as HCV, is the most common chronic bloodborne infection in the United States, according to the CDC. Injecting drug use is the most common cause of HCV. The rates of HCV are lower than the rates of HAV or HBV. Males have a greater risk for contracting HCV. The rate in 2001 was 0.8 per 100,000 males, compared with 0.4 per 100,000 females. There were about 3,197 cases of acute HCV in 2000, according to the CDC. (Complete data was not available for 2001.)

Symptoms of Viral Hepatitis

Some forms of hepatitis have many symptoms, while others have only a few indicators. With HAV, the most common symptom is jaundice (yellow skin), and this symptom is experienced by the majority of patients. Patients may also experience nausea, abdominal pain, diarrhea, lack of appetite, headache, and fever.

HBV often causes no symptoms when the disease is initially contracted, but patients later develop jaundice and abdominal pain when the disease is more advanced.

HCV is a very serious illness that often leads to liver failure and the need for liver transplantation in order to survive. Symptoms usually do not occur until the disease is advanced and may include such vague symptoms as abdominal pain and fatigue.

Treatment for Viral Hepatitis

No treatment is available for HAV. Patients infected with HBV should see their physicians every six months to determine if any liver disease is present. Patients with chronic HBV may receive medications to boost the immune system, such as alpha-interferon, lamivudine, and adefovir. Patients must completely avoid alcohol to avoid damaging the liver. If liver damage does occur, a liver transplant may be needed.

Patients infected with HCV should see their physicians every six months. Doctors may treat them with interferon, pegylated interferon, and ribavirin. They may be given interferon alone or in combination with ribavirin.

See also ALCOHOLIC HEALTH PROBLEMS; FATTY LIVER DISEASE/STEATOSIS.

For further information on hepatitis, contact the following organizations:

American Liver Foundation
75 Maiden Lane
Suite 603
New York, NY 10038
(888) 443-7872 (toll-free) or (212) 668-1000
http://www.liverfoundation.org

Centers for Disease Control and Prevention (CDC)
Division of Viral Hepatitis

1600 Clifton Road
Mail Stop C-14
Atlanta, GA 30333
(800) 443-7232 (toll-free) or (404) 371-5900
http://www.cdc.gov/hepatitis

Hepatitis Foundation International
504 Blick Drive
Silver Spring, MD 20904
(800) 891-0707 (toll-free) or (301) 622-4200
http://www.hepatitisfoundation.org

Immunization Action Coalition
1573 Selby Avenue
St. Paul, MN 55104
(651) 647-9009
http://www.immunize.org

Centers for Disease Control and Prevention. *Hepatitis Surveillance,* Centers for Disease Control and Prevention, Report No. 58. Washington, D.C.: U.S. Department of Health and Human Services, 2003.

Minocha, Anil, M.D., and Christine Adamec. *The Encyclopedia of Digestive Diseases and Disorders.* New York: Facts On File Inc., 2004.

heredity See GENETIC PREDISPOSITIONS.

heroin An illegal and heavily addictive drug that is derived from opium poppies grown in South America, Mexico, and Southwest and Southeast Asia. Experts report that South American heroin is the most common form in the United States, primarily managed and dominated by criminals in Colombia. It is estimated that between 750,000 and 1 million individuals in the United States are addicted to heroin.

Heroin was first synthesized in the United States in 1874. It was first used as a pain medication in 1898. Doctors continued to use the drug as an analgesic until 1914, when heroin was named as a controlled substance under the Harrison Narcotic Act. It was not difficult for individuals to obtain heroin on their own, without a prescription, until heroin was criminalized in 1914.

Today, heroin is a Schedule I drug under the CONTROLLED SUBSTANCES ACT of 1970, which means that it is considered to be among drugs that have the highest potential for abuse and dependence and it has no valid medical use in the United States. (Other drugs under the Schedule I category are MARIJUANA, LSD, and ECSTASY.) In some other parts of the world, such as in the United Kingdom, heroin is prescribed to treat pain in terminally ill patients and physicians may prescribe the drug to other patients. There are strict consequences for the illegal use of the drug, however, and particularly for the selling of heroin.

Heroin is considered a dangerous drug, not only because of its addictive qualities but also because, more than with most other street drugs, individuals can easily overdose on the drug and die of a fatal overdose. The LD50, a term that refers to the dose that would kill 50 percent of the subjects in a laboratory setting, is exceptionally close to the therapeutic dose in the case of heroin.

In addition, in countries like the United States where heroin is illegal, the addict is at the mercy of the drug dealer with regard to the purity and the potency of the drug.

Heroin is often a white or off-white powder, although some forms of heroin are black and may be sticky like tar. Heroin can also be brown. The drug is smoked, snorted, or injected intravenously. When heroin is sniffed or smoked, the effects are felt within about 10–15 minutes. When it is used intravenously, the effects occur within about eight seconds. Users report feeling a pleasurable rush of sensation from the drug, and they may also have a flushing of the skin. They may experience nausea and vomiting as well as severe itching. Breathing can become very slowed to the point of respiratory failure and death.

If individuals who have tried heroin continue to use the drug, they will develop both a physical dependence and a physical tolerance. A physical dependence means that the body will need heroin to function normally and avoid withdrawal symptoms, which can be severe. A physical tolerance means that greater amounts of the drug will be required to achieve the same effect as was experienced when the drug was first taken and to avoid withdrawal symptoms. The heroin habit becomes increasingly expensive and dangerous as higher and higher doses are required.

Experts report that many individuals have the misconception that they can avoid addiction by smoking or snorting the drug rather than by injecting it. The reality is that any form of heroin delivery into the body can cause addiction.

Heroin Users

The National Household Survey on Drug Abuse has estimated that about 3 million people in the United States ages 12 and older have used heroin at least once in their lives. The largest age group of people who have used heroin at least once are people between the ages of 18 and 25 years, and about 1.6 percent of people in this age group have used the drug. The next largest group includes those who are 35 and older, and 1.5 percent of this group have used heroin at least once.

Experts report that heroin addicts are usually not violent, although they may become involved in criminal acts in order to obtain the money they need to buy their heroin. In general, the crimes they may commit are nonviolent.

Most heroin users began abusing other drugs before using heroin, such as marijuana, COCAINE, and other substances. Some users combine heroin with cocaine, which is referred to as speedballing.

Health Risks of Heroin Use

In addition to the health risk of addiction and the risk of death from overdosing on heroin, numerous other health risks are involved with heroin use. Heroin users who inject the drug and share needles with others may contract the human immunodeficiency virus, hepatitis of various types, and other serious illnesses. Heroin users are also more likely to develop sexually transmitted diseases. The constant injecting of the drug may cause significant and life-threatening skin infections, skin scarring, and collapse and occlusion of the veins. Injections from dirty needles can cause bloodborne infections with multiple body sites affected, including infections of the heart valves.

As repeated injections are required to maintain a heroin habit and veins are increasingly damaged or cannot be found, heroin addicts resort to injections in their veins in places such as under the tongue or in the penis. Infections in these areas can be life threatening and can also cause permanent damage to these parts of the body.

Heroin addicts may also suffer from pneumonia, tuberculosis, and liver and kidney disease. They may experience slowed mental functioning and extreme fatigue.

Pregnant women who use heroin may have a miscarriage or a premature delivery. Heroin exposure in utero can increase the risk of sudden infant death syndrome in the newborn that survives the delivery. Infants who are born to addicted mothers will undergo withdrawal symptoms.

Another risk for heroin users is that heroin is often adulterated with other substances, some of which can be very dangerous, such as strychnine and other poisons or drugs. These drugs may clog the blood vessels when the heroin is injected and can lead to cell death and organ damage.

Even if the heroin is not adulterated, the strength of the drug is highly variable, which is another risk. An inadvertent overdose is a frequent cause of death in heroin users as individuals inject too much of the drug, causing rapid death due to respiratory failure.

Treatment for Heroin Addiction

According to the *National Survey on Drug Use and Health, 2002* (published in 2003), an estimated 277,000 people were treated for heroin addiction in the United States in 2002.

Most patients who are treated for heroin and enter treatment programs are white (47.3 percent), followed by Hispanic patients (24.7 percent), and African-American patients (24.2 percent). In addition, about two-thirds of the heroin addicts that are admitted for treatment are males.

Many patients who are addicted to heroin are given METHADONE, which is also a scheduled drug under the Controlled Substances Act. Some experts believe the use of methadone involves simply exchanging one addictive substance for another. Others, however, believe that methadone is a better choice because the purity of the drug is known and the drug is managed by physicians in conjunction with drug treatment programs. Another benefit is that patients in methadone maintenance programs do not have to engage in illegal and/or unsafe acts in order to obtain their methadone.

Another drug that may be effective in treating heroin addiction is NALTREXONE, particularly if the patient has an alcohol dependence as well as an addiction to heroin. Naltrexone blocks the effects of OPIATES such as heroin, making the use of the street drug ineffective and unsatisfying to the drug user.

Another medication, Naloxone, may be used to treat some heroin addicts. BUPRENORPHINE is another drug used in the treatment of patients addicted to heroin.

Withdrawal from heroin is potentially dangerous and should be performed only under a doctor's supervision, preferably in a hospital or treatment center for addicted individuals. It is not, however, as dangerous as withdrawal from alcohol or BENZODIAZEPINES. Withdrawal symptoms from heroin include nausea, vomiting, lack of body temperature control, diarrhea, and a profound craving for the drug. Due to the severity of the nausea and vomiting, the patient may also experience severe dehydration and an electrolyte imbalance.

Once the patient has overcome DETOXIFICATION, most methadone patients can be treated on an outpatient basis.

See also DRUG ENFORCEMENT ADMINISTRATION; INTRAVENOUS DRUG USE, ILLEGAL; NARCOTICS; SCHEDULED DRUGS.

Executive Office of the President, Office of National Drug Control Policy, "ONDCP Drug Policy Information Clearinghouse Fact Sheet: Heroin, June 2003," Available online. URL: http://www.whitehousedrugpolicy.gov/publications/factsht/heroin. Accessed on March 11, 2005.

Fiellin, David A., M.D., and Patrick G. O'Connor, M.D. "Office-Based Treatment of Opiod-Dependent Patients," *New England Journal of Medicine* 347, no. 11 (September 12, 2002): 817–823.

National Drug Intelligence Center, *National Drug Threat Assessment 2003.* U.S. Department of Justice Product No. 2003-Q0317-001. Washington D.C.: U.S. Department of Justice, January 2003.

homelessness   The state of not having a residence and living on the streets, in automobiles, or in temporary shelters. Many people who are homeless are addicted to drugs and/or alcohol and/or they are mentally ill, with severe illnesses such as SCHIZOPHRENIA, psychotic depression, or BIPOLAR DISORDER. For example, in their study on the prevalence of SUBSTANCE ABUSE disorders and mental illness among 216 homeless women, published in a 1998 issue of the *American Journal of Psychiatry*, Dr. Ellen Bassuk and her colleagues found that over two-thirds of the women had been diagnosed with at least one lifetime diagnosis of a serious psychiatric

disorder. About one-third of the women had been diagnosed with three or more disorders.

The researchers compared the rates of substance abuse and lifetime diagnoses of psychiatric disorders of the homeless women with a group of low-income mothers who were housed and on public assistance. They found similar rates of substance abuse and psychiatric disorders, although there were some differences. For example, both the homeless (45 percent) and the nonhomeless women (42.8 percent) had lifetime diagnoses of major depressive disorders. Both groups also had very high rates of posttraumatic stress disorder (PTSD), and 36.1 percent of the homeless women had been diagnosed with PTSD, as had 34.1 percent of the low-income women who were not homeless. Bipolar disorder was more common (1.9 percent) among the homeless women than the nonhomeless women (0.9 percent).

Both groups had problems with "any alcohol or drug abuse or alcohol dependence," but it was a larger problem for the homeless women (41.1 percent) than for the housed women (34.7 percent). When considering the substances that were abused, the homeless women were most likely to abuse alcohol (31.7 percent) as were the nonhomeless group (28.7 percent). However, the second most abused substance differed between the two groups. Among the homeless women, cocaine led, at 25.1 percent. Among the low-income women who were not homeless, though, the second most abused substance was marijuana (14.8 percent).

It should also be noted that the prevalence of depression and substance abuse was significantly higher among both groups of women than among all women in the National Comorbidity Survey, according to the authors. Thus the rate of such disorders may be higher among poor women than among women in the general population.

Characteristics of Homeless People Admitted for Substance Abuse Treatment

According to a 2003 *DASIS Report*, published by the Substance Abuse and Mental Health Services Administration on the characteristics of homeless people admitted for substance abuse treatment in 2000 in the United States, more than 120,000 people admitted for treatment or 10 percent of all recorded admissions were of homeless people. Homeless people were more likely to self-refer for treatment (43 percent) than people who were not homeless (30 percent). The majority (51 percent) of the homeless people were admitted for alcohol abuse, followed by opiates (18 percent) and smoked cocaine (17 percent).

The average age of homeless patients who were admitted for treatment was 38 years, which was older than the 33 years average age of the non-homeless population who were admitted for treatment. Most of the homeless admissions were male (76 percent) compared with the 70 percent of non-homeless patients who were admitted for treatment.

When considering race, most of the homeless patients who were admitted were white (53 percent), compared with the 59 percent of admissions of nonhomeless patients. Of the homeless patients who were admitted, 30 percent were African American, compared with the nonhomeless patient admissions, or 24 percent. Thus there was an increase in the percentage of African-American patients among the homeless, although white patients still represented the majority. No significant differences occurred in the admissions of other racial and ethnic groups between homeless and nonhomeless patients.

See also DEPRESSION; DUAL DIAGNOSIS.

Bassuk, Ellen L., M.D., et al. "Prevalence of Mental Health and Substance Use Disorders Among Homeless and Low-Income Housed Mothers," *American Journal of Psychiatry* 155, no. 11 (November 1998): 1,561–1,564.

Office of Applied Studies, Drug and Alcohol Services Information System. "Characteristics of Homeless Admissions to Substance Abuse Treatment: 2000," *The DASIS Report.* Washington, D.C.: Substance Abuse and Mental Health Services Administration, August 8, 2003.

homicide   The intentional taking of another person's life. Homicide is also known as murder. Although individuals addicted to drugs or alcohol usually do not commit homicides, the risk for committing violent acts is greatly increased when they are under the influence of such substances. Some drugs, such as COCAINE and METHAMPHETAMINE, increase the risk of homicide because they may induce aggressive behavior and paranoia in users.

See also VIOLENCE.

illegal drugs and health problems See DRUG ABUSE/ADDICTION AND HEALTH PROBLEMS.

impulse control disorder A type of psychiatric problem characterized by the inability to cease from performing actions that are harmful to oneself or to others. One of the most common forms of impulse control disorders, which is also an additive behavior, is compulsive GAMBLING. Other examples of impulse control disorders are trichotillomania (the constant pulling out of the hair), intermittent explosive disorder (periods of extreme rage and/or physical violence), kleptomania (stealing items), and pyromania (setting fires). Some experts consider COMPULSIVE SHOPPING to be a form of impulse control disorder. Because some of the acts that people with impulse control disorder commit are by their very nature criminal, such as setting fires or stealing items, individuals with impulse control disorder are often caught in the act and subsequently charged with crimes and prosecuted.

Individuals with impulse control disorder are more likely to abuse alcohol and drugs. For example, in one small study of compulsive buyers, reported in the *American Journal of Psychiatry* in 1998, 18 percent of compulsive buyers either used or were dependent on alcohol, compared with about 9 percent of a control group. In addition, about 12 percent of the compulsive buyers either used or were dependent on drugs, compared with only about 5 percent of the control group subjects.

Some experts also consider individuals with compulsive sexual habits, also known as sex addicts, to have a form of impulse control behavior. They may engage in promiscuous sexual behavior and may be obsessed with reading and thinking about pornography. They may become involved with individuals engaged in PROSTITUTION because purchasing sex may seem easier and quicker than obtaining intimacy through a normal relationship.

See also ATTENTION DEFICIT HYPERACTIVITY DISORDER; IMPULSIVITY; SEXUAL ADDICTION.

Black, Donald W., M.D., et al. "Family History and Psychiatric Comorbidity in Persons with Compulsive Buying: Preliminary Findings," *American Journal of Psychiatry* 155, no. 7 (July 1998): 960–963.

impulsivity Reacting with little or no conscious thought. Some individuals are more prone to exhibiting impulsivity on a regular or frequent basis, such as those with ATTENTION DEFICIT HYPERACTIVITY DISORDER. Impulsivity may also be a trait exhibited among people with some addictive behaviors, such as GAMBLING and the abuse of alcohol or illegal drugs, as well as less common behaviors, such as a perceived necessity to engage in EXTREME SPORTS or other risk-taking ventures.

Some individuals with severe and chronic problems with impulsivity are said to have an IMPULSE CONTROL DISORDER, such as those with compulsive gambling or COMPULSIVE SHOPPING. Other individuals with impulsivity may be diagnosed with psychiatric disorders, such as antisocial personality disorder, conduct disorder, BIPOLAR DISORDER, or borderline personality disorder.

See also CREDIT CARD OVERSPENDING.

Moeller, F. Gerard, M.D. "Psychiatric Aspects of Impulsivity," *American Journal of Psychiatry* 158, no. 11 (November 2001): 1,783–1,793.

incarceration Confinement to a jail or prison as punishment for a crime or while awaiting trial for the alleged commission of a criminal act. Some addictive behaviors lead to arrest and incarceration, particularly the selling of illegal drugs.

Incarceration can be very dangerous for some addicts, particularly those addicted to some prescription drugs or to illegal addicting drugs, because they are unable to obtain the substance while incarcerated. In some cases, individuals are jailed for a relatively minor offense and may undergo withdrawal from substances to which they are addicted. This withdrawal can be extremely difficult for the addicted person and can even lead to death if the prisoner is untreated.

See also HOMICIDE; VIOLENCE.

inhalants, abuse of   Abuse of common household and commercial products by individuals who purposely sniff or inhale these substances for the purpose of self-intoxication and/or to induce a state of EUPHORIA. Another apparent motivation of using inhalants, particularly among younger adolescents, is to impress others. Inhalant abuse is also called *huffing*. Male adolescents in the 12–14 age group appear to be at the greatest risk for using inhalants, although some females and individuals of other age groups also do so. Continued abuse of inhalants can lead to addiction as well as to brain damage and even death.

Some products used as inhalants are GLUE, cleaning solvents, commercial adhesives, paint products, gasoline, lighter fluid, nail polish remover, vegetable cooking spray, dessert topping spray (such as whipped cream), and other sprayed or volatile substances. Nitrates, such as amyl nitrates (also known as *poppers*) are drugs that fall into the inhalant category, as are butyl nitrates. In addition, chlorofluorohydocarbons (freons) fall into the category of inhalants when they are abused. (Freon is a substance used in air-cooling machinery, such as air conditioners.)

It is estimated that more than a thousand household products can be misused as inhalants. Inhalants may be inhaled directly from the container, or they may be placed into plastic bags, sniffed from saturated cloths, or used in other ways.

Some abusers develop a TOLERANCE to the product and need greater amounts to achieve the same effects. However, inhaling any amount of inhalants

is very dangerous because of the unpredictability of their effects. The very first use of an inhalant may be fatal.

Attraction to Risky Behaviors and Inhalant Abuse

The abuse of inhalants may be tied to an increased attraction that some individuals have toward performing risky behaviors. A study of GAMBLING and other risk behaviors among students in grades eight to 12 in the United States was reported in *Pediatrics* in 1998. The researchers studied risk behaviors in 21,297 students in 79 public and private schools in Vermont. They found that inhalant use was reported at 10 percent among students who said they did not gamble, but the rate doubled to 20 percent among those who said that they did gamble. In addition, among the students who gambled and who said they had problems related to gambling, one-third of them said that they used inhalants.

Inhalant Abusers

According to the 2002 National Survey on Drug Use and Health, an estimated 180,000 people abused or were dependent on inhalants in 2002. Youth risk behavior surveillance studies have shown that about 15 percent of students in the United States have used inhalants at least once.

In general, white (16 percent) and Hispanic (15 percent) students are more likely than African-American students (about 6 percent) to report inhalant use. About 5 percent of students have used inhalants more than once. Younger students in grades 9 and 10 are significantly more likely to use inhalants than students in grade 12. In 2002, only about 1.5 percent of high school seniors in the United States reported using inhalants in the past month, compared with 2.4 percent of 10th graders and 3.8 percent of eighth graders.

Some individuals try inhalants one time, while others use them repeatedly in an addictive fashion. Individuals may select inhalants because they are products that are easy to buy or are readily available in their own homes, in contrast to the difficulty adolescents would experience in purchasing alcohol or illegal drugs.

Emergency Department Treatment for Inhalants

In 2002, the number of patients treated in hospital emergency rooms for inhalant abuse increased.

EMERGENCY DEPARTMENT VISITS FOR INHALANT ABUSE, COTERMINOUS UNITED STATES

1995	1996	1997	1998	1999	2000	2001	2002
736	1,030	1,539	1,735	650	1,141	522	1,496

Source: Substance Abuse and Mental Health Services Administration (SAMHSA), Office of Applied Studies. *Emergency Department Trends from the Drug Abuse Warning Network, Final Estimates 1995–2002.* DAWN Series: D-24, DHHS Publication No. (SMA) 03-3780, Md.: SAMHSA, July 2003.

This information was provided by the Drug Abuse Warning Network, a database of major hospital emergency rooms in 48 states and Washington, D.C. (not including Alaska and Hawaii). This statistical data is significant because it involves people who are suffering from the medical complications of drug abuse.

The numbers of admissions for inhalant abuse increased from 522 patients in 2001 to 1,496 in 2002. This is not as high as the level seen in 1998 (1,735 patients). However, an upward trend is a matter for policy makers, researchers, and others to evaluate to determine possible causes and solutions.

Effects of Inhalants

Experts report that a heavy use of inhalants over a short period of time, such as hours or days, can create a physical tolerance, requiring greater quantities of the substance to achieve the same effect. Addicted individuals who stop using inhalants will go through WITHDRAWAL. They may experience a rapid pulse, sweating, insomnia, nausea and vomiting, and even HALLUCINATIONS and grand mal seizures. Some individuals die instantly from inhalant abuse, usually because this action triggers erratic heart rhythms (arrhythmias), which then lead to heart stoppage.

Inhalant abuse may cause serious long-term health problems, such as memory loss, apathy, and learning problems caused by permanent brain damage. Inhalant abuse may also cause damage to other major organs, such as the lungs, kidneys, liver, and heart.

Indicators of Inhalant Abuse

Signs of inhalant abuse include unexplained paint or stains on an individual's clothing, sores around the mouth, constant red eyes and nose, a chemical smell on the person's breath, a loss of appetite, and irritability. Users may have slurred speech and appear drunk. Some users may become belligerent or violent, while others may appear apathetic. These signs may also indicate other health problems that should be investigated by a physician.

Admissions for Substance Abuse Treatment

According to the Treatment Episode Data Set database of information collected by the Substance Abuse and Mental Health Services Administration, 1,199 patients were admitted for treatment of inhalant abuse in 2002 in the United States. This is less than 1 percent of all patients admitted for SUBSTANCE ABUSE treatment nationwide. The number of patients treated for inhalant abuse or addiction has been steadily declining since a high of 2,918 patients treated in 1992. Why fewer patients are being treated for inhalant abuse in the face of a continuing problem with inhalants is unknown.

Of all the patients who were admitted for substance abuse treatment for inhalants in 2002, nearly 19 percent were under age 15 and nearly 22 percent were ages 15–17 years old. Nearly half (49 percent) were treated as outpatients rather than hospitalized. Of all the patients treated for abuse of inhalants, the largest percent, 33 percent, were referred by the criminal justice system for driving under the influence of substances; 30 percent were individual referrals, although it is unknown by whom they were referred.

Laws to Protect Minors

Most states (46 states as of this writing, according to the National Drug Intelligence Center) have passed laws related to the use of inhalants by minors. For example, in Massachusetts, before selling the product retailers must obtain an identification from any minor seeking to purchase glue or cement, and they must keep a written record of the purchase that can be examined by the police. Only a glue or cement that contains oil of mustard or another deterrent that prevents the inhalation of fumes is exempt from this requirement. Glue is one of the most commonly used inhalants of abuse among youths. State laws vary considerably in how they address the legalities of and punishments for inhalant abuse.

See also EMERGENCY TREATMENT; TEENAGE AND YOUTH DRUG ABUSE; TEENAGE AND YOUTH GAMBLING.

For further information on inhalant abuse, contact the following organizations:

National Drug Intelligence Center
319 Washington Street
Fifth Floor
Johnstown, PA 15901
(814) 532-4690
http://www.usdog.gov/ndic

National Inhalant Prevention Coalition
2904 Kerbey Lane
Austin, TX 78703
(800) 269-4237 (toll-free)
http://www.inhalants.org

Substance Abuse and Mental Health Services
     Administration (SAMSHA)
Department of Health and Human Services
5600 Fishers Lane
Rockville, MD 20857
(800) 729-6686 (toll free) or (800) 487-4889
     (TTY)

Grunbaum, Jo Anne, et al. "Youth Risk Behavior Surveillance—United States, 2001," *Morbidity and Mortality Weekly Report* 51, no. SS-4 (June 28, 2002): 32.

Office of National Drug Control Policy. "Inhalants." February 2003, Available online. URL: http://www.whitehousedrugpolicy.gov/publications/factsht/inhalants/index.htm. Downloaded on March 29, 2005.

Proimos, Jenny, et al. "Gambling and Other Risk Behaviors Among 8th to 12th-Grade Students," Available online. URL: http://www.pediatrics.org/cgi/content/full/102/2/e23 Accessed on March 15, 2004.

Substance Abuse and Mental Health Services Administration (SAMHSA). *Results from the 2003 National Survey on Drug Use and Health: National Findings.* Office of Applied Studies, NHSDA Series H-22, DHHS Publication Number SMA 03-3836. Rockville, Md.: SAMHSA, 2003.

Substance Abuse and Mental Health Services Administration (SAMHSA), Office of Applied Studies. *Emergency Department Trends from the Drug Abuse Warning Network, Final Estimates 1995–2002.* DAWN Series: D-24, DHHS Publication No. (SMA) 03-3780, Rockville, Md.: SAMHSA, July 2003.

Substance Abuse and Mental Health Services Administration (SAMHSA), Office of Applied Studies. *Treatment Episode Data Set (TEDS) Highlights—2002: National Admissions to Substance Abuse Treatment Services.* DASIS Series: S-22, Department of Health and Human Services Publication No. (SMA) 04-3946, Rockville, Md.: SAMHSA, May 2004.

Internet An electronic interconnection of an assortment of research and informational sites, originally set up by the federal government of the United States and now available to millions of researchers, students, and everyday users in the United States and countries throughout the world. The Internet was originally called the Defense Advanced Research Projects Agency-Network, or DARPA-Net, when it was created in the 1960s. It was a system used by the federal government and by universities performing research for the government. As time passed, increasing numbers of corporations, and eventually individuals, began to request access to the use of the online services, which ultimately became known as the Internet in the 1990s.

Today the Internet is also used in commerce, and many large and small companies sell their goods and services on their Web sites. Many individuals also use the Internet to exchange electronic messages about work or daily events in their lives. Some people use the Internet as a vehicle to engage in addictive behaviors. For example, some individuals purchase illegal drugs or buy prescribed drugs without a prescription through online Web sites that are sometimes known as Internet pharmacies. Others who are addicted to pornographic material may view or purchase such materials on a plethora of such sites on the Internet. Whether an item is legal or not, or harmful or not, it may be available for sale on the Internet.

Drug Use

Although there is an increasingly strict oversight by federal agencies in the United States, such as the DRUG ENFORCEMENT ADMINISTRATION and the Food and Drug Administration (FDA), some Web sites on the Internet offer prescribed drugs for sale to individuals without prescriptions, including NARCOTICS, DIET PILLS, ANABOLIC STEROIDS, and other drugs. These drugs may be available from countries such as Mexico or Thailand, and it is unknown if they are safe and/or unadulterated. In other cases, the drugs are sold through online Web sites in the United States by physicians, pharmacists, and other individuals. Fatalities and nonfatal drug overdoses have resulted from patients who abused drugs that were purchased online.

Law enforcement authorities are seeking to stop abuses with criminal prosecutions. In one case, cited in a statement in 2004 before Congress by William K. Hubbard, the associate commissioner for policy and planning for the FDA, the owner of Genapharm.com, an online pharmacy, pled guilty to possessing controlled drugs and admitting that he had engaged in a conspiracy to sell counterfeit, misbranded, and Schedule I drugs from 1999–2001 over the Internet. Some of the drugs that he sold included methylenedioxymethamphetamine (ECSTASY) and 1,4-butanediol, a substance that converts to gamma-hydroxybutyrate inside the body. He had also sold counterfeit human growth hormone and other drugs.

In 2004, the General Accounting Office (GAO) released testimony of their report on Internet pharmacies, in which they concentrated on online pharmacies in the United States that sold hydrocodone, an addictive medication, to consumers without prescriptions. The investigators were able to purchase hydrocodone from eight different online pharmacies, each time with no prescription required. Such purchases are very expensive. For example, in one case, the fees for 60 days of hydrocodone were $190, which is significantly higher than the cost of this drug when purchased in a local pharmacy with a legitimate prescription. It is a very lucrative business for the illicit pharmacies—unless they are identified and prosecuted by federal and state authorities. Physicians and pharmacists who have been prosecuted for selling drugs over the Internet without prescriptions have been fined, lost their licenses, and served jail time.

In some cases of online pharmacies, several questions may be asked about a patient's medical history, usually on a form that is provided. However, these questions, if asked, are usually cursory. There is no verification of the responses through the patient's primary care physician or any other doctor and there is rarely any follow-up. Investigations have shown that sometimes no physicians review the responses to these forms. As a result, individuals can obtain dangerous drugs that are not only harmful by themselves but are also dangerous for people who take other medications or who have some illnesses.

Without the constraints of medical oversight, people who are addicted to drugs (or who are at risk for addiction), those who wish to experiment with drugs, or those who genuinely suffer from pain or other medical problems but for some reason do not wish to see a doctor are all potential markets for illicit online pharmacies. As long as the consumer has a valid credit card, in most cases, their request for drugs will be filled with few or no questions asked.

Some minors have purchased illegal drugs over the Internet by using their parents' credit card without their knowledge. According to the GAO report, in discussing an investigator's interview with a doctor who prescribed hydrocodone to consumers over the Internet, "When asked about the possibility of children buying narcotics through him, the physician claimed that the need for a credit card is the 'safeguard' to prevent that from happening and that 'a kid shouldn't have a credit card.' However, he admitted that 'parents call [him] all the time saying that their children have gotten hold of their credit cards.' " It seems that this doctor knew that some children had obtained narcotics illegally.

It is important to keep in mind and should also be emphasized that many pharmacies do legitimate business online and save patients considerable time and money. For example, they help many disabled people who cannot easily travel to local pharmacies by delivering needed medications and medical devices directly to their homes. Legitimate pharmacies require prescriptions from the patient's physician.

According to the FDA, the Verified Internet Pharmacy Practice Sites or VIPPS system, which was developed by the National Association of Boards of Pharmacy (NABP), is one way that consumers in the United States can choose a legitimate online pharmacy. The organization offers a seal of approval to member pharmacies they have checked to verify that they meet state licensure standards and NABP standards. Consumers can call the NABP at (847) 698-6227 or go to their Web site (http://www.nabp.net) to discover whether a Web site is a licensed pharmacy in good standing.

Consumers should avoid buying medications from Web sites that do not post an address and a phone number in the United States where someone can be contacted if there were a problem. The FDA advises against purchasing drugs from foreign

Web sites because of the inherent risks and because importing drugs from other countries into the United States in this manner is usually illegal.

Pornography

The free viewing, as well as the buying and selling of pornography, are burgeoning activities on the Internet. In fact, many individuals receive unsolicited offers by electronic mail or in pop-up messages during their Internet use, urging them to buy pornographic materials or to engage in phone sex, for which a credit card will be billed.

Federal and state laws in the United States have attempted to restrict the number of such unsolicited messages. Many online services, such as America Online and Yahoo! have created active antispam programs to prevent pornography purveyors from contacting private users of online services. In addition, individuals and corporations purchase programs to block these services from their personal or corporate use of the Internet.

When pornography is viewed and/or purchased by adults and it does not involve the sexual abuse of minor children, it is generally a lawful act. However, some individuals engage in an addictive use of pornography over the Internet, spending many hours compulsively seeking out and viewing explicit material and neglecting their personal, work, and family life.

One major concern among many groups is that pornography should not be available to children. Despite federal and state efforts in the United States to limit the Internet sales of videos, photographs, and other sexually explicit materials only to adults over age 18, in many cases, individuals need only assert that they are older than age 18. After having asserted that they are 18 or older, no further attempts to restrict access are undertaken by the site owners. At that point, an underage person may view sexually explicit material on a Web site and/or use a credit card to purchase a video or other material.

Child Pornography

Sometimes children under age 18 are used in the creation of pornography that is sold over the Internet, including very young children. Some children are lured by pedophiles (adults who are sexually attracted to children) who lurk on various sites on the Internet, pretending to be teenagers or children themselves and well aware of the anxieties, fears, and insecurities of many adolescents. These adults may enter chat rooms and other sites where they can communicate with adolescents or children and prey on their insecurities. Sometimes they are successful in convincing children to meet them and to pose for pornographic photographic sessions.

The creation and the possession of child pornography is a crime in the United States. It does not matter whether the buyer is aware that the people depicted in the scenes are children, although often it is obvious and it is advertised that the individuals are under age 18, which is largely the appeal of the material to pedophiles and to some others.

The purchase of child pornography may be an addictive behavior that is related to pedophilia. Experts disagree on whether buying child pornography will prevent an individual from abusing a child or will inflame an individual to act out on a child rather than to fantasize with child pornography. In any case, the child who was depicted in the pornography was used as an object of sexual abuse. Some pedophiles may use such pictures to show children and try to convince them that because other children have posed or behaved in such a manner, it is acceptable or normal to act in this way and that the children should also emulate this behavior.

Some Internet purveyors of pornography are very prolific. In one study, described in a 2002 issue of the *American Journal of Psychiatry*, researchers studied the descriptions of the incidents of 10 children who were known to have been sexually abused. The abuse ranged from exposing the children's genitals to oral/anal/vaginal intercourse and forced urination and defecation. The average age of the victims was 5.6 years at the time of the last abuse and 6.9 years when they were interviewed by the police.

Said the authors, "He [the perpetrator] was convicted on numerous charges of child sexual abuse as well as illegal Internet distribution of some 47,000 pictures and 800 films featuring child pornography. He was sentenced to psychiatric care."

The researchers were interested that most of the abused children denied or belittled their experiences, despite the taped evidence, possibly because of childhood amnesia, their active attempts to forget, or avoidance of the abusive memories. In spite of not remembering or minimizing the experience, mental health professionals conclude that these children will experience significant aftereffects in later life.

Compulsive Shopping

Some people with a COMPULSIVE SHOPPING disorder use the Internet to make their numerous purchases, spending many hours on a variety of shopping sites that may also send them electronic mail informing them of the latest sales or newest items. The vast quantity of Web sites and products may increase the level of addictiveness. The availability of the Internet at any time of the day or night, and the privacy generally experienced by the shopper, may also promote out of control behaviors, although research has not confirmed this.

Compulsive Gambling and Role Playing

Individuals with a gambling disorder sometimes use the Internet to gamble compulsively on games of chance. Compulsive gambling may be triggered by Internet access, with its ease of use and reliance on credit cards. Some types of computcrizcd gambling may even have a special impact on the central nervous system due to the visual/television component of the activity.

Some people spend many hours on role-playing games, where they assume alternate identities that are far different from their everyday roles in life. These games can become obsessive or addictive activities, with an individual becoming focused on the activity to the detriment of other aspects of ordinary life, such as work and family.

Sexual Addictions

Some individuals develop sexual relationships with individuals whom they encounter in online chatrooms or through other means on the Internet. Some of these relationships would be described as aberrant or destructive, although others are ordinary sexual relationships. Some people divorce their spouses because of these relationships. Although in some cases, the marriages or long-term relationships may have been shaky before the sexual exploration on the Internet occurred, experts report that even stable marriages have been destroyed by these encounters.

A substantial amount of literature suggests that many of these compulsive and addictive behaviors, such as addiction to Internet pornography or sexual relationships on the Internet, are related to depression, loneliness, and social isolation in the addicted individual.

Combinations of Addictive Behaviors

Sometimes individuals exhibit combinations of addictive behaviors that they use the Internet to facilitate. For example, in a 2001 issue of the *American Journal of Psychiatry*, the authors described a patient who spent several hours a day downloading pornography from the Internet, spending more money than he could afford. Although this incident described only one patient (who was actually a composite of several patients of the doctors), he is sufficiently typical to illustrate a common problem.

In this case, the patient was addicted to pornography and he was also engaged in compulsive shopping for the pornographic materials. The patient was also in denial about his behavior, believing that it was not affecting his marital relationship at all. However, when he masturbated to orgasm as a result of using downloaded pornographic materials, he was unable to have an orgasm with his wife later that day.

The patient had masturbated to orgasm often in the past. According to the authors, this behavior had not affected his social or work functioning until he gained easy access to Internet pornography. He worked at a university and spent a great deal of time looking for particular pornographic photographs.

Said the authors, "It is interesting to note that cultural factors—development of the Internet—seem to have markedly contributed to the pathogenesis of this patient's symptoms. Although the Internet may offer clinicians and their patients valuable opportunities for psychoeducation and support, it may also provide an opportunity for pathological gambling and other kinds of dysfunctional behavior."

Other Addictive Behaviors

Many addictive behaviors that can be identified can also be practiced or exploited on the Internet. It is important to note that there are many sites on the Internet that offer helpful advice for individuals who suffer from a wide variety of medical problems and to their family members. There are also sites that can be used in a destructive manner. For example, individuals with problems such as ANOREXIA NERVOSA or BULIMIA NERVOSA can learn how to become more efficient at dieting and purging through Web sites that are run by individuals who will enable them and also teach them to hide their medical symptoms from others who are worried about them. As a result, the Internet can be used as a valuable tool or it can be a harmful device, depending upon the individual and the services that are used.

See also GHB; INTERNET ADDICTION DISORDER; SEXUAL ADDICTION.

Sjoberg, Rickard L., and Frank Lindblad, M.D. "Limited Disclosure of Sexual Abuse in Children Whose Experiences Were Documented by Videotape," *American Journal of Psychiatry* 159, no. 2 (2002): 312–314.

Stein, Dan J., M.D., et al. "Hypersexual Disorder and Preoccupation with Internet Pornography," *American Journal of Psychiatry* 158, no. 10 (2001): 1,590–1,594.

U.S. Food and Drug Administration. "Statement of William K. Hubbard, Associate Commission for Policy and Planning Before the Committee on Government Reform, U.S. House of Representatives Hearing on Internet Drug Sales, March 18, 2004," Available online. URL: http://www.fda.gov/ola/2004/internetdrugs0318.html. Accessed on September 8, 2004.

U.S. General Accounting Office. "Internet Pharmacies: Hydrocodone, an Addictive Narcotic Pain Medication Is Available Without a Prescription Through the Internet: Statement of Robert J. Cramer, Managing Director, Office of Special Investigations", Available online. URL: http://www.gaogov/new.items/d04892t.pdf. Downloaded on March 28, 2005.

Internet addiction disorder   Constant use of the INTERNET to the extent that an individual ultimately suffers emotional, financial, and/or personal consequences at work as well as in his or her personal and family life. Internet addiction disorder is not a clinically recognized entity by the AMERICAN PSYCHIATRIC ASSOCIATION as of this writing.

New York psychiatrist Ivan Goldberg first jokingly asserted the possibility of Internet addiction disorder in 1995. Psychologist Kimberly Young of the University of Pittsburgh was the first to write about Internet dependence in 1998, based on her 1996 study of nearly 400 obsessive Internet users.

Dr. David Greenfield subsequently surveyed 18,000 people on their Internet use in conjunction with ABC News.com in 1998. His respondents were primarily male (71 percent), and most were college educated (87 percent). He found that 6 percent of the respondents were compulsive users of the Internet. According to Greenfield, over 29 percent used the Internet as a means to escape or alter their mood. Greenfield also found that many of the addicted users reported a feeling of timelessness during their use of the Internet nearly all the time, as opposed to 39 percent among the nonaddicts who reported feeling that way.

Timelessness is a feeling of losing track of time to the extent that hours can slip away without the individual's awareness. This feeling of timelessness can be very seductive and appealing and in itself provides an element of addictiveness to the experience of spending time on the Internet.

Dr. Dawn Heron and Dr. Nathan Shapira at the University of Florida created an acronym (MOUSE) to describe the symptoms of excessive Internet use, which included the following items:

- More than the time intended is spent online.
- Other responsibilities are neglected.
- Unsuccessful attempts are made at cutting down on Internet use.
- Significant relationship problems have occurred.
- Excessive thoughts or anxiety occurs when the person is not on the Internet.

Types of Excess Use of the Internet

There are several key types of excessive uses of time on the Internet. They largely fall into the following categories:

- Sex/pornography
- Friendship/shared interests (which may transform into sexual relationships)
- Gaming (gambling, stock trading)
- Compulsive shopping

Cybersex and Pornography

The largest category of abusive use of the Internet is the perusal of sex Web sites and chat rooms. Some individuals become addicted to the consumption of Internet pornography to the extent that they ignore real-life sexual opportunities with their own partners or other individuals that they know, instead seeking virtual liaisons with strangers online.

They may engage in chat room communication and may masturbate in front of their computers to the point of orgasm, rationalizing to themselves that since the other party is not physically present, it cannot be considered to be "real" sex. However, sometimes these online encounters progress further to phone sex and/or then to true sexual encounters. Mental health professionals disagree on whether virtual sex is a betrayal of marital intimacy. In contrast, some family law attorneys believe that this activity should be legally defined as infidelity.

In Greenfield's study, he found that 38 percent of the Internet addicts engaged in explicit sex talk in their online encounters, and 37 percent said they engaged in masturbation while online. In addition, 42 percent admitted to having an online affair.

Changed Relationships Over the Internet

Many people meet others on the Internet through shared interests or hobbies. Said Dr. Gwinnell in her book, *Online Seductions: Falling in Love with Strangers on the Internet*, "It is clear that for many people Internet relationships can provide experiences of intimate communication, intimate connections that are not available in face-to-face interactions in daily life. To some degree it's simply a matter of numbers—as millions of people take to the Internet, joining online services and sending messages, their opportunities to get to know one another increase exponentially. No other place, outside school, allows so many people to meet on common ground. With *millions* of people leaving notes for each other in cyberspace, friends (and enemies) are made. Some people find love, some find sex and some find the intellectual stimulation they haven't had since midnight conversations in the campus coffee shop."

Dr. Gwinnell says that the relationship may progress as a casual interchange, which may then lead to private electronic mail. The private e-mails may become more personal and then more and frequent. Eventually, they may also lead to phone conversations and to a meeting.

Many people wonder how strangers can become attached to each over the Internet. One key reason is because of the false sense of intimacy and the breaking down of boundaries and barriers that the medium of the Internet achieves. As described by Dr. Gwinnell in her book, a key element in the unique medium of the Internet is that the normal screening by all the senses is absent. Individuals cannot see, hear, or touch each others.

Unless individuals provide valid photographs of themselves, as they often fail to do, the only way to evaluate each other in chat rooms or other areas where individuals meet is through the words that they share. As a result, individuals may begin to imagine and to attribute desirable qualities to the other person with whom they are communicating. Later, if they decide to meet, the emotional investment they have already made may have become a major one to the extent that they are almost preprogrammed to like or even love each other. Some individuals marry people they meet online, although whether these relationships are lasting is unknown.

Gaming

Some individuals are fascinated by role-playing games that can be played online. It can be a rush for a mild-mannered accountant to play the role of an aggressive warrior or other completely different person from the daily life of the individual. Sometimes this alternate identity can become a very powerful persona that becomes extremely important to the individual and the role-playing and gaming is addictive.

Some individuals also engage in online gambling, engaging in games of chance, and gambling compulsively.

Compulsive Shopping

Some users are mesmerized by eBay while others love to search the Internet for many different shopping sites. Some compulsive shoppers move from link to link. They may gain a feeling of power and control from clicking and ordering items to be shipped to their home.

Possible Reasons for Excessive Use of the Internet

Some experts consider excessive Internet use as a form of an IMPULSE CONTROL DISORDER. It is also likely that many individuals who use the Internet to excess have an underlying problem with DEPRESSION. Some may have other serious emotional problems.

Symptoms of Excessive Use of the Internet

There are both physical and psychological symptoms of excessive use of the Internet. Physical symptoms may include severely dry eyes, chronic headaches, and changes in sleeping and eating patterns. Psychological symptoms are self-isolation, severe distress if the Internet is unavailable for some reason, and difficulty or inability to control the use of the time that is spent on the Internet.

Work and Internet Abuse

Some employees get into trouble on the job with their abuse of the Internet, whether it is with downloading obscene photographs, sending them by electronic mail to coworkers, or many other actions that are grounds for getting fired, such as playing games or making fun of the boss in an e-mail. Many employees do not realize that when they are on the job, their use of the Internet can be monitored around the clock and often it is. When inappropriate use is observed, their services may be terminated.

Children and Internet Abuse

Children and adolescents can become addicted to the Internet, and this can be dangerous in many different ways. For example, they may become involved in dangerous relationships with sexual predators who manipulate them and convince them to run away from home and engage in sordid behaviors and crimes. Children and adolescents may also engage in gambling and become enthralled by pornography online. Although it is illegal for children under age 18 to view such sites, they can lie and attest that they are of legal age and view such material. Some adolescents steal their parents' credit cards to pay for the material.

Treatment of Internet Addiction Disorder

Although it sounds ironic, some Web sites on the Internet purport to help individuals to curb their dependence on using the Internet. However, most experts agree that it is probably best for most people to see a therapist in person who understands the problem and who can use therapy to help people to disengage from their overly intense dependence on the Internet. Any underlying emotional disorders, such as depression, obsessive-compulsive disorder, or other emotional problems, should also be dealt with.

See also COMPULSIVE SHOPPING; SEXUAL ADDICTION.

Greenfield, David N. "The Net Effect: Internet Addiction and Compulsive Internet Use," Available online. URL: http://www.virtual-addiction.com/a_neteffect.com Accessed on June 12, 2004.

Greenfield, David N. *Virtual Addiction: Help for Netheads, Cyberfreaks, and Those Who Love Them.* Oakland, Calif.: New Harbinger Publications, Inc., 1999.

Gwinnell, Esther, M.D. *Online Seductions: Falling in Love with Strangers on the Internet.* New York: Kodansha, 1998.

Heron, Dawn, M.D., and Nathan A. Shapira, M.D. "Time to Log Off: New Diagnostic Criteria for Problematic Internetic Use," 2, no. 4. Available online. URL: http://www.psychiatry.com/2003_04/0403_internet.asp Accessed on October 22, 2003.

Mitchell, Peter. "Internet Addiction: Genuine Diagnosis or Not?" *Lancet* 355, no. 9204 (February 19, 2000): 632.

Young, Kimberly S. "Internet Addiction: The Emergence of a New Clinical Disorder," Available online. URL: http://www.netaddiction.com/articles/newdisorder.htm Accessed June 13, 2004.

intervention   A staged action that is taken by immediate relatives and/or friends of alcoholics and/or addicted persons, usually in concert with a trained mental health professional, in order to confront them with the fact of their addiction and also the consequences of this addiction, as perceived by the people who are performing the intervention. In general, the goal of the intervention is to encourage the persons to enter a rehabilitation facility immediately after the confrontation.

intravenous drug use, illegal   Injection of illegal drugs directly into the vein. Although many medications are legally injected into individuals by physicians and other health professionals, illegal intravenous drug use involves the nonmedical injection of drugs such as COCAINE, HEROIN, and other substances. Individuals who self-inject drugs illegally may share needles with others, increasing the risk of contracting the human immunodeficiency virus, HEPATITIS, sexually transmitted diseases, and other diseases. Continued injection into one area of the body may cause a collapse of the veins. Toxic additives or unclean needles can lead to infections of the injection site as well as widespread infection of the blood or severe infections of the skin (cellulites), which can lead to infections in other sites in the body and even to death.

ketamine   A drug that is a combination of codeine and ANABOLIC STEROIDS; its primary legal use is as an anesthetic for animals and humans. Ketamine is a Schedule III prescription drug under the CONTROLLED SUBSTANCES ACT. It is sometimes obtained illegally from another individual or stolen from a legitimate user, such as a veterinarian, and used as a drug of abuse because of its hallucinogenic qualities, which are similar to those of phencyclidine.

Ketamine also has amnesiac qualities and has been used as a DATE RAPE DRUG by sexual predators; it is colorless, odorless, and has a rapid effect on the victim, who may appear intoxicated to others. Ketamine is sometimes added to marijuana by drug abusers. In addition, it may also be included in a tablet containing other illegal drugs such as methylenedioxymethamphetamine (ECSTASY).

According to the National Drug Intelligence Center in 2003, ketamine is a drug of concern among high school students, and an estimated 3 percent of all high school seniors have used ketamine at least once. Most ketamine users (74 percent) who were treated in emergency departments of hospitals in 2000 were ages 12–25 years old according to the Drug Abuse Warning Network.

Effects of Ketamine

Ketamine causes users to have impaired judgment and coordination for as long as 24 hours or more after it has been taken. It can cause delirium, depression, high blood pressure, and amnesia, and sometimes it leads to fatal respiratory problems.

See also DATE/ACQUAINTANCE RAPE; PCP; SCHEDULED DRUGS.

liver The organ in the body that metabolizes alcohol and many different types of foods and medications. Chronic excessive use of alcohol may lead to CIRRHOSIS (severe inflammation) of the liver. Some individuals with ALCOHOLISM have such damaged livers that they require a liver transplantation in order to stay alive.

The regular use of substances such as alcohol or BENZODIAZEPINES increases the level of the liver enzymes responsible for detoxifying the body of these substances. This can lead to requirements for higher doses of many drugs that are used in the treatment of other serious medical conditions because the liver breaks down these drugs. For example, individuals taking antiseizure medications may find that the blood levels of their medications drop as their liver enzymes increase, requiring them to take higher dosages of the medication.

See also ALCOHOLIC HEPATITIS; FATTY LIVER DISEASE/STEATOSIS; HEPATITIS.

LSD (lysergic acid diethylamide) A hallucinogenic drug derived from the ergot rye fungus. Albert Hofmann, a chemist in Switzerland, first synthesized the drug in 1938. Several years later, he accidentally consumed a small amount of the drug and reportedly was terrified by the hallucinogenic effects he experienced.

In the mid-20th century, some scientists used LSD in their research. Timothy Leary, a Harvard psychology professor in the 1960s, was a proponent of LSD use. He coined the phrase, "Tune in, turn on, and drop out," encouraging others to try LSD. The use of LSD was subsequently made illegal and LSD is now a drug of abuse. It is a Schedule I drug under the CONTROLLED SUBSTANCES ACT.

LSD is a clear white drug that is odorless and extremely powerful. A dose of only 30 micrograms

can last from 6 to 12 hours. Because so little of the drug is needed to have an effect, the drug is often crushed into powder and mixed with binding agents. It is often made into microdot tablets, put into sugar cubes, and applied to paper from where it can be licked off.

Decline in Popularity of LSD

No longer a popular drug of abuse, the numbers of emergency room mentions of LSD continues to decline. In 2002, there were 891 mentions of emergency department visits nationwide in the United States related to LSD, down from 2,821 in 2001, according to the Drug Abuse Warning Network.

This declining popularity of LSD is supported by surveys of youths, such as the Monitoring the Future study on drug use of students in grades eight, 10, and 12. The National Institute on Drug Abuse analyzed this data and reported that LSD use among adolescents has been declining since 1996 at all three grade levels. The use declined dramatically from 2001–03. For example, among students in grade 12, annual prevalence dropped from 6.6 percent in 2001 to 1.9 percent in 2003. Among 10th graders, prevalence dropped from 4.1 percent in 2001 to 1.7 percent in 2003. Among eighth-graders, the annual prevalence dropped from 2.2 percent in 2001 to 1.3 percent in 2003.

LSD Users

Of the few LSD users, most are ages 18–25 years old and Caucasian. In one report of lifetime hallucinogen use among youths ages 12–17 in 2001, based on data from the National Household Survey on Drug Abuse, 3.9 percent of Caucasian adolescents had used LSD, compared with 2.3 percent of Asian adolescents, 2.1 percent of Hispanics, and 0.5 percent of African-American adolescents.

Effects of LSD

The drug begins to work in 30–90 minutes. Users may refer to their hallucinogenic experiences with LSD as trips. The experiences are entirely unpredictable and may be pleasurable or terrifying. The physiological experiences may include increased blood pressure and heart rate, appetite loss, nausea, and sweating. The primary effects of the drug, however, are the sensory and emotional effects, which may range from euphoria to deep depression. Users may experience a dissociative feeling of being outside their body while under the influence of the drug as well as when they later experience flashbacks from the drug.

LSD users may develop a psychological TOLERANCE for the drug and need greater amounts in subsequent uses to achieve the same effect. However, if users stop taking LSD for several days, this tolerance is apparently lost. There is no physical tolerance, and there are no withdrawal symptoms if chronic users stop taking LSD. However, psychological aftereffects may occur, such as a drug-induced psychosis and flashbacks of prior experiences when under the influence of the drug.

Drug-Induced Psychosis

Some users of LSD experience a PSYCHOTIC BREAK; their mental illness may last for years, and they may not recover. This problem has occurred in individuals who had no prior history of mental illness or any previous symptoms of any emotional disorders. Some users of LSD have experienced severe physical injuries because of the actions they took while under a drug-induced psychosis. For example, in one case, a man assumed that he could fly while under the influence of LSD and he jumped from a very high point. He survived, but broke his back and became paralyzed for life.

Flashbacks

Some users of LSD report reexperiencing LSD perceptual disorders when they are not taking LSD, months or even years later. Experts call such experiences "hallucinogen persisting perception disorder," but most people refer to them simply as flashbacks. Flashbacks may occur as long as five years after the LSD was used. They generally consist of seeing bright flashes of light or colors. Some-

times physicians who are unaware of the patient's prior use of LSD may misdiagnose the condition as a stroke or a brain tumor. ANTIDEPRESSANT medications may help reduce the flashback symptoms.

See also ECSTASY; HALLUCINATIONS; PCP.

National Institute on Drug Abuse. "High School and Youth Trends" in *NIDA InfoFacts.* Washington, D.C.: National Institutes of Health, January 2004.

Office of Applied Studies, Substance Abuse and Mental Health Services Administration (SAMHSA). "Racial and Ethnic Differences in Youth Hallucinogen Use" in *The NHSDA Report.* Rockville, Md.: SAMHSA, August 15, 2003.

Substance Abuse and Mental Health Services Administration (SAMHSA), Office of Applied Studies. *Emergency Department Trends from the Drug Abuse Warning Network, Final Estimates 1995–2002.* Rockville, Md.: DAWN Series: D-24, DHHS Publication No. (SMA) 03-3780, Rockville, Md.: SAMHSA, July 2003.

lung cancer   A malignant tumor in the lungs, most often caused by many years of smoking cigarettes. Experts estimate that about 90 percent of all cases of lung cancer are caused by smoking. Other less common causes of lung cancer are asbestos exposure or exposure to other industrial toxins, tuberculosis, metastatic cancer from other areas of the body, or a prior occurrence of lung cancer.

According to the authors of an annual report on cancer, published in the *Journal of the National Cancer Institute* in 2003, the prevalence of smoking in 2001 was highest in Kentucky (30.9 percent) and was lowest in Utah (13.3 percent). The authors said, "Lung cancer deaths were lowest in Utah, the state with the lowest adult smoking prevalence, and highest in Kentucky, the state with the highest adult smoking prevalence."

Lung cancer is the leading cause of cancer deaths. Cancer is the second leading cause of death in the United States, after heart disease. In 2004, the American Cancer Society estimated that 91,930 men and 68,510 women would die of lung cancer in 2004. African Americans with lung cancer have a higher death rate than whites, or 66.4 deaths per 100,000 African Americans compared with 56.7 deaths per 100,000 for whites, although the reason for this difference is unknown.

The American Cancer Society estimated that about 93,000 new cases of lung cancer in men and 81,000 new cases in women would be diagnosed in 2004. The survival rate after five years from the diagnosis of lung cancer is only about 14 percent. Many patients are not diagnosed until they are already in the late stages of the disease.

Lung cancer is also the leading cause of cancer deaths in Canada. According to the National Cancer Institute of Canada, an estimated 18,800 people died of lung cancer in 2003, including 10,900 men and 7,900 women.

There are two main types of lung cancer: nonsmall cell lung cancer (which is the more common form) and small cell lung cancer. Small cell lung cancer is more dangerous and aggressive than nonsmall lung cancer.

Risk Factors for Developing Lung Cancer

Although adults of any age can contract lung cancer, those who are the most at risk are as follows:

- People who were exposed to high-risk substances such as asbestos at work and who also smoke
- African-American men
- Males over age 60
- People who have smoked a pack or more of cigarettes a day for 20 years or more
- People exposed to smoke from other smokers

Symptoms of Lung Cancer

Most people with lung cancer have symptoms of the disease, although they may not consider their symptoms as serious or see the doctor until they become very ill. Some key symptoms of lung cancer are:

- A chronic cough
- Chronic chest pain
- Vomiting of blood
- Bloody or rust-colored spit
- Constant shortness of breath or hoarseness
- Frequent infections with pneumonia or bronchitis
- Facial or neck swelling
- Appetite loss and weight loss
- Chronic fatigue

Other diseases may also cause these symptoms. Only a physician can accurately determine whether or not a person has lung cancer.

Diagnosis and Treatment

If doctors suspect the presence of lung cancer, they employ various tests to determine the diagnosis. First, the doctor may order a chest X-ray, computerized tomography (CT) scan, or magnetic resonance imaging (MRI) scan of the chest to determine if any mass is on the lung. An analysis of the sputum (spit) may also be performed. Three samples of morning sputum can be analyzed to determine if cancer cells are present.

The doctor may also order a test that employs the use of a bronchoscope, which is a device that is inserted into the breathing passages to inspect them. The patient is sedated during this procedure. This bronchoscopy also allows the doctor to collect tissue samples for a biopsy. The biopsy determines if cancer is present.

Biopsy tissue can also be removed with a needle that is inserted directly into the chest.

The doctor may perform a bone scan to determine if cancer has advanced into the bones. A CT scan or MRI scan may also provide further information to the doctor that will help with diagnosis. A special procedure called a mediastinoscopy can determine whether cancer is present in the lymph nodes of the neck. An incision is required for this procedure, which is performed under anesthesia.

Once cancer is identified, it is staged. This means that the doctor determines how advanced the cancer is and whether it has spread to other parts of the body, such as the bones or lymph nodes. This staging is important in order to help the doctor determine the best treatment for the individual patient.

Anyone diagnosed with lung cancer must stop smoking immediately and permanently in order to improve their survival odds and lengthen their lives. (All others are also well advised to quit smoking, to avoid developing lung cancer and other smoking-related cancers and illnesses in the future.)

In many cases, surgery will be recommended for patients with lung cancer. The surgeon will remove all or part of the lung under a general anesthesia while the patient is in the hospital. Sometimes surgery cannot be done because reaching the tumor is too difficult or the patient is too ill to undergo surgery. Surgery for lung cancer is a major procedure, and most patients need weeks and sometimes months to recover.

If the tumor is very small (less than 4–5 centimeters), some surgeons may use video-assisted thoracic surgery to remove the tumor. This procedure uses a tiny camera to enable the surgeon to see the tumor. This procedure should be done only by a very experienced and specially trained surgeon because it is technically more difficult than removing all or part of the lung.

Radiation therapy may be recommended. In most cases, the patient receives radiation from a special machine that irradiates the cancerous area. Radiation therapy for lung cancer may cause a sore throat, trouble with swallowing, tiredness, and appetite loss.

Chemotherapy is another treatment option for patients with lung cancer. Cancer-killing drugs are introduced into the body intravenously or with a catheter. Some oral anticancer drugs are also available. Chemotherapy often causes nausea, fatigue, and hair loss, among other side effects.

Cryosurgery is another option sometimes used to treat nonsmall cell lung cancer. In this procedure, the area that includes the cancer cells is frozen so that they are destroyed.

See also CANCER; EMPHYSEMA; ORAL CANCER; SECONDHAND SMOKE; SMOKING, CIGARETTE; SMOKING AND HEALTH PROBLEMS.

For further information on lung cancer or other forms of cancer, contact the following organizations:

American Cancer Society
1599 Clifton Road NE
Atlanta, GA 30329
(800) 227-2345 (toll-free) or (404) 320-3333
http://www.cancer.org

National Cancer Institute
Division of Cancer Epidemiology and Genetics
6120 Executive Boulevard, MSC-7234
Executive Plaza South, 7th Floor
Rockville, MD 20852
(301) 496-1691

Weir, Hannah K., et al. "Annual Report to the Nation on the Status of Cancer, 1975–2000, Featuring the Uses of Surveillance Data for Cancer Prevention and Control," *Journal of the National Cancer Institute* 95, no. 17 (September 3, 2003): 1,276–1,299.

marijuana Plant-based drug that is illegal to use in the United States, although some states have passed laws allowing for the medicinal use of marijuana in some patients. Heavy users of marijuana may develop an addiction to the drug, experiencing withdrawal symptoms when they do not use marijuana. As of this writing, the federal DRUG ENFORCEMENT ADMINISTRATION does not acknowledge or accept the validity of these laws. Thus marijuana continues to be classified as a Schedule I drug nationwide under the CONTROLLED SUBSTANCES ACT. In 2005, the U.S. Supreme Court held in *Gonzales v. Raich* that the federal Controlled Substances Act can be enforced despite some state laws allowing marijuana to be prescribed by doctors for patients with medical problems. Patients who use "medical marijuana" include those with cancer, severe chronic back pain, muscle spasms due to multiple sclerosis, and other painful conditions. Angel Raich, a California woman, challenged the federal law, and she lost her case. The ruling has broad implications because several states, including Alaska, California, Colorado, Hawaii, Maine, Montana, Nevada, Oregon, and Washington, have laws on medical marijuana. It is possible that the U.S. Congress may enact a law allowing the use of medical marijuana, but as of this writing, such a law has not been passed.

The U.S. Supreme Court ruling does not invalidate existing medical marijuana laws in the states that have them. The ruling does state, however, that people who smoke marijuana can be prosecuted under federal laws, despite state laws on medical marijuana. After the Supreme Court decision, some doctors said they would no longer write authorizations for marijuana until they determined the effect of the Supreme Court ruling. Most arrests for medical marijuana have occurred in California.

The key psychoactive ingredient in marijuana is a chemical called tetrahydrocannabinol (THC), which is the ingredient responsible for its intoxicating effects. THC is most appropriately described as a hallucinogen. In the mid-1970s, the THC level of most marijuana was about 1 percent. In 2002, the level is greater than 6 percent. Thus the marijuana of the 21st century is far more potent than the drug experienced by some middle-aged or older Americans when they used marijuana in their youth.

Cannabis is a term that applies to marijuana as well as other drugs that come from the same plant, *Cannabis sativa.* Another form of cannabis is sinsemilla, which may have 9 percent THC or as high as 25 percent THC. Sinsemilla is made from the buds and flowering tips of the plants. HASHISH is a strong form of cannabis. It contains from 9 percent to as high as 19 percent THC.

Marijuana is a drug that is primarily smoked, either in rolled-up cigarette papers (referred to as a joint) or in a pipe. A bong is a water pipe that is used to smoke marijuana. Some users smoke crack cocaine that is mixed with the marijuana. Marijuana can also be eaten. Traces of the drug (metabolites) usually stay in the body for several days. However, heavy users of marijuana may have traces of the drug in their bodies for weeks after they have ceased using marijuana.

Users of Marijuana

Marijuana is the most commonly used illegal drug among youths and adults and is used by an estimated 75 percent of all illegal drug users. An estimated 4 million youths in the United States (16 percent of all youths), ages 12–17, reported using marijuana in the past year in 2002. Of all the youths ages 12–17 years who were in drug treatment in 2000, about 62 percent had a primary marijuana

PERCENTAGES OF MARIJUANA USE IN LIFETIME AMONG PERSONS AGES 12 TO 17 YEARS AND PERSONS AGES 18 TO 25 YEARS, DURING THE YEARS 1992 TO 2002, BY GENDER, UNITED STATES.

	Ages 12 to 17 Years			Ages 18 to 25 Years		
Year	Total	Male	Female	Total	Male	Female
1992	11.8	14.1	9.7	44.5	49.4	39.6
1993	12.4	14.6	10.3	43.4	48.4	38.6
1994	13.9	15.6	12.1	43.5	48.4	38.6
1995	16.4	18.1	14.6	44.1	48.0	40.3
1996	17.9	19.5	16.3	44.3	48.3	40.4
1997	18.6	19.6	17.5	45.7	49.8	41.9
1998	19.9	21.4	18.3	47.0	51.0	43.2
1999	19.7	21.4	18.0	50.3	54.1	46.6
2000	20.4	22.2	18.6	51.8	54.9	48.7
2001	21.9	23.1	20.7	53.0	56.4	49.7
2002	20.6	21.5	19.7	53.8	56.2	51.3

Source: Office of Applied Studies, Substance Abuse and Mental Health Services Administration (SAMHSA), *Results from the 2002 National Survey on Drug Use and Health: National Findings,* Table 4.58B National Survey on Drug Use and Health Series: H-22. Rockville, Md.: SAMHSA, September 2003. Available online at URL: http://www.oas.samhsa.gov/nhsda/2k2nsduh/html/Sect4peTabs1to76.htm#tab4.46a, downloaded January 15, 2004.

diagnosis. Approximately half of them were referred to treatment from the criminal justice system, and the other half were referred from other sources.

According to the *2002 National Survey on Drug Use and Health,* there were 14.6 million marijuana users of all ages in 2002. Of these individuals, 4.8 million were heavy users and reported using marijuana for 20 or more days in a month. There were about 2.6 million new marijuana users in 2002.

Males generally use marijuana more than females. For example, in 2002, 56.2 percent of males 18–25 years old had ever used marijuana compared with 51.3 percent of females of the same age. (See table above.)

Most people obtain their marijuana from a friend, whether they receive it for free or they purchase the drug. The National Survey on Drug Use and Health found that 79 percent of marijuana users received the drug at no cost from a friend and 81.8 percent purchased their marijuana from a friend.

Most young marijuana users (about 56 percent) who purchased marijuana bought it inside their own home or dormitory, although 9 percent of youths bought their marijuana on school property.

Marijuana use has somewhat declined among youths ages 12–17, from 21.9 percent who had ever used marijuana in 2001 to 20.6 percent in 2002. However, among young adults ages 18–25, the rate slightly increased from 53.0 percent in 2001 to 53.8 percent in 2002.

Delivery of Marijuana

Most of the marijuana used by people in the United States is smuggled in from Mexico, but some enters from Canada and from the Caribbean. Marijuana is usually transported for sale by criminal organizations, outlaw motorcycle gangs, and independent smugglers for profit. Some marijuana is also smuggled from Colombia and Jamaica, particularly marijuana that is transported to be sold to users on the East Coast of the United States.

The primary areas for receiving marijuana for resale in the United States, according to the National Drug Intelligence Center, are central Arizona; Chicago, Illinois; Los Angeles, California; Miami, Florida; New York City, New York; and Seattle, Washington. Other areas that receive large quantities of marijuana are Dallas and Houston, Texas, and San Diego, California.

Use of Marijuana and Other Drugs

Individuals who use marijuana are more likely to use other addictive substances, such as tobacco, alcohol, and illegal drugs. Although much maligned, the gateway theory does appear to have some validity. This is the theory that users of marijuana will become bored with the drug and seek greater thrills by using cocaine, heroin, and other illegal drugs.

A second theory is that individuals who use marijuana have less resistance to trying or using other illegal drugs. Of course, not everyone who uses marijuana starts using other illegal drugs. However, using the drug does increase the risk for such behavior.

According to the Office of National Drug Control Policy, adults who used marijuana as youths were found to be eight times more likely to use cocaine and 15 times more likely to use heroin than non-users.

Early Use of Marijuana Is Predictive of Later Use

In one unique study of 311 monozygotic (identical) and dizygotic (nonidentical) twins in Australia, the researchers analyzed the risk of using illegal drugs as adults in individuals who started using cannabis (marijuana) by the age of 17 years. The researchers found that when only one twin used marijuana as an adolescent, that twin had about a twofold to sixfold increased risk of using illegal drugs or having an alcoholism problem as an adult compared with the twin who did not abuse marijuana as an adolescent. This was true whether the twins were identical or not.

Effects and Risks of Marijuana Use

Marijuana has an intoxicating effect on the user, which is the key reason why it is used. Regular users of marijuana may develop bronchitis and poor lung function. They may also develop problems with short-term thinking and memory, which is one of the reasons why students who start using marijuana usually experience a significant drop in their school performance and their grades. In addition, regular users may develop an increased heart rate and even have a doubling of their normal rate. They may also experience panic attacks and anxiety attacks.

Marijuana impairs alertness and concentration, and thus users of the drug should not drive. A study of reckless drivers in the United States revealed that about a third of the subjects who were not under the influence of alcohol tested positive for marijuana use.

Because marijuana contains NICOTINE, experts believe that it causes lung cancer. However, many marijuana users also smoke cigarettes, according to the National Institute on Drug Abuse. Teenage tobacco smokers are 14 times likelier to try marijuana than those who have never smoked (84 percent v. 6 percent). In addition, a majority (57 percent) of teenagers who have tried marijuana smoked cigarettes first. As a result, isolating the carcinogenic effect of marijuana from the effect of cigarettes has been impossible. However, it is known that marijuana smokers are prone to lung infections, and long-term use increases the risk of chronic cough, bronchitis, and EMPHYSEMA.

Because marijuana lowers inhibitions, users are more likely to engage in risky sexual behavior. Marijuana users are more likely to have multiple sexual partners and to fail to engage in safe sex.

Chronic marijuana users may develop problems with DEPRESSION and ANXIETY DISORDERS. However, whether the marijuana causes mood disorders or if it is used more frequently by individuals who are already depressed, anxious, and unconsciously seeking to self-medicate their distressing emotions is unclear. As with the use of other hallucinogens, heavy users of marijuana can also develop psychotic disorders. In individuals who are already severely mentally ill, such as those with SCHIZOPHRENIA, marijuana can exacerbate psychotic symptoms.

Effects on Children of Users

Marijuana can be harmful to the developing fetus. Some studies have shown that children of mothers who smoked marijuana during their pregnancy had greater attention and behavioral problems in their preschool and early school years.

Marijuana also affects the nursing baby, and THC is heavily concentrated in the breast milk. Some experts report that marijuana use in the first month of pregnancy can impede the muscle movement of the newborn infant.

Law Enforcement

Using marijuana is illegal in the United States. However, most drug arrests are for selling the drug rather than for using it. An estimated 98 percent of about 8,000 offenders sentenced for marijuana crimes were found guilty of trafficking (selling) the drug rather than using it. Many states and localities treat marijuana use as a misdemeanor offense, for which the violator must pay a fine. However, law enforcement agencies regard selling marijuana in a much more serious way. Unfortunately, people who use marijuana on a regular basis have an increased likelihood of selling the drug as well.

According to the National Drug Threat Assessment 2003, published by the National Drug Intelligence Center, 97.1 percent of all federal sentences for marijuana were for selling marijuana. Of course, states and cities have their own laws against marijuana use too, and thus marijuana users may be arrested for violating the laws of the state or city even if they are not arrested for a federal offense.

Marijuana and Delinquent Behavior

Youths ages 12–17 years who use marijuana have twice the risk of stealing, destroying property, or attacking others as do nonmarijuana users of the same age. The frequency of delinquent acts increases with the frequency of marijuana use. For example, when considering youths who had not used marijuana in the past year, 18.2 percent of this group had engaged in serious fighting at school or work. If the individual used marijuana on one to 11 days in the past year, the percentage of fighting rose to 25.5 percent. Among those individuals who used marijuana on 300 or more days in the past year, 42.2 percent of this group had engaged in serious fighting.

There is also an increased risk for selling illegal drugs with the use of marijuana among youths. For example, among youths who had not used marijuana in the past year, less than 1 percent sold illegal drugs. Among individuals who used marijuana on from one to 11 occasions, the percentage of those selling illegal drugs rose to 6 percent. Among those who used marijuana for 300 or more days in the past year, the majority (57.3 percent) were selling illegal drugs. (See figure below.) The numbers of thefts or attempted thefts rose with marijuana use, to a high of 31.7 percent among heavy marijuana users. (See figure on page 161.)

PERCENTAGES OF YOUTHS AGES 12 TO 17 WHO SOLD ILLEGAL DRUGS IN THE PAST YEAR, BY FREQUENCY OF PAST-YEAR MARIJUANA USE: 2002

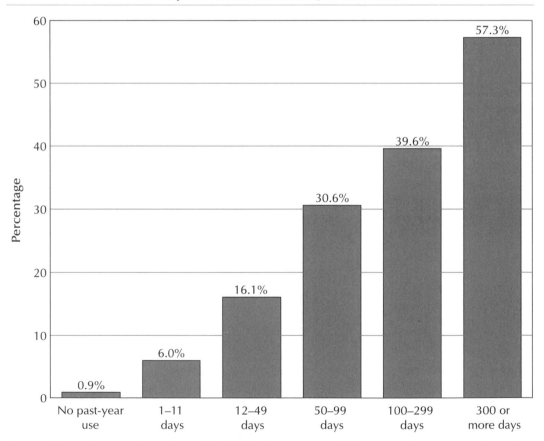

Source: National Survey on Drug Use and Health, "Marijuana Use and Delinquent Behaviors Among Youths," *The NSDUH Report*. Rockville, Md.: Office of Applied Studies, Substance Abuse and Mental Health Services Administration, January 9, 2004.

PERCENTAGES OF YOUTHS AGES 12 TO 17 WHO STOLE OR TRIED TO STEAL ANYTHING WORTH MORE THAN $50 IN THE PAST YEAR, BY FREQUENCY OF PAST YEAR MARIJUANA USE, 2002

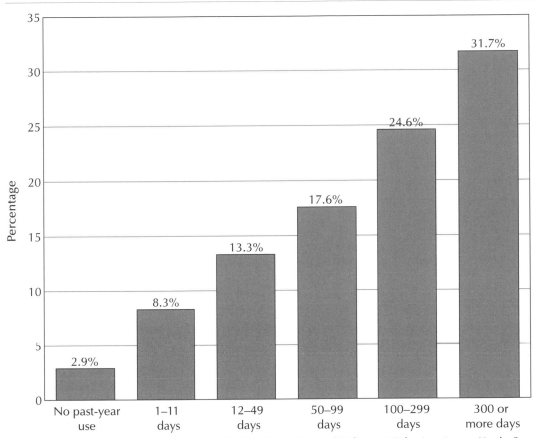

Source: National Survey on Drug Use and Health, "Marijuana Use and Delinquent Behaviors Among Youths," *The NSDUH Report*. Rockville, Md.: Office of Applied Studies, Substance Abuse and Mental Health Services Administration, January 9, 2004.

The percentage of youths who attacked someone with the intent to hurt them rose with increased marijuana use. For example, among youths age 12–17 years old who had not used marijuana in the past year, about 6 percent had attacked someone. When marijuana was used from one to 11 times in the past year, the attack percentage increased to about 11 percent. Among youths using marijuana for 300 or more days in the past year, about 33 percent had attacked someone. (See figure on page 162.) The common belief about marijuana is that users of this drug are peaceful and nonviolent. The statistics prove that this belief is false.

The pattern of increased risk of delinquent behaviors also continued with youths stealing items valued at more than $50, those who took part in a group-against-group (gang) fights, and those who carried handguns. (See figure on page 162.) For example, about 3 percent of youths who had not used marijuana carried handguns. With marijuana use of 300 or more days, 22 percent of youths carried handguns. (See figure on page 163.)

Treatment for Marijuana Abuse or Addiction
Patients who are treated for the chronic abuse of marijuana and/or addiction can recover with hard

PERCENTAGES OF YOUTHS AGES 12 TO 17 WHO ATTACKED SOMEONE WITH THE INTENT TO SERIOUSLY HURT THEM IN THE PAST YEAR, BY FREQUENCY OF PAST YEAR MARIJUANA USE: 2002

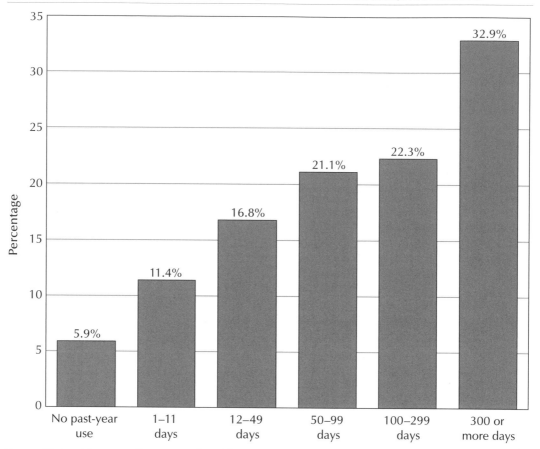

Source: National Survey on Drug Use and Health, "Marijuana Use and Delinquent Behaviors Among Youths," *The NSDUH Report*. Rockville, Md.: Office of Applied Studies, Substance Abuse and Mental Health Services Administration, January 9, 2004.

work. According to the Drug and Alcohol Services Information System in *The DASIS Report,* researchers analyzed the treatment outcomes for 117,000 patients nationwide. Patients received treatment for a variety of addiction problems, including alcohol, opiates, cocaine, marijuana/hashish, and stimulants. The outpatient treatment completion rate was the highest for patients whose problem was with alcohol (41 percent), followed by marijuana (32 percent).

See also DRUG COURTS; SMOKING, CIGARETTE.

Drug and Alcohol Services Information System. "Discharges from Outpatient Treatment: 2000," *The DASIS Report*. Rockville, Md.: Office of Applied Studies, Substance Abuse and Mental Health Services Administration, (November 21, 2003). Available online. URL: http://www.oas.samhsa.gov/2k3/outpatientDischarges/outpatientDischarges.htm. Accessed on January 30, 2004.

Gfoerer, Joseph C., Li-Tzy Wu, and Michael Penne. *Initiation of Marijuana Use: Trends, Patterns, and Implications*. Rockville, Md.: Substance Abuse and Mental Health Services Administration, Office of Applied Studies, July 2002.

Lynskey, Michael T., et al. "Escalation of Drug Use in Early-Onset Cannabis Users vs. Co-twin Controls," *Journal of the American Medical Association* 289, no. 4 (January 22/29, 2003): 427–433.

PERCENTAGES OF YOUTHS AGES 12 TO 17 WHO CARRIED A HANDGUN IN THE PAST YEAR, BY FREQUENCY OF PAST YEAR MARIJUANA USE: 2002

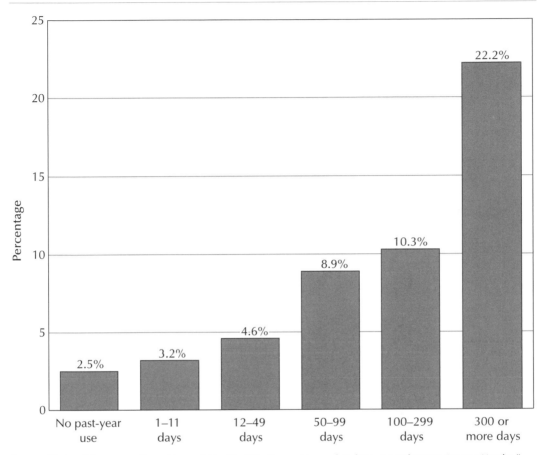

Source: National Survey on Drug Use and Health, "Marijuana Use and Delinquent Behaviors Among Youths," *The NSDUH Report*. Rockville, Md.: Office of Applied Studies, Substance Abuse and Mental Health Services Administration, January 9, 2004.

National Drug Intelligence Center. *National Drug Threat Assessment 2003*. U.S. Department of Justice (DOJ) Product No. 2003-Q0317-001. Washington, D.C.: DOJ, January 2003.

National Institute on Drug Abuse (NIDA). *Marijuana: Facts Parents Need to Know*. National Institutes of Health, NIH Publication No. 02-4036. Washington, D.C.: NIDA, 2002.

National Survey on Drug Use and Health. "Marijuana Use and Delinquent Behaviors Among Youths," *The NSDUH Report* (January 9, 2004). Available online. URL: http://www.oas.samhsa.gov/2k4/MJdelinquency/MJdelinquency.pdf. Accessed on March 16, 2004.

Office of National Drug Control Policy. *What Americans Need to Know about Marijuana: Important Facts About Our Nation's Most Misunderstood Illegal Drug*. Washington, D.C.: Office of the President, 2003.

Master Settlement Agreement (MSA) A pact made in 1998 between the major tobacco companies and the attorneys general in 46 states in the United States, the District of Columbia, and the five U.S. territories to settle lawsuits filed by states throughout the United States against the tobacco companies.

In 1994, the attorney general of Mississippi, Michael Moore, and the attorney general of Minnesota, Hubert Humphrey III, had both filed lawsuits against the large tobacco companies in order to recover the state costs of Medicaid to patients with tobacco-related illnesses. By 1996, every state had filed a lawsuit against the tobacco companies.

In 1997, a global settlement was proposed to Congress, but Congress failed to implement the legislation sponsored by Senator John McCain (R-Arizona). In 1998, the attorneys general of the 46 states that had not settled with the tobacco companies did reach agreement, which was the MSA. This agreement did not require congressional approval.

The MSA does not stipulate how the money from the tobacco companies is to be spent. According to Dr. Schroeder in his article in the *New England Journal of Medicine* in 2004, "In the current climate of fiscal crises, the MSA funds have become an irresistible target from the perspective of state policymakers to help address budget deficits and avert new taxes. In many states, important tobacco-control activities—such as the landmark antismoking programs in Minnesota, Massachusetts, and Florida—are being dismantled. For example, in 2003 state antitobacco budgets were slashed by 99 percent in Florida and by 92 percent in Massachusetts. Even before the current fiscal crisis, less than 5 percent of state funds from the MSA was spent on tobacco control, and some states spent essentially nothing." The MSA allows for payment from the tobacco companies of nearly $206 billion spread out to the year 2025. (Florida, Minnesota, Mississippi, and Texas had previously made separate settlements with the tobacco industry.)

The MSA has a variety of stipulations, including the restriction against advertising that targets individuals under the age of 18 years old. For example, the R. J. Reynolds company agreed to stop using cartoons to advertise their products, and the MSA specifically prohibits the use of Joe Camel, the cartoon character. In addition, the tobacco companies agreed to stop using most outdoor billboard advertisements, strictly limit brand-name sponsorships of events (such as sporting events, concerts, and so forth) to one per manufacturer, end the sale of merchandise with brand names on it (such as T-shirts and hats with tobacco company names on them), and other provisions.

One of the stated goals of the MSA was that states would spend at least some of the funds they received on tobacco control programs. In one analysis of how the tobacco settlement funds have been spent so far, reported in 2002 in the *New England Journal of Medicine*, researchers found that very little of the settlement money had been spent on tobacco control programs and that, in fact, only six states—Arizona, Massachusetts, Hawaii, Vermont, Mississippi and Maine—had exceeded the nationwide average per capita recommendation made by the Centers for Disease Control and Prevention of $7.47.

Instead, the actual nationwide average per capita funding was $3.59 per person, ranging from spending lows of $0.10 in Pennsylvania and $0.13 per person in Ohio to highs of $12.82 in Mississippi per person and $15.47 per capita in Maine.

The CDC had set desired expenditure goals for each state; for example, the per capita spending goal set for Pennsylvania was $5.46 per person, compared to the 10 cents per person that was actually spent in Pennsylvania on tobacco control programs. The goal for Ohio was $5.52 per person for tobacco control programs, compared to the 13 cents per capita that was actually spent. However, since the MSA did not stipulate how the funds were to be spent, states made their own decisions.

Researchers found that of the $6.5 billion settlement funds distributed in 2001, only about 6 percent actually was spent on tobacco control programs. The rest of the money had gone to health care (41 percent), long-term care (3 percent), a category called other (40 percent), aid to tobacco-growing communities (5 percent), and research (4 percent). The researchers also found that 20 states invested the settlement money in trust funds.

In general, the researchers found that the states with the highest smoking rates (which were also often states that were tobacco producing) had the lowest expenditures on tobacco control programs.

The researchers concluded, "State health needs appear to have little effect on the funding of state tobacco-control programs. Because only a very small proportion of the tobacco settlement is being used for tobacco-control programs, the settlement represents an unrealized opportunity to reduce morbidity [illness] and mortality [death] from smoking."

See also SMOKING AND HEALTH PROBLEMS; SMOKING, CIGARETTE.

Gross, Cary P., M.D., et al. "State Expenditures for Tobacco-Control Programs and the Tobacco Settlement," *New England Journal of Medicine* 347, no. 14 (October 8, 2002): 1,080–1,086.

Schoeder, Steven A., M.D. "Tobacco Control in the Wake of the 1998 Master Settlement Agreement," *New England Journal of Medicine* 350, no. 3 (January 15, 2004): 293–301.

MDMA (methylenedioxymethamphetamine)
See ECSTASY.

mental illness/psychiatric problems   Serious problems with thinking and behavior, such as BIPOLAR DISORDER, DEPRESSION, ANXIETY DISORDER, OBSESSIVE-COMPULSIVE DISORDER, SCHIZOPHRENIA, or other illnesses that make it difficult and sometimes impossible for the individual to function normally in society.

Mentally ill people are at greater risk for abusing drugs and alcohol than their peers without mental illness. Addictive substances, including some prescribed drugs, illegal drugs, or alcohol, may sometimes trigger or exacerbate psychiatric symptoms.

See also AMPHETAMINE PSYCHOSIS; ATTENTION DEFICIT HYPERACTIVITY DISORDER; BENZODIAZEPINES; COCAINE; DUAL DIAGNOSIS; GAMBLING, PATHOLOGICAL; HOMELESSNESS; IMPULSE CONTROL DISORDER; IMPULSIVITY; MOODS; MOOD STABILIZERS; POSTTRAUMATIC STRESS DISORDER; PSYCHIATRIC MEDICATIONS; PSYCHIATRISTS.

methadone   A synthetically made narcotic used to treat individuals addicted to HEROIN as well as some patients who have developed an addiction to oxycodone, especially OXYCONTIN, Percodan, and Percocet. There are alternative treatments for opiate addiction, such as BUPRENORPHINE or levomethadyl acetate. Some patients with severe chronic pain take methadone that is prescribed for PAIN MANAGEMENT.

Methadone comes in tablet, oral, or injectable liquid forms. It has been available in the United States since 1947. It is a Schedule II drug under the CONTROLLED SUBSTANCES ACT. It is considered to have a high potential for abuse. Other Schedule II drugs are COCAINE and METHAMPHETAMINE.

Heroin and opiate addicts can obtain methadone legally in a controlled program through a physician. It can suppress withdrawal symptoms from opiates for about 24 hours, and it does not provide the euphoric rush that heroin gives to users. Most patients receive the drug on a daily basis, although some patients are given take-home doses for a longer period. According to the National Drug Intelligence Center, treatment programs are allowed to dispense up to a 30-day supply of methadone to long-term patients. One problem is that some methadone patients illegally sell the drug.

methadone as a drug of abuse   Some individuals obtain methadone illegally and abuse the drug, causing serious health risks. The Drug Abuse and Warning Network reported that methadone was involved in nearly 11,000 emergency room visits in 2001, which was a 37 percent increase from the number reported in 2000. Some states have also found an increased rate of death from illicit methadone use. For example, in Florida, drug-related deaths involving methadone increased from 357 deaths in 2001 to 556 deaths in 2002, a 56 percent increase and a greater percentage increase than for any other drug.

According to the National Drug Intelligence Center, some users take dangerously high doses of methadone in an attempt to attain the euphoric rush. How much methadone is taken does not matter, it will never provide the euphoria that heroin gives users. However, these illegal high doses may cause an OVERDOSE. Symptoms of a methadone overdose include severe respiratory depression, decreased heart rate and blood pressure, and, in the worst cases, coma and death.

Efficacy of Methadone
Methadone has been found to be an effective drug to treat individuals addicted to heroin and other opiates. It does not cure them of their dependency on opiate drugs but can prevent addicts from taking more dangerous drugs, such

as heroin and opiates. Administering methadone to addicted individuals is also less costly than the expenses that would be incurred in incarcerating addicts for crimes they committed to obtain drugs illegally.

Another reason that methadone is used is that it has a very long duration of action, unlike opiates such as heroin or oxycodone. Opiate addicts frequently require multiple doses of opiates each day. In contrast, methadone can be used once daily with durable effect. This same advantage can also complicate withdrawal in patients who are addicted to methadone because methadone symptoms can persist far longer than is commonly seen with withdrawal from heroin or oxycodone.

In a study reported in a 2000 issue of the *New England Journal of Medicine,* researchers did a 17-week randomized study of 220 patients, placing them on levomethadyl acetate (75–115 mg), buprenorphine (16–32 mg), low-dose methadone (20 mg), or high-dose methadone (60 to 100 mg). They found that high-dose methadone, levomethadyl acetate, and buprenorphine all had a major effect in reducing the use of opioid drugs. Low-dose methadone, however, was not as effective.

Concluded the researchers, "As compared with low-dose methadone, levomethadyl acetate produced the longest duration of continuous abstinence; buprenorphine administered three times weekly was similar to that of levomethadyl acetate in terms of study retention and was similar to high-dose methadone in terms of abstinence."

Side Effects

Patients taking methadone may experience some side effects, such as dizziness, sedation, constipation, and nausea.

Counseling Is Important

Studies of patients taking methadone have shown that the combination of methadone and counseling was more effective in reducing opiate use than taking methadone alone.

Methadone for Pain Management

In recent years, methadone has also been used to treat patients with chronic severe pain who have never been addicted to heroin or other illegal drugs in the past.

Methadone is far less expensive than some pain medications, such as OxyContin, and it may be as efficacious in combating pain. However, the social stigma against taking methadone remains strong. Many people with chronic pain are resistant to taking methadone, fearing that others will think that they are drug addicts rather than using the drug as a pain medication.

See also DETOXIFICATION; OPIATES; PAIN MANAGEMENT CENTERS.

For further information on methadone, contact the following organization:

National Drug Intelligence Center
319 Washington Street
Fifth Floor
Johnstown, PA 15901
(814) 532-4601
http://www.usdoj.gov/ndic

Johnson, Rolley E., et al. "A Comparison of Levomethadyl Acetate, Buprenorphine, and Methadone for Opioid Dependence," *New England Journal of Medicine* 343, no. 18 (November 2, 2000): 1,290–1,297.

National Drug Intelligence Center. "Methadone Abuse Increasing." *Information Bulletin,* Product no. 2003-L0424-004. Washington, D.C.: U.S. Department of Justice, 2003.

methamphetamine A humanmade stimulant that is addictive to the central nervous system and is derived from AMPHETAMINE. Methamphetamine abuse and addiction is a problem in the United States and in many other countries worldwide. For example, according to a 2003 issue of the *Lancet,* in Thailand about 800 million tablets of "yaba" (a Thai word meaning crazy medicine) are consumed each year, making Thailand the world's largest per capita consumer of methamphetamine. In some psychiatric hospitals in Thailand, 30–50 percent of the beds are taken by patients with methamphetamine psychosis. This is a problem against which the Thai government is actively working to combat.

Methamphetamine is a Schedule II drug under the CONTROLLED SUBSTANCES ACT of 1970, and thus it is considered a drug with a high potential for abuse. Other Schedule II drugs include COCAINE and OxyContin. Methamphetamine can be detected in the urine if DRUG TESTING is ordered by a court, as a requirement to obtain a job, or is performed for another purpose.

Illegally used methamphetamine can be taken orally, nasally, by smoking, or by injecting the drug. It comes in a powder that resembles crystals. When it appears in a rock form, some individuals refer to the drug as crank, ice or crystal meth, and it is smoked or injected.

Lawful Medical Uses

Methamphetamine has some legitimate medical uses in the United States, such as when it is prescribed for the treatment of narcolepsy or ATTENTION DEFICIT HYPERACTIVITY DISORDER. For example, Desoxyn (methamphetamine tablets) are prescribed to some patients to treat their attention deficit hyperactivity disorder. In those cases of medical therapies, the drug is made legally by pharmaceutical companies. Sometimes legally produced methamphetamine is illegally sold to others, such as when the prescribed drug is freely obtained from or sold by someone with a prescription or the medication is stolen from them.

Illegal Manufacturing of Methamphetamine

In cases in which methamphetamine is produced illegally for consumption in the United States, the drug is manufactured in clandestine laboratories within the United States or other countries, such as MEXICO, China, and Thailand.

Manufacturers use commonly available chemicals or even other drugs, such as over-the-counter cold remedies. These are called precursor chemicals. Manufacturing methamphetamine is a dangerous process because some of the chemicals used are highly volatile and even explosive as well as severely toxic to humans. Severe burns or death can result from manufacturing the drug in clandestine laboratories.

In 2000, the Methamphetamine Anti-Proliferation Act was passed by the federal government. This act provides for training to state and federal law enforcement officers on methamphetamine investigations and the chemicals used to create methamphetamine in clandestine laboratories.

Some states have passed laws trying to limit the illegal manufacture of methamphetamine in different ways. For example, in 2003, Indiana created a program to help retailers identify individuals who may be purchasing large quantities of common household chemicals in order to make illicit drugs. Retailers are given civil immunity if they make a good faith effort to report these sales to law enforcement personnel. In North Dakota, possession of more than 24 grams of a methamphetamine precursor is regarded as an intent to violate the controlled substance manufacturing laws of the state.

Because it is so dangerous, producing methamphetamine may also be regarded as a form of CHILD ABUSE. In some states (Alaska, Arizona, Colorado, Iowa, Minnesota, Montana, North Dakota, Utah, and Washington), manufacturing a controlled substance while a child is present is legally considered either child abuse or child endangerment.

Abusers of Methamphetamine

According to results from the *2002 National Survey on Drug Use and Health: National Findings,* more than 12 million people ages 12 and older in the United States have used methamphetamine at least once in their lifetime. About 597,000 people ages 12 and older (less than 1 percent of the population) said they had used methamphetamine in the past month in 2002. When considering high school students only, an estimated 4 percent of students in the 10th and 12th grades had used methamphetamine within the past year.

Most methamphetamine abusers in the United States are white or Hispanic males, although females and individuals of other races and ethnicities sometimes abuse methamphetamine. The drug is readily available in most regions of the United States. According to the 2004 National Drug Threat Assessment produced by the National Drug Intelligence Center, "Methamphetamine availability is very high in the Pacific, Southwest, and West Central regions. In the Great Lakes and Southeast regions, methamphetamine availability has increased to such a level that most state and local law enforcement agencies now report that availability of the drug is either high or moderate in their areas. Methamphetamine availability in the Northeast/Mid-Atlantic region is low but increasing."

Effects of Methamphetamine

Use of methamphetamine quickly gives the user a rush of energy and euphoria, and methamphetamine also decreases appetite. The injected or snorted (taken intranasally) forms of the drug work more rapidly than the oral tablets. When methamphetamine is taken orally, it takes about 20 minutes for the effects to be felt. When it is snorted, the effects occur in about five minutes. The effects of methamphetamine use may last for up to 12 hours.

Chronic use of methamphetamine can lead to auditory and visual HALLUCINATIONS. Insomnia is also a common problem. Paranoia and extreme rages may also occur, precipitating VIOLENCE. Some people suffer from the delusion that bugs are crawling under their skin, and they may develop body sores from their extreme scratching. If individuals use crystal methamphetamine, which is typically more pure and thus more powerful than the powdered form of methamphetamine, they risk developing psychotic symptoms that may persist for months or years after the drug has been used.

Hyperthermia (an excessively high body temperature) may occur after use, as may convulsions. If the patient is not treated, death can occur. According to the Drug Abuse Warning Network in the United States, 17,696 people nationwide sought emergency help because of a reaction to taking methamphetamine in 2002. A sharp upward trend occurred each year from 1999, when 10,447 emergency mentions were related to the abuse of methamphetamine.

The chronic use of methamphetamine can cause inflammation of the lining of the heart. If users inject the drug, they may damage their blood vessels and cause skin abscesses. Some users suffer from acute lead poisoning because many producers of methamphetamine use lead acetate as a reagent to make the drug.

Regular users of methamphetamine who inject the drug have an increased risk of contracting the human immunodeficiency virus as well as hepatitis B and C. In addition, they may develop pneumonia, tuberculosis, and diseases of the kidneys and the liver. Withdrawal symptoms from the drug may include DEPRESSION, paranoia, aggression, and fatigue as well as an intense CRAVING for more methamphetamine.

Treatment for Methamphetamine

Although no medications can directly treat methamphetamine addiction, such as ANTABUSE or NALTREXONE is used for alcoholism or METHADONE for heroin addiction, antidepressants are often used to combat the clinical depression that frequently occurs with withdrawal, and other medications are used to treat the symptoms of withdrawal from methamphetamine. Counseling is also an important treatment option for patients who are withdrawing from methamphetamine.

When patients present to the emergency room of a hospital with possible methamphetamine toxicity, they often require urgent treatment. In his Internet article, Dr. Robert Derlet, chief of emergency medicine at the University of California (Davis), described the diagnosis and treatment of individuals with suspected methamphetamine toxicity. (He also noted that children who present with first-time seizures to the emergency room should be evaluated for methamphetamine abuse.)

According to Dr. Derlet, patients who may have methamphetamine toxicity need a complete blood count and chemistry panel to evaluate their condition. In addition, he advised a computerized tomography scan of patients who presented to the emergency room with altered mental status in order to rule out intracranial bleeding. This type of bleeding could occur from methamphetamine-induced hypertension or from head trauma related to taking the drug. Patients should also have an electrocardiogram because of the cardiac risks associated with the drug.

Dr. Derlet advised droperidol or haloperidol, both antipsychotic medications, to treat hyperactivity or agitation. Sometimes BENZODIAZEPINES are used for these symptoms, although antipsychotics apparently work faster and more effectively. Benzodiazepines may be needed to terminate amphetamine-induced seizures. Other medications should be used to correct hypertension, hypotension, hyperthermia, and metabolic and electrolyte abnormalities.

See also AMPHETAMINE PSYCHOSIS; OVEREATING/OBESITY.

Khabir Ahmad. "Asia Grapples with Spreading Amphetamine Abuse," *The Lancet* 361, no. 9372 (May 31, 2003): 1,878–1,879.

National Drug Intelligence Center. *National Drug Threat Assessment 2004.* U.S. Department of Justice (DOJ) Product No. 2003-Q0317-001. Washington, D.C.: DOJ, April 2004.

Robert Darlet, M.D. "Toxicity, Methamphetamine," Available online. URL: http://www.emedecine.com/EMERG/topics859.htm. Accessed on April 26, 2004.

Sanchez, Devonne R., and Blake Harrison. "The Methamphetamine Menace," *Legisbrief* 12, no. 1 (January 2004): 1–2.

Mexico A country south of the United States and a major supplier of and conduit for illegal drugs that are transported into the United States. According to a country profile on Mexico published by the United Nations Office on Drugs and Crime in 2003, "Mexico has been important not only for cocaine consignments originating in Colombia, but also for home-produced cannabis [marijuana] and heroin, mainly to be sent to consumer markets in the United States of America and Canada."

A 2003 report from the DRUG ENFORCEMENT ADMINISTRATION (DEA) confirms the impact of Mexico on drug trafficking to the United States and says that about 70 percent of all the cocaine destined for the United States travels through the Mexico–Central America corridor. In addition, Mexico is the number one foreign supplier of marijuana to the United States and is also a major supplier of HEROIN and METHAMPHETAMINE.

One concern is that at least some of the Mexican methamphetamine is highly pure, which also means that it is a far more powerful drug than users may anticipate. For example, according to the DEA's Special Testing and Research Laboratory, the average purity for methamphetamine in the United States was 48 percent in 2003. In contrast, during the same period, methamphetamine seized from Mexico was 83 percent pure.

Mexico is also a source country for the illegal use of other drugs, such as OXYCONTIN, KETAMINE, ROHYPNOL, and ANABOLIC STEROIDS. According to the DEA, nearly all the opium that is converted to heroin in Mexico is destined for the United States.

Most of the marijuana and opium grown in Mexico is cultivated in the northern and western Sierra Madre states, particularly in the states of Chihuahua and Sinaloa. The Mexican government has an active program to seize illegal drugs as well as to eradicate drugs that are cultivated for illegal sales. According to the DEA's 2003 report, "The Mexican Government's eradication program is one of the largest and most aggressive in the world."

Despite these efforts, however, organized drug traffickers are still successful.

Drugs are smuggled out of Mexico in many different ways, including sometimes inside the bodies of humans. Some Mexican drug traffickers have created tunnels to transport illegal drugs into the United States. Tunnels from Mexico have been discovered in Arizona and California. These tunnels have ranged from very simple ones to those equipped with electricity, ventilation, and even rail systems.

It is believed that most of the illegal drugs sold from Mexico are managed by only a handful of organized crime syndicates. Despite numerous arrests of key people in these groups, the drug cartels continue to operate and are often violent. They are also involved with an associated criminal trafficking of humans, particularly females from Central America who are brought to the United States for PROSTITUTION. Drug-related crime is a serious problem in Mexico.

Drug Addiction in Mexico

In recent years, drug abuse and addiction have become an internal problem to Mexico as increasing numbers of Mexican citizens have abused and have become addicted to drugs. The government in Mexico is working to reduce the demand for illegal drugs among its citizens through prevention programs. In 2001, 86 committees against drug dependency were opened in cities in Mexico, for a total of 328 committees. Mexico's first lady Marta Sahagún de Fox led the opening of another 168 municipal centers in 2002. However, centers for drug treatment and rehabilitation are also available in Mexico.

See also COCAINE; COLOMBIA; ECSTASY; MARIJUANA; VIOLENCE.

Drug Enforcement Administration. *Mexico: Country Profile for 2003*, FRS-03047. Washington, D.C.: U.S. Department of Justice, November 2003.

United Nations Office on Drugs and Crime. "Mexico 2003: Country Profile," Available online. URL: http://www.unodc.org/pdf/mexico/country_profile_mexico.pdf. Accessed on March 29, 2005.

moods Overall feelings, such as general happiness, sadness, anxiety, and so forth. Addiction can affect moods in many ways. For example, the use of some addictive substances may cause depression or EUPHORIA. In addition, the deprivation of or the WITHDRAWAL from a substance to which a person is addicted can cause the person to feel anger, distress, panic, and many other emotions in addition to the physical symptoms that withdrawal can cause. Some people with addictive behaviors also have a mood disorder, such as clinical DEPRESSION, BIPOLAR DISORDER, an anxiety disorder, or other emotional disturbances.

See also ANXIETY DISORDERS; DUAL DIAGNOSIS; MOOD STABILIZERS; PSYCHIATRIC MEDICATIONS; PSYCHIATRISTS.

mood stabilizers Medications used to treat patients who experience extremes of moods, such as patients with BIPOLAR DISORDER. Studies have shown that individuals with bipolar disorder are more likely to abuse illegal drugs as well as to relapse after addiction treatment. With appropriate treatment, however, patients with mood disorders can significantly decrease their likelihood of relapse. Mood stabilizers are also being tested to assess their effect in preventing relapse in patients who do not have clear-cut affective (mood) disorders.

Typical mood stabilizers include drugs such as lithium carbonate or lithium citrate as well as many anticonvulsant medications that were originally used to treat seizure disorders. Valproate is an anticonvulsant drug that was approved by the Food and Drug Administration to treat the mania associated with bipolar disorder. Other antiseizure drugs used to treat bipolar disorder include carbamazepine (Tegretol) and gabapentin (Neurontin).

See also ANXIETY DISORDERS; DEPRESSION; DUAL DIAGNOSIS; MENTAL ILLNESS/PSYCHIATRIC PROBLEMS; MOODS; OBSESSIVE-COMPULSIVE DISORDER.

morphine An opiate painkiller used by some patients with advanced cancer or with intractable or severe chronic pain. Morphine, a SCHEDULED DRUG, is derived from the opium poppy and is a powerful anesthetic, although most anesthesiologists in the United States rely upon other more modern drugs. Elderly people may be particularly sensitive to the side effects from this drug, such as HALLUCINATIONS.

Patients who take morphine will build up a tolerance to the drug. Consequently, it should be taken only under the care of an experienced physician. If morphine is used illegally, patients can become addicted to the drug rapidly. Drugs such as morphine or any other scheduled drugs should never be purchased from others or through the Internet. Some individuals have died from taking drugs they purchased in this manner.

Morphine can be taken in an oral form. It is also given in the form of an injection. Some chronic pain patients use an implanted morphine pump in which the drug can be delivered directly into their bloodstream. Because of the nature of the delivery system, the drug delivered by a morphine pump is covered by Medicare.

Morphine was first manufactured as an anesthetic and/or a painkiller in the United States in 1832. During the Victorian era of the late 19th century, morphine use was commonplace. The drug was used or included in remedies to treat headaches, menstrual cramps, colic, diarrhea, and many other illnesses as an over-the-counter drug. At that time, many people self-medicated their illnesses and thus did not need a doctor's prescription for morphine or other drugs.

See also CONTROLLED SUBSTANCES ACT; HEROIN; NARCOTICS; OPIATES; PAIN; PAIN MANAGEMENT.

Meldrum, Marcia L. "A Capsule History of Pain Management," *Journal of the American Medical Association* 290, no. 18 (November 12, 2003): 2,470–2,475.

multiple addictions The presence of two or more addictions. Many addicted individuals are addicted to more than one substance. For example, most people who abuse alcohol and/or illegal drugs are also smokers. Individuals who use illegal drugs such as COCAINE or MARIJUANA are also often alcohol abusers. Treatment can be complicated for patients with multiple addictions. Experts may decide to concentrate on helping a patient deal with the one or two most destructive addictions, such as concentrating on the abuse of illegal drugs combined with alcohol abuse, while dealing with a nicotine addiction at a later date.

See also DUAL DIAGNOSIS.

mushrooms/psilocybin Specific mushrooms, such as *Psilocybe caerulipes* or *Psilocybe cubensis,* that grow in areas of tropical and subtropical areas of South America, Mexico, and the United States and that contain psilocybin, a hallucinogen. The mushrooms contain from 0.2–0.4 percent psilocybin. The drug, which is illegal to use in the United States, is a Schedule I drug under the CONTROLLED SUBSTANCES ACT. It is very bitter in taste and is often consumed in teas and added to other foods to hide the unpleasant flavor. Some users coat it with chocolate.

Psilocybin is used for religious or spiritual purposes by some groups, especially in Central America.

Users of Drug

According to the National Household Survey on Drug Abuse in 2001, the percentages of youthful users of this drug are low. An estimated 2.7 percent of whites ages 12–17 years old have ever used psilocybin, compared with 1.4 percent of Hispanic youths of the same age. Less than 1 percent, or 0.7 percent of Asians and 0.4 percent of African Amer-

icans have ever used this drug. However, older individuals are much more likely to use the drug. According to the National Household Survey on Drug Abuse, 12.2 percent of surveyed individuals ages 18–25 years said they had ever used psilocybin. In addition, 6.3 percent ages 26 and older said they had ever tried the drug.

Effects of Psilocybin

When ingested, the effects of the drug occur within about 20 minutes and may last as long as six hours. Users may experience nausea and vomiting, weakness, lack of coordination, and sleepiness. They may also experience HALLUCINATIONS. Panic may occur or even a psychotic reaction, especially if high doses are ingested. Another risk with mushrooms is that poisoning may occur because the user may mistakenly consume a poisonous mushroom rather than a mushroom containing psilocybin.

See also LSD; TEENAGE AND YOUTH DRUG ABUSE.

naltrexone A medication used to treat individuals addicted to alcohol. Naltrexone is also an opiate antagonist and is used to treat patients who are addicted to narcotics. In addition, naltrexone has been shown to be effective in some patients with problems with pathological gambling, according to a study reported in the *Journal of the American Medical Association* in 2001.

Naltrexone blocks certain receptors in the brain. If a person who has taken naltrexone also drinks alcohol, he or she will not experience euphoria or any of the desired effects that drinking has provided in the past.

In previous years, disulfiram (ANTABUSE) was the primary drug used to treat ALCOHOLISM. However, many alcoholics refused to take the drug because it caused extreme vomiting when even a tiny amount of alcohol was accidentally or unknowingly ingested. Naltrexone does not have this side effect, and hence compliance should be greater.

Naltrexone should not be used in patients with liver disease, such as HEPATITIS or CIRRHOSIS of the liver, which may mean that it must be ruled out for patients with long-term alcoholism who have already sustained damage to their livers. High doses of the drug, such as a dose of 300 mg, may cause liver toxicity in otherwise healthy people. Thus liver enzymes should be monitored in patients taking higher doses.

Most patients take 50 mg of naltrexone per day. However, some studies have shown that higher doses of 100–150 mg per day may be effective in patients who do not respond to 50 mg.

About 10 percent of patients who take naltrexone may develop nausea, which usually goes away in time. Some patients may experience headaches. Others may experience abdominal pain or anxiety. Most patients do not experience these side effects.

Rapid Detoxification with Naltrexone

Some physicians have used naltrexone as a medication to detoxify patients rapidly who are addicted to opiates. The drug is administered over a three to seven day period (rapid detoxification) in combination with clonidine. Some doctors have used other drugs in rapid detoxification instead of naltrexone, such as BUPRENORPHINE. Patients usually need to take a maintenance dose of naltrexone for a time after the rapid detoxification period. Some studies have shown the mildest withdrawal symptoms from rapid detoxification with a combination of clonidine, naltrexone, and buprenorphine.

Rapid detoxification is complex and difficult. According to Dr. Thomas Kosten and Dr. Patrick O'Connor in their 2003 article in the *New England Journal of Medicine,* "Rapid detoxification is a very intensive intervention, however, and should only be undertaken by clinicians who have had substantial experience working with simpler approaches to withdrawal, such as using clonidine alone or tapering the dosage of methadone in an inpatient setting."

A controversial use of naltrexone is that of ultrarapid detoxification. This procedure is performed under a general anesthetic and is meant to detoxify patients who are addicted to opiates in a very short period—within one to two days—and in a hospital setting. There is insufficient data on ultrarapid detoxification to evaluate it, although experts say that it is best done on younger patients rather than on long-term addicts. Said Dr. Kosten and Dr. O'Connor, "Withdrawal symptoms persisting for a week or longer, high cost, and safety are noteworthy problems with this method."

See also ANTABUSE; CAMPRAL; DETOXIFICATION; GAMBLING, PATHOLOGICAL; NARCOTICS; WITHDRAWAL.

Kosten, Thomas, R., M.D., and Patrick G. O'Connor, M.D. "Management of Drug and Alcohol Withdrawal," *New England Journal of Medicine* 348, no. 18 (May 1, 2003): 1,786–1,795.

Krystal, John H., M.D., et al. "Naltrexone in the Treatment of Alcohol Dependence," *New England Journal of Medicine* 345, no. 24 (December 13, 2001): 1,734–1,739.

O'Connor, Patrick G., M.D. and Richard S. Schottenfeld, M.D. "Patients with Alcohol Problems," *New England Journal of Medicine* 338, no. 9 (February 26, 1998): 592–602.

O'Connor, Patrick G., M.D., and Thomas R. Kosten, M.D. "Rapid and Ultrarapid Opioid Detoxification Techniques," *Journal of the American Medical Association* 279, no. 3 (January 21, 1998): 229–234.

Potenza, Marc N., M.D., Thomas R. Kosten, M.D., and Bruce J. Rounsaville, M.D. "Pathological Gambling," *Journal of the American Medical Association* 286, no. 2 (July 11, 2001): 141–144.

narcotics Legal and illegal opioid-based drugs. In the United States, the DRUG ENFORCEMENT ADMINISTRATION (DEA) has imposed special controls on narcotics, set by the CONTROLLED SUBSTANCES ACT.

There are five categories of drugs that are regulated by the DEA. They are called schedules. Most narcotics fall under Schedule II, such as most oxycodone drugs, including OXYCONTIN. Schedule I drugs are illegal drugs for which there is no medical purpose, such as HEROIN and MARIJUANA. (The DEA does not acknowledge any medical use for marijuana.) Schedule II drugs are those for which there is a medical purpose, but the drugs are deemed as having a high risk of abuse. COCAINE is also a Schedule II drug.

See also MORPHINE; OPIATES; SCHEDULED DRUGS.

Narcotics Anonymous A self-help organization for people addicted to drugs that is loosely based on the 12-step model of ALCOHOLICS ANONYMOUS, GAMBLERS ANONYMOUS, and related organizations. It is an organization for individuals addicted to narcotics (opiate-based drugs, such as HEROIN) as well as to other drugs or a combination of drugs, rather than to alcohol.

According to Narcotics Anonymous information, the first Narcotics Anonymous meeting occurred in 1947 in a federal public health hospital in Lexington, Kentucky. In 1953, an independent, community-based group in Los Angeles adopted these principles and this group later evolved into the nationwide Narcotics Anonymous organization. Today Narcotics Anonymous is an international organization with an estimated 20,000 registered weekly meetings in 70 countries around the globe. Narcotics Anonymous informational books and pamphlets are published in 23 languages.

Membership in the organization is open to all drug addicts. Members must admit they have a problem, seek help, work on self-examination, and take other basic steps. Some meetings are open to the community, while others are closed and only addicts may attend.

A 1996 survey of the members indicated that the average age of members was 37 years, with a range of 16–69 years. About 60 percent of the members were male. Almost half (48 percent) learned about Narcotics Anonymous when they were in a treatment facility or incarcerated.

For further information, contact the organization at:

Narcotics Anonymous World Services, Inc.
P.O. Box 9999
Van Nuys, CA 91409-9099
(818) 773-9999
http://www.na.og

National Institute on Alcohol Abuse and Alcoholism (NIAAA) An organization created by Congress in 1970 under the National Institutes of Health for the purpose of working toward solving problems related to alcohol abuse and alcoholism. The NIAAA provides research-based information on the broad array of issues that affect individuals with alcohol abuse and alcoholism, such as epidemiology, genetics, neuroscience, health risks, prevention, and treatment. The NIAAA collaborates with international, federal, state, and local organizations, agencies, and programs that are involved with alcohol-related issues.

According to the NIAAA Strategic Plan 2001–2005, the organization defined seven key goals:

Goal 1: Identify genes that are involved in alcohol-associated disorders.

Goal 2: Identify mechanisms associated with neuroadaptation at multiple levels of analysis (molecular, cellular, neural circuits, and behavior).

Goal 3: Identify additional science-based preventive interventions (such as drinking during pregnancy and college age drinking).

Goal 4: Further delineate biological mechanisms involved in the biomedical consequences associated with excessive alcohol consumption.

Goal 5: Discover new medications that will diminish cravings for alcohol, reduce the likelihood of posttreatment relapse, and accelerate recovery of alcohol-damaged organs.

Goal 6: Advance knowledge of the influence of environment on expression of genes involved in alcohol-associated behavior, including the vulnerable adolescent years and in special populations.

Goal 7: Further elucidate the relationships between alcohol and violence

For further information, contact the NIAAA at:

National Institute on Alcohol Abuse and
  Alcoholism
5635 Fishers Lane, MSC 9304
Bethesda, MD 20892
http://www.niaaa.nih.gov

National Institute on Drug Abuse (NIDA) An organization originally formed in 1974 that became a part of the National Institutes of Health in 1992. NIDA provides information on scientific research on drug addiction and supports over 85 percent of the world's research on health aspects of drug abuse and drug addiction.

For more information, contact the NIDA at:

National Institute on Drug Abuse
National Institutes of Health
6001 Executive Boulevard
Room 5313
Bethesda, MD 20892
(301) 443-1124
http://www.nida.nih.gov

nicotine An addictive substance found in cigarettes, cigars, pipe tobacco, and SMOKELESS TOBACCO. When a smoker inhales the smoke from a cigarette, the nicotine speeds to the brain within about 10 seconds, causing it to release epinephrine (also known as adrenaline). This epinephrine release creates a rush type of feeling in the user. Although the effect is nearly immediate, the nicotine continues to act on the body for as long as 30 minutes. The nicotine also causes the release of dopamine from the brain, a neurochemical that causes pleasure. On average, a person who smokes 40 cigarettes a day will receive 400 hits of nicotine to the brain.

The addiction to nicotine is also the reason why it is so difficult for many smokers to stop smoking. When the body is used to receiving nicotine on a regular basis, and it is not provided, for whatever reason, then the individual will experience WITHDRAWAL symptoms, such as irritability, insomnia, and difficulty in paying attention to anything else. Other symptoms, such as headaches and stomach pain, may also occur. The withdrawing smoker may also experience some psychiatric symptoms, such as DEPRESSION or anxiety.

Some individuals who stop smoking will also experience an increased appetite, which is a key reason why many people, especially women, fear giving up smoking; they think they will gain a great deal of weight. Some people do gain about five pounds or so, and a few people gain a significant amount of weight. An additional consideration is that nicotine may boost the basal metabolic rate, leading to a slowing of the metabolism during an unknown period following nicotine cessation.

Stress or anxiety also affects the action of nicotine on the body, causing the tobacco user to need greater quantities of nicotine to achieve the same effect. Thus the smoker who is under stress and says that he or she has a need to smoke more is reporting a common reaction. Unfortunately, a sustained increased level of smoking will create a greater need for nicotine, even when the person is no longer in a stressful environment or situation.

Because of the intense hold that nicotine has on many smokers, one therapy that works for some individuals is NICOTINE REPLACEMENT THERAPY. This provides a decreasing amount of nicotine and enables a withdrawal from smoking. Smokers, however, must keep in mind that using a nicotine replacement therapy—such as a skin patch, gum, or another form of nicotine replacement—while also continuing to smoke is very dangerous. Even among people who have smoked for years, the combination of cigarettes and the nicotine replacement therapy can cause nicotine poisoning.

Bupropion (ZYBAN or Wellbutrin) is another form of treatment for people who wish to quit smoking. It is not a nicotine replacement therapy but, instead, is a drug that is also used to treat people with depression and anxiety disorders. It has been found to be very effective in many people who wish to quit smoking.

Note that cigarettes also include other substances in addition to nicotine, such as tar and the carbon monoxide that is released during smoking. The amount of tar in cigarettes ranges from a low of about 7 mg in a low-tar cigarette to 15 mg in an average cigarette. The ingested tar increases the risk of developing LUNG CANCER, EMPHYSEMA, and bronchitis. The carbon monoxide increases the risk of developing cardiovascular diseases, such as stroke.

See also CARCINOGENS; SMOKING AND HEALTH PROBLEMS; SMOKING CESSATION; SMOKING, CIGARETTE; TEENAGE AND YOUTH SMOKING.

National Institute on Drug Abuse. "Cigarettes and Other Nicotine Products," *NIDA Info Facts* Available online. URL: http://www.ci.barrington.ri.us/government/prevention/nicotine%20facts.pdf. Accessed on March 15, 2005.

Nicotine Anonymous A self-help support group for people who want to end their addiction to tobacco, loosely modeled on the ALCOHOLICS ANONYMOUS framework of TWELVE STEPS for people who want to stop abusing alcohol. According to the organization, there are about 550 groups worldwide.

For further information, contact the organization at:

Nicotine Anonymous World Services
419 Main Street
PMB Number 370
Huntington Beach, CA 92648
(415) 750-0328
http://nicotine-anonymous.org

nicotine replacement therapy A treatment used to help smokers quit smoking by substituting nicotine in the form of a gum, lozenge, or transdermal (skin) patch for the nicotine from cigarettes. Nicotine gum, patches, and lozenges are available as over-the-counter drugs. Experts report that heavy smokers (those who are used to smoking more than 25 cigarettes per day) do better with gum containing 4 mg of nicotine rather than 2 mg.

Nicotine replacement therapy is also available in other forms, such as a nicotine inhaler and a nasal spray. Both of these are prescribed items.

Because the nicotine is the addictive substance in tobacco products, the theory behind nicotine replacement therapy is that the tobacco user can gradually reduce the level of nicotine that is consumed over time, with the end goal of eliminating nicotine altogether. The broad majority of nicotine replacement therapy users are people who wish to give up cigarette smoking.

Precautions
People who use nicotine replacement therapy should avoid smoking altogether. However, if they relapse and smoke one or two cigarettes in the course of using the therapy, continuing the therapy is generally safe. Avoiding acidic foods and drinks within a half hour of using the nicotine gum, lozenge, or inhaler is also best because acidic foods and drinks prevent the drug from working.

Some people including pregnant women, people who are prone to seizures, those with eating disorders, and individuals with ALCOHOLISM or alcohol abuse disorders, should consult with their physicians before using nicotine replacement therapy, as nicotine replacement can have negative effects which complicate these conditions.

Effectiveness of Therapy
Some individuals combine nicotine replacement therapy with other choices that help with smoking cessation, such as the prescribed medication bupropion (ZYBAN or Wellbutrin), or counseling, or hypnosis. Bupropion is also used as an antidepressant.

In a study reported in a 1999 issue of the *New England Journal of Medicine*, researchers compared the smoking cessation rates of subjects who were given a placebo (sugar pill), those given a nicotine patch, subjects given bupropion alone, and those given a combination of both bupropion and the nicotine patch. The researchers found that treatment with the bupropion alone or together with the nicotine patch resulted in significantly higher rates of smoking cessation than with the patch or the placebo alone.

The combination therapy, with bupropion and the patch, gave the best results. After one year, the placebo group were an average of 15.6 percent abstinent from smoking and the nicotine patch group were 16.4 percent abstinent. In contrast, the bupropion group was 30.3 percent abstinent and the bupropion and nicotine patch group was 35.5 percent abstinent.

In another study, reported in a 2004 issue of *Annals of Internal Medicine,* researchers sought to find if one form of nicotine replacement therapy worked better for some groups than others. Said the researchers, "Smokers who started out highly dependent on nicotine, obese smokers, and members of minority groups achieved higher quit rates with nasal spray. Smokers with lesser initial nicotine dependence, nonobese smokers, and white smokers achieved higher quit rates with transdermal nicotine."

Support Groups

Support groups, such as NICOTINE ANONYMOUS, provide an opportunity for some individuals to end their smoking habit. The National Cancer Institute's Smoking Quitline may offer further suggestions at their toll-free number: 877-448-7848.

See also NICOTINE; SMOKING AND HEALTH PROBLEMS; SMOKING CESSATION; SMOKING, CIGARETTE; TEENAGE AND YOUTH SMOKING; TOBACCO.

For further information on nicotine replacement therapy and smoking cessation, contact the following organizations:

American Cancer Society
1599 Clifton Road NE
Atlanta, GA 30329
(800) 227-2345 (toll-free)
http://www.cancer.org

American Lung Association
61 Broadway
6th Floor
New York, NY 10006
(800) 586-4872 (toll-free)
http://www.lungusa.org

Centers for Disease Control and Prevention (CDC)
Office on Smoking and Health
Mail Stop K-50
4770 Buford Highway, NE
Atlanta, GA 30341
(800) 311-3435 (toll-free)
http://www.cdc.gov

National Cancer Institute
Cancer Information Service
Suite 3036A
6116 Executive Boulevard
MSC 8322
Bethesda, MD 20892
(800) 422-6237 (toll-free)

Jorenby, Douglas E., et al. "A Controlled Trial of Sustained-Release Bupropion, A Nicotine Patch, or Both for Smoking Cessation," *New England Journal of Medicine* 340, no. 9 (March 4, 1999): 685–691.

Lerman, Caryn, et al. "Individualizing Nicotine Replacement Therapy for the Treatment of Tobacco Dependence," *Annals of Internal Medicine* 14, no. 6 (March 16, 2004): 426–433.

Rigotti, Nancy A., M.D. "Treatment of Tobacco Use and Dependence," *New England Journal of Medicine* 346, no. 7 (February 14, 2002): 506–512.

nonnarcotic pain relievers Drugs that can be used instead of narcotics to combat pain. Nonnarcotic pain relievers include such common analgesics as aspirin or acetaminophen as well as nonsteroidal anti-inflammatory drugs and other medications such as Ultram (TRAMADOL) and CARISOPRODOL. However, narcotic painkillers such as MORPHINE, OXYCONTIN, and other forms of opioids are the most powerful medications that are available for patients with moderate-to-severe pain.

obsessive-compulsive disorder (OCD)   A form of anxiety disorder in which a person suffers from frequent unwanted thoughts and also feels compelled to repeat unnecessary actions, such as washing the hands over and over, counting items, or performing other ritualistic acts. The upsetting thoughts are obsessions, and the actions that the person feels compelled to take repeatedly are compulsions. Some experts believe that addictive behaviors such as ANOREXIA NERVOSA or BULIMIA NERVOSA may be a subset of OCD. People with OCD are at risk for developing DEPRESSION and other anxiety disorders.

About 3.3 million people in the United States have OCD, according to the National Institute of Mental Health (NIMH). Males and females are equally likely to develop OCD. In most cases, people with OCD are aware that their behavior is irrational, but despite this, they find changing their behavior difficult or impossible. Medications and therapy often help the patient with OCD. Without treatment, many patients have a low quality of life.

Interestingly, one study in Sweden found that patients with OCD had a lower rate of smoking than the general population. According to the researchers in their 1999 article in *Comprehensive Psychiatry*, only 14 percent of the patients with OCD were current smokers, compared with 25 percent in the general population. Of the patients with OCD, 72 percent had never smoked. Rates of smoking among patients with other illnesses, such as SCHIZOPHRENIA, were very high in Sweden, in a range of 74–88 percent.

The researchers said, "Since a decreased smoking rate among OCD subjects was confirmed, the smoking prevalences in schizophrenia and OCD, respectively, seem to represent either end of a con-tinuum, and OCD may also differ significantly from other anxiety disorders in this respect."

Possible Causes

It is unknown what causes OCD, although the onset is often in childhood or adolescence. There may be a genetic cause for OCD since the problem seems to run in families. In a 2002 issue of the *American Journal of Medical Genetics*, researchers found suggestive evidence for a genetic linkage for OCD on chromosome 9p on a sample size of 56 people diagnosed with OCD.

In another study, published in the *Archives of Pediatric and Adolescent Medicine*, researchers studied adolescents in Hawaii to determine if race and ethnicity affected the prevalence of OCD. The researchers studied 619 high school students and found a significantly high rate of OCD among some racial groups. For example, among the 25 students who were either Samoan or part Samoan, 20 percent had OCD. Of the students who were native Hawaiian or part Hawaiian, the prevalence was 14.9 percent. The prevalence rates of OCD were lower for all other groups. For example, none of the 19 white students had OCD and 10.3 percent of the Filipino students were diagnosed with OCD.

The researchers speculated that the high rate of OCD among some ethnic groups might be due to a combination of genetic and environmental risk factors, such as an increased risk for rheumatic fever and an autoimmune response to streptococcus infection.

Other researchers also believe that OCD may be an autoimmune disease, which means that the immune system attacks the body. Preliminary research from the NIMH has indicated that in a few cases, infection with streptococcus has apparently led to the development of OCD in some children and adolescents. Eradication of the bacteria resolved the problem.

It is also possible that SUBSTANCE ABUSE may trigger the development of OCD. Some studies have found that subjects using both COCAINE and MARIJUANA have an increased risk for the subsequent development of OCD.

Indicators of OCD

According to the NIMH in their patient booklet on OCD, a positive response to some of the following questions may indicate that a person has OCD, although only a psychiatrist can diagnose the illness:

- I have upsetting thoughts or images enter my mind again and again.
- I feel like I cannot stop these thoughts or images even though I want to.
- I have a hard time stopping myself from doing things again and again, like counting, checking on things, washing my hands, rearranging objects, doing things until it feels right, and/or collecting useless objects.
- I worry a lot about terrible things that could happen if I am not careful.
- I have unwanted urges to hurt someone but know I never would.

Diagnosis and Treatment

Physicians diagnose OCD based on the patient's medical history and symptoms. A careful diagnosis is needed because some symptoms that may appear to be OCD can be part of another disorder, such as Tourette's syndrome. As a result, a psychiatrist or neurologist is the best specialist to diagnose a person with symptoms that present as OCD.

OCD can usually be treated with medications. Some medications that have been proven helpful have been antidepressants, such as clomipramine (Anafranil), fluoxetine (Prozac), fluvoxamine (Luvox), sertraline (Zoloft), citalopram (Celexa), and paroxetine (Paxil). The physician selects the medication that is most likely to be effective. If it does not help the patient, usually another medication will work. Some patients are treated with BENZODIAZEPINES or beta blocker drugs. Combination therapy may be best for some patients; for exam-

ple, some physicians supplement clomipramine or fluoxetine with clonazepam.

Patients may also benefit with therapy provided by a psychologist. Some psychologists use behavior therapy in which the person may be exposed to objects about which they are obsessed. For example, individuals obsessed with cleanliness would be encouraged to touch something that they believe is dirty and then prevented from washing their hands. The therapist should be someone who is trained and experienced in this form of therapy.

Cognitive-behavioral therapy, in which the patient describes the thought processes and the therapist helps the patient learn to challenge irrational thoughts actively, may help some patients with OCD. According to Dr. Michael Jenike in his 2004 article on OCD for the *New England Journal of Medicine,* most patients benefit from a combination of medication and cognitive-behavioral therapy.

See also ANXIETY DISORDERS; BIPOLAR DISORDER; DUAL DIAGNOSIS; PSYCHIATRIC MEDICATIONS; PSYCHIATRISTS.

For further information on OCD, contact the following organizations:

Anxiety Disorders Association of America
8730 Georgia Avenue
Suite 600
Silver Spring, MD 20910
(240) 485-1001
http://www.adaa.org

National Alliance for the Mentally Ill (NAMI)
Colonial Place Three
2107 Wilson Boulevard
Suite 300
Arlington, VA 22201
(703) 524-7600
http://www.nami.org

National Institute of Mental Health (NIMH)
6001 Executive Boulevard
Room 8184, MSC 9663
Bethesda, MD 20892
(888) 826-9438

Obsessive-Compulsive Foundation
676 State Street
New Haven, CT 06511
(203) 401-2070
http://www.ocfoundation.org

Arnold, Paul D. and Margaret A. Richter. "Is Obsessive-Compulsive Disorder an Autoimmune Disease?" *Canadian Medical Association Journal* 165, no. 10 (2001): 1,353–1,358.

Bejerot, S. and M. Humble. "Low Prevalence of Smoking Among Patients with Obsessive-Compulsive Disorder," *Comprehensive Psychiatry* 40, no. 4 (July/August 1999): 268–272.

Crum, R. M. and J. C. Anthony. "Cocaine Use and Other Suspected Risk Factors for Obsessive-Compulsive Disorder: A Prospective Study with Data from the Epidemiologic Catchment Area Surveys," *Drug Alcohol Dependence* 31, no. 3 (1993): 281–295.

Guerrero, Anthony P. S., M.D., et al. "Demographic and Clinical Characteristics of Adolescents in Hawaii with Obsessive-Compulsive Disorder," *Archives of Pediatric and Adolescent Medicine* 157, no. 7 (July 2003): 663–670.

Hanna, Gregory L., et al. "Genome-Wide Linkage Analysis of Families with Obsessive-Compulsive Disorder Ascertained through Pediatric Probands," *American Journal of Medical Genetics* 114 (2002): 541–552.

Jenike, Michael, M.D. "Obsessive-Compulsive Disorder," *New England Journal of Medicine* 350, no. 3 (January 15, 2004): 259–265.

National Institute for Mental Health. *A Real Illness: Obsessive-Compulsive Disorder* (OCD), National Institutes of Health, NIH Publication No. 00-4676. Washington, D.C.: NIH, n.d.

opiates Medications derived from opium or synthesized from opium-like chemicals, such as HEROIN, METHADONE, MORPHINE, OxyContin, hydrocodone, and oxycodone. Opiates are the oldest forms of prescribed analgesics. In the early 20th century, they were available as over-the-counter drugs and were included in many nonprescribed preparations for adults and children. When opiates are taken continuously, patients develop a TOLERANCE to them, which means that they need a greater dose to achieve the same effect.

In the past, it was believed that a majority of those addicted to opiates were also those who took these medications for severe chronic pain; however, the National Cancer Institute reports otherwise. They maintain that the large percentage of individuals who develop a drug addiction problem are those who seek to gain an artificial high or EUPHORIA from drug abuse rather than a respite from severe pain. In any event, many people are addicted to opiates and need treatment.

The treatment for opiate addiction varies, depending on the opiate to which the patient is addicted. If the patient is addicted to heroin, the therapy may be methadone maintenance. Patients addicted to heroin or other forms of opiates may also be treated with BUPRENORPHINE. Some patients are treated with DETOXIFICATION within hospital settings. It is dangerous and even life-threatening for anyone addicted to opiates to attempt to end the addiction without any medical assistance.

See also ADDICTION MEDICINE; CANCER; NARCOTICS; PAIN; PAIN MANAGEMENT; PAIN MANAGEMENT CENTERS.

oral cancer Cancer of the lips, mouth, or pharynx (part of the throat), primarily caused by any form of tobacco use. Cigar smokers and users of SMOKELESS TOBACCO have an increased risk of developing oral cancer. Experts estimate that at least 90 percent of all oral cancers are linked to tobacco use, including cigarettes, pipe tobacco, cigars, chewing tobacco, and any other form of tobacco that individuals may use. In addition, patients who use both tobacco and alcohol have an increased risk of developing oral cancer. Oral cancers are more likely to occur in middle-aged or elderly adults, although they can develop in younger individuals.

People who smoke cigarettes, cigars, or pipes may develop oral cancer at any location within the oral cavity or the oropharynx, as well as developing cancer in the esophagus, the larynx, the lungs, the bladder, the kidneys, and other organs in the body. Pipe smokers are at risk for cancers of the lips. Individuals who use smokeless tobacco (snuff or chewing tobacco) have an increased risk of developing oral cancers of the gums, cheek, and the inner surface of their lips. According to the American Cancer Society, this risk is increased by 50 times over non-users.

Sometimes dentists discover an oral cancer during a routine oral examination of the mouth and teeth. This is another reason why most individuals should see their dentists at least once a year.

According to the American Cancer Society, about 28,000 new cases of oral cancer were diagnosed in 2003. An estimated 7,200 people, including 4,800 men and 2,400 women, died of oral cancer in 2003. The five-year survival rate for all types of oral cancers is 56 percent, and the 10-year survival rate is 41 percent. Patients who are diagnosed with oral cancer must immediately give up smoking to avoid any exacerbation or recurrences of the cancer.

Some symptoms of oral cancer are as follows (although the person may have a noncancerous ailment and only a physician can determine if cancer is present):

- A sore that does not heal
- Difficulty swallowing
- White or red patches in the mouth
- A hoarse voice
- Swelling of the jaw that causes dentures to fit poorly
- Numbness in the tongue or other parts of the mouth

Diagnosis and Treatment

The doctor will determine how advanced the oral cancer is and whether it has spread (metastasized) to other tissues. Depending on the stage of the cancer, the treatment may include surgery, radiation therapy, and chemotherapy.

For further information on oral cancer, contact the following organizations:

American Cancer Society
1599 Clifton Road NE
Atlanta, GA 30329
(800) 227-2345 (toll-free) or (404) 320-3333
http://www.cancer.org

National Cancer Institute
Division of Cancer Epidemiology and Genetics
6120 Executive Boulevard
MSC-7234
Executive Plaza South, 7th Floor
Rockville, MD 20852
(301) 496-1691

National Institute of Dental and Craniofacial
Research
National Oral Health Information Clearinghouse
31 Center Drive MSC 2290
Bethesda, MD 20852
(301) 402-7364
http://www.nidcr.nih.gov

See also CANCER; CARCINOGENS; LUNG CANCER; NICOTINE; SMOKING AND HEALTH PROBLEMS.

overdose Excessive consumption of a drug or alcohol, which can cause serious health problems or even death. Some individuals take an overdose of their medication as a means to commit SUICIDE, while for most people, the overdose is accidental. Many people do not realize that taking prescribed or illegal drugs along with alcohol is dangerous and can be fatal, nor do they realize taking certain drugs together is dangerous and they risk adverse reactions.

Some individuals, particularly adolescents, have suffered from accidental overdoses of INHALANTS they have ingested.

See also ACCIDENTAL OVERDOSE.

overeating/obesity Eating more food than is healthy for one's body frame, which results in excessive weight or obesity. This behavior may occur as a result of an eating disorder, such as BINGE EATING DISORDER, or from chronic heavy eating. Obesity may also result from extremely sedentary behavior. Most people are overweight or obese as a result of a combination of eating too much and exercising too little. However, obesity is a more complex problem than is acknowledged by some physicians, and many people have an extremely difficult time with losing weight. In general, the greater the amount of weight they need to lose, the more that individuals struggle with weight loss.

Some experts refer to the problem of overeating as a food addiction. Overeating may also be associated with other addictions, such as GAMBLING. It is often associated with psychiatric disorders (which are often undiagnosed), such as DEPRESSION or ANXIETY DISORDERS.

Overeating is a very common problem in the United States. As a result, about two-thirds of American adults (65.7 percent) were overweight in 2002 and nearly a third (30.6 percent) of Americans were obese, according to a 2004 report in the *Journal of the American Medical Association.* In addition, 5.1 percent were extremely obese, or more than 100 pounds overweight. The World Health Organization estimates that about 300 million people worldwide are obese. Obesity is not limited to wealthy people; in fact, those who are poor are more likely to be overweight or obese.

Overeating and Children and Adolescents

Many children and adolescents have a problem with overeating and the resulting problems of overweight and obesity. According to a policy statement from the Committee on Nutrition of the American Academy of Pediatrics, published in a 2003 issue of *Pediatrics,* 15.3 percent of children ages six to 11 years old in the United States were obese (above the 95th percentile for body mass index [BMI] on standard growth charts), as were 15.5 percent of children ages 12–19 years old.

The statement noted the sedentary behavior of many children as well as a national survey that reported that more than 25 percent of children in the United States watch four hours or more of television each day. Hours of television watching among children (as with adults) is associated with an increased risk for obesity. The report also noted that a television sited inside the child's bedroom increased the risk for overweight, even among preschool children. One of the recommendations of the report was to limit television watching to no more than two hours a day. Some other recommendations included encouraging parents and caregivers to provide children with healthy snacks and to promote physical activity.

Overweight children have an increased risk of becoming overweight or obese as adults. In addition, overweight or obese children are at risk for developing illnesses during childhood, such as type 2 diabetes, hypertension, dyslipidemia, and other medical problems that are not common in children.

Rarely, children may have diseases that directly cause obesity, such as Prader-Willi syndrome. This medical condition, which is usually a genetic disorder, is characterized by mental developmental delays, behavioral problems, decreased muscle mass, short stature, genital abnormalities, and obesity. It causes patients afflicted with the condition to have an insatiable appetite. Their parents sometimes have to place a lock on the refrigerator and food supply cabinets to limit the extreme binge eating. Studies on patients with Prader-Willi syndrome indicate an abnormality of ghrelin, a hormone associated with satiety (a feeling of fullness). Some experts believe that if researchers could find the cause of the extreme appetite experienced by patients with Prader-Willi syndrome, this information may provide many answers for the millions of people who suffer with obesity.

Other Causes of Overeating and Obesity

Many people have a genetic predisposition toward overweight and obesity. Some researchers have found a genetic link to both type 2 diabetes and obesity on chromosome 18p11, as described in the March 2001 issue of the journal *Diabetes.* Further genetic research may lead to greater breakthroughs and help for patients with obesity problems.

In some cases, medications can cause a temporary obesity, such as with steroid medications that are taken on a regular basis for severe pain. Illnesses may also lead to obesity as individuals with severe arthritis, back pain, or other painful chronic medical problems may radically decrease their level of physical activities even if they do not increase the amount of food that they eat. The sedentary behavior requires few calories, and thus the individual gains weight.

Many experts believe that obesity is primarily caused by a lack of exercise and too great a reliance on driving cars to work and other places rather than walking to their destinations. Others say that the supersizing of portions in restaurants is a contributing cause of obesity.

For many individuals, obesity is likely caused by a combination of factors, some of which they can control. For example, although individuals cannot control their genetic heritage, they can work with their physician to identify any existing illnesses that are causing or contributing to the obesity so that they can be treated and so that their physician can help them to create an exercise and diet plan to resolve their weight problem.

Measuring Obesity

Overweight and obesity is measured in terms of the BMI, which is derived from a person's weight in kilograms divided by the height in meters squared. The average healthy person has a BMI that is within the range of 18.5–24. Because most people do not wish to perform the calculations needed to determine their own BMI, they can find their height and weight on charts listing BMIs and discover if they are underweight, of normal weight, overweight, obese or severely obese. Severely obese people are about 100 pounds greater than their ideal weight, and they have the most severe health risks.

According to the National Heart, Lung, and Blood Institute of the National Institutes of Health, weight categories of BMI are as follows:

Underweight: Less than 18.5
Normal weight: 18.5–24.9
Overweight: 25.0–29.9
Obesity: 30–39.9
Severe obesity: 40.0 and greater

Food as a Substance Abuse Issue

Some experts, such as Dr. Mark Gold at the University of Florida, believe that overeating should be considered another form of SUBSTANCE ABUSE. Dr. Gold, a psychiatrist, says that the brain responds to excessive eating and excessive drinking in a similar way.

Said Dr. Gold in the *Journal of Addictive Diseases* in 2004, underlining his view of overeating as an addictive disorder, "Treatment of obesity, from surgery to medications, often involves 12-step meetings. Overeating and obesity are increasing in prevalence and public health significance. Applying research methodologies applied to addictions may offer hope for understanding and the development of common treatments."

Weight Gain Associated with Resolving Other Addictive Behaviors

Researchers have noted that when individuals give up one addictive behavior, sometimes they turn to another type of addictive behavior. For example, smokers may gain an average of six to eight pounds when they stop smoking. Other studies have indicated that when individuals resolve problems of substance abuse, they may increase their food intake and consequently gain weight.

In a study reported in the *Journal of Addictive Diseases* in 2004 on adolescents who underwent treatment for substance abuse, the researchers analyzed the subjects' BMI after undergoing abstinence from drug use. The subjects were 215 males and 67 females between the ages of 13 and 17 years. They were either self-referred, civilly committed by their parents, or sent to the treatment center by the court system. The adolescents were supervised constantly, and their average stay in the facility was 168 days.

According to the researchers, "There was a substantial weight gain and BMI increase from admittance to 60 days. Participants gained an average of about 11 pounds and increased their BMI by 1.58 during this time."

The researchers also found that about 6 percent of the population was overweight upon admission to the treatment facility. By the 90-day point, 10.3 percent were overweight. By the time of discharge, 13.5 percent were overweight. In addition, the researchers found that patients who smoked had a greater weight gain than nonsmokers. Said the researchers, "These data suggest that adolescents who smoke are at greater risk of weight gain during supervised abstinence from drugs, including tobacco and alcohol, increasing their propensity to become at risk of becoming overweight."

The researchers also noted, "Food, tobacco, and illicit drugs are all reported to be addictive or stimulating to the brain reward system. Food ingestion, as well as smoking and other drug self-administration, is linked to the neurotransmitter dopamine and is the subject of current studies." The researchers said that some have suggested that a dopamine deficiency may be a factor in individuals who have a problem with drug addiction or food addiction. Further research is needed on this subject.

Health Risks of Overeating

Whatever the primary cause (or multiple causes) of obesity, many overweight and obese people are at risk for developing many health problems, including type 2 diabetes, hypertension, heart disease, stroke, and some forms of cancer, such as colorectal cancer and liver cancer. In addition, according to the surgeon general in the United States, obese people have a 50 percent or greater risk of premature death from all causes compared with nonobese individuals, and as many as 300,000 deaths per year may be attributable to obesity. For these reasons, overweight and obese people should work with their physicians and nutritionists to lose weight.

In a study reported in a 2003 issue of the *Journal of the American Medical Association,* the researchers did a telephone survey of over 195,000 adults ages 19 and older in 2001 in the United States, seeking to estimate the prevalence of obesity and diabetes in adults. The researchers found that 20.9 percent of the subjects were obese in 2001, up from 19.8 percent in 2000. With regard to diabetes, the prevalence had also increased, from 7.3 percent in 2000 to 7.9 percent in 2001. In addition, the researchers found a significant correlation between overweight and obesity and the incidence of diabetes, high blood pressure, high cholesterol blood levels, asthma, arthritis, and poor health status.

Many patients who suffer from hypertension (high blood pressure), type 2 diabetes, and other ailments that are often associated with overweight and obesity will see an improvement or even a remission of these problems if they lose weight.

Obesity Among High School Students in the United States

Although adolescents tend to be concerned about their personal appearance and their weight, overweight is still a problem for many high school students. According to researchers from the Centers for Disease Control and Prevention, an estimated 10.5 percent of high school students in the United States in 2001 were overweight, with the largest percentage of overweight adolescents residing in Texas (14.2 percent), Mississippi (14.0), and Arkansas (13.8 percent). In contrast, the following states have low percentages of overweight students: Montana (6.1 percent), Utah (6.2 percent), and Colorado (7.1 percent).

African-American and Hispanic students had a higher percentage of overweight students than other racial or ethnic groups, and about 16 percent of African-American students nationwide are overweight, as are 15.1 percent of Hispanic students. (See the table on page 186.)

Treatment for Obesity

Some patients who have problems with overweight or obesity take prescribed or over-the-counter DIET PILLS in order to lose weight, and these medications have been effective for some people. Often, however, when people stop taking the drug, they regain the weight. Many years ago, AMPHETAMINES were used for weight loss, but these drugs can be addictive and are no longer

legally prescribed for weight loss in the United States.

Prescribed diet pills that are available to patients in the United States include sibutramine (Meridia), orlistat (Xenical), and phentermine (Fastin, Adipex-P). Other diet drugs are in development.

In the past, an herbal remedy known as ephedra was used. In 2004, however, the Food and Drug Administration banned the use of ephedra as a diet drug in the United States because several individuals died from using it. Ephedra is also known as ma huang.

Many people continue to seek out a quick fix diet pill that they can purchase over the counter and that will cause a very rapid weight loss; consequently, many sites on the INTERNET as well as on television programs make such promises to dieters. However, rapid weight loss is generally ineffective and may be unsafe. Drugs that induce a quick weight loss often do so by causing diarrhea and water loss. The diarrhea causes malabsorption of nutrients and can lead to malnutrition. The water loss can lead to clinically significant dehydration. Weight lost due to dehydration is regained when water is replenished.

Some individuals use other methods to lose weight, such as hypnosis, self-hypnosis, or acupuncture. In general, studies have not proven these methods to be effective.

Some individuals who are severely obese undergo weight reduction surgery, also known as bariatric surgery. In this surgery, which is usually a gastric bypass procedure, the patient undergoes elective surgery to decrease the size of the stomach in order to limit the amount of food that can be consumed. The procedure is generally not reversible. It is also difficult for many patients to adjust to because they must eat many very small meals throughout the day, and if they eat more than their reduced stomach can handle, they will vomit.

The gastric bypass (or any other means of bariatric surgery) is a dangerous operation, and the risks should be taken seriously. However, gastric bypass can extend life for morbidly obese patients as most lose greater than 20 percent of their body weight. Although some insurance companies will pay for this surgery if patients have a BMI of 40 or greater, many insurance companies will not pay for this procedure.

PERCENTAGE OF HIGH SCHOOL STUDENTS WHO REPORTED BEING OVERWEIGHT, BY SEX, RACE AND ETHNICITY, 2001

State	Total	Male	Female	White	African American	Hispanic
Alabama	12.3	16.9	7.6	10.3	16.3	—
Alaska (not available)						
Arizona (not available)						
Arkansas	13.8	18.7	8.7	12.4	18.6	—
California (not available)						
Colorado	7.1	11.1	2.5	5.6	—	12.8
Connecticut (not available)						
Delaware	10.8	12.9	8.9	8.7	15.7	12.9
District of Columbia (not available)						
Florida	10.4	13.6	6.8	9.5	11.7	11.3
Georgia (not available)						
Hawaii	12.1	16.6	8.3	6.7	—	—
Idaho	7.2	9.7	4.5	7.0	—	8.8
Illinois	9.5	15.3	5.4	8.6	—	—
Indiana	11.4	15.2	8.0	10.5	—	—
Iowa	9.8	12.8	6.7	9.1	—	—
Kansas (not available)						
Kentucky	12.3	16.0	8.9	12.2	—	—
Louisiana	13.0	17.0	9.8	11.7	15.6	—
Maine	10.4	14.8	5.5	10.3	—	—
Maryland (not available)						
Massachusetts	10.0	13.5	6.3	8.9	16.9	13.6
Michigan	10.7	14.0	7.2	9.6	16.8	17.2
Minnesota (not available)						
Mississippi	14.0	18.4	9.9	12.8	15.3	—
Missouri	12.8	17.0	8.5	11.6	18.6	—
Montana	6.1	8.3	3.7	5.6	—	—
Nebraska	9.0	12.2	5.6	8.3	—	—
Nevada (not available)						
New Hampshire	8.6	12.0	5.3	8.7	—	—
New Jersey	10.1	14.0	6.1	9.0	13.6	13.1
New Mexico (not available)						
New York	10.6	16.1	4.5	9.5	—	—
North Carolina	12.9	16.6	9.0	11.9	15.5	9.1
North Dakota	9.2	13.8	4.2	7.9	—	—
Ohio (not available)						
Oklahoma (not available)						
Oregon (not available)						
Pennsylvania (not available)						
Rhode Island	9.2	14.8	3.5	8.6	15.2	10.6
South Carolina	12.9	16.3	9.4	10.7	16.3	—
South Dakota	7.6	10.7	4.7	6.9	—	—
Tennessee	13.2	16.3	10.1	11.9	19.1	—
Texas	14.2	19.4	8.7	10.9	17.3	17.6
Utah	6.2	9.6	2.6	6.0	—	—
Vermont	9.7	14.0	5.1	—	—	—
Virginia (not available)						

State	Total	Male	Female	White	African American	Hispanic
Washington (not available)						
West Virginia (not available)						
Wisconsin	9.6	13.3	5.6	8.9	14.2	—
Wyoming	6.6	9.3	3.7	6.2	—	7.8
United States	10.5	14.2	6.9	8.8	16.0	15.1

Source: Centers for Disease Control and Prevention, *The Burden of Chronic Diseases and Their Risk Factors: National and State Perspectives*. Washington, D.C.: U.S. Department of Health and Human Services, February 2004.

Psychological Aspects of Weight Gain and Loss

For many individuals, food is used in an emotional manner, and overeating often occurs as a response to stress. For example, if a person is upset about a problem, she may eat a piece of chocolate cake (or an extra piece) or another favorite food. Food may also be used in an attempt to self-medicate untreated depression, anxiety, or other emotional problems. Identifying and changing problematic behavior patterns related to overeating are both integral to succeeding with weight loss.

In order to lose a significant amount of weight and keep it off, patients who are overweight or obese must also change their views toward food. For example, individuals who use food as a reward for virtually every major or minor event in their lives or as the consolation prize for every loss will need to find alternative means of positive reinforcement or solace. Even individuals who have bariatric surgery must make a psychological transition in their attitude toward food and their own self-image in order to maintain the weight loss.

A psychologist who is experienced in weight loss issues may be able to assist individuals with this task, as may support groups such as Overeaters Anonymous (OA). This group assists individuals with meetings based on the TWELVE STEPS concept loosely adapted from ALCOHOLICS ANONYMOUS. They charge no dues. An estimated 7,000 or more OA groups are in 52 countries that offer OA meetings.

OA seeks to help people determine if they are compulsive overeaters by asking such questions as "Do you have feelings of guilt and remorse after overeating?" and "Do you eat to escape from worries or trouble?"

Many people tie their self-esteem to their weight and assume that if they are slender, they are good, and if they are overweight or obese, they are bad. Such issues need to be carefully thought through by the person who is seeking to lose weight. It is healthier to realize that an individual is still valuable to himself or herself and the world whether the person weighs 185 pounds or 285 pounds. Depression and self-hatred over obesity tend to lead to further overeating and comfort eating and thus, to further weight gain.

See also ANOREXIA NERVOSA; BULIMIA NERVOSA.

For more information about OA, contact them at:

The World Service Office of Overeaters Anonymous
P.O. Box 44020
Rio Rancho, NM 87174-4020
(505) 891-2664
http://www.oa.org/ws

Committee on Nutrition, American Academy of Pediatrics. "Prevention of Pediatric Overweight and Obesity," *Pediatrics* 112, no. 2 (August 2003): 424–430.

Hedley, Allison A., et al. "Prevalence of Overweight and Obesity and U.S. Children Adolescents, and Adults, 1999–2002," *Journal of the American Medical Association* 291, no. 23 (2004): 2,847–2,850.

Gold, Mark S., M.D. "Introduction," *Journal of Addictive Diseases* 23, no. 3 (2004): 1–3.

Hodgkins, Candace C., et al. "Adolescent Drug Addiction Treatment and Weight Gain," *Journal of Addictive Diseases* 23, no. 3 (2004): 55–65.

Hu, Frank B., M.D., et al. "Television Watching and Other Sedentary Behaviors in Relation to Risk of Obesity and Type 2 Diabetes Mellitus in Women," *Journal of the American Medical Association* 289, no. 14 (April 9, 2003): 1,785–1,791.

Minocha, Anil, M.D. and Christine Adamec. *The Encyclopedia of the Digestive System and Digestive Disorders.* New York, N.Y.: Facts On File, Inc., 2004.

Mokdad, Ali H., et al. "Prevalence of Obesity, Diabetes, and Obesity-Related Health Risk Factors, 2001," *Journal of the American Medical Association* 289, no. 1 (January 1, 2003): 76–79.

Parker, Alex, et al. "A Gene Conferring Susceptibility to Type 2 Diabetes in Conjunction with Obesity is Located on Chromosome 18p11," *Diabetes* 50 (March 2001): 675–680.

Petit, William, M.D. and Christine Adamec. *The Encyclopedia of Endocrine Diseases and Disorders.* New York, N.Y.: Facts On File, Inc., 2005.

over-the-counter medications   Drugs that do not require a prescription and that can be purchased at many pharmacies or supermarkets. Examples of such medications are cold preparations, cough syrups, and painkillers such as aspirin, ibuprofen, and acetaminophen and laxatives. Some individuals, particularly adolescents, abuse over-the-counter medications, such as cough syrup. People with ANOREXIA NERVOSA or BULIMIA NERVOSA may abuse laxatives.

See also COUGH SYRUP.

OxyContin   A timed-release form of oxycodone hydrochloride that is produced by Purdue Pharma, L.P. OxyContin was originally approved by the Food and Drug Administration in 1995 for the treatment of chronic moderate or severe non-cancer pain and the pain associated with cancer.

Oxycodone is a narcotic that is also found in drugs such as Percocet, Percodan, and Tylox, but these drugs must be taken more frequently, such as every four to six hours rather than every 12 hours, as with OxyContin. As a result, OxyContin is more convenient for many patients with chronic severe pain. OxyContin is prescribed for people with moderate-to-severe pain resulting from injuries, arthritis, back pain, sickle cell anemia, cancer, and other conditions that result in chronic moderate or severe pain that lasts more than a few days.

The drug was immediately popular when it was introduced, in part because of reports about the undertreatment of pain patients as well as an aging population that was increasingly prone to back pain, cancer, injuries, and arthritis. According to a 2003 report from the United States General Accounting Office (GAO), a federal governmental agency, in 1996 about 317,000 prescriptions for OxyContin were written in the United States and sales to Purdue were about $45 million. Sales rapidly grew; by the year 2002, about 7 million pre-scriptions were written for OxyContin and sales of the drug were about $1.5 billion. OxyContin is available in dosages of 10 mg, 20 mg, 40 mg, and 80 mg tablets. A 160 mg tablet was produced, but it was voluntarily withdrawn from the market by the manufacturer in 2001.

Abuse and Misuse of OxyContin

OxyContin is a Schedule II narcotic under the CONTROLLED SUBSTANCES ACT. It is also a drug that has been abused by some people for its euphoric effect. Abusers of the drug chew or crush the tablets to obtain the effect all at once rather than over time (which is very dangerous), and sometimes they inject the drug. Some individuals have died in cases involving OxyContin; deaths were first documented in Kentucky, Ohio, Virginia, and West Virginia.

When the drug is used as it was intended, OxyContin is highly efficacious at controlling moderate to severe pain, according to both physicians and patients. It does not create any euphoria in patients. The problem arises when the drug is used illegally or when it is abused, for example, if patients take higher doses than prescribed or if they see several doctors to obtain multiple prescriptions.

Some people steal OxyContin from pharmacies while others illegally write their own prescriptions by stealing prescription pads from doctors. A few physicians are careless in their own prescribing of pain medications, prescribing overly high doses of drugs, although the DRUG ENFORCEMENT ADMINISTRATION maintains a watchful eye for problematic prescribing patterns. As a result, some patients develop an addiction, although patients with true pain, on low doses of the drug, should not usually become addicted.

An estimated 1 million people in the United States ages 12 and older have abused OxyContin at least once in their lifetime. Individuals who abuse OxyContin develop a tolerance to the drug and need higher doses to achieve the same euphoric result. New or inexperienced users of the drug who take a large dose can experience a severe respiratory depression that leads to death. OxyContin abusers who inject the drug with shared needles risk contracting diseases such as the human immunodeficiency virus, HEPATITIS B and C, and other bloodborne viruses.

Actions to Stop or Prevent Abuse

According to the GAO, Purdue, the pharmaceutical company that produces OxyContin, has tracked the potential abuse and misuse of OxyContin through information from its sales representatives. Purdue sales representatives receive extensive reports on physician prescribing practices. The information is usually used for marketing purposes. However, the company was apparently concerned about abuse of the drug and decided to take what may have been an unprecedented action, as described in a GAO report that was released in 2003, "Although this [prescribing] information has always been available for use by Purdue and its sales representatives, it was not until fall 2002 that Purdue directed its sales representatives to begin using 11 indicators to identify possible abuse and diversion and to report the incidents to Purdue's General Counsel's Office for investigation. Among the possible indicators are a sudden unexplained change in a physician's prescribing patterns that are not accounted for by changes in patient numbers, information from credible sources such as a pharmacist that a physician or his or her patients are diverting medications, or a physician who writes a large number of prescriptions for patients who pay with cash. As of September 2003, Purdue—through its own investigations—had identified 39 physicians and other health care professionals who were referred to legal, medical, or regulatory authorities for further action. Most of the 39 referrals stemmed from reports by Purdue's sales force."

The company also created tamper-proof prescription pads for OxyContin prescriptions. These actions, however, could not stop some people from stealing the drug or buying it from illegal sources.

As a result of concern over abuse and safety problems, some states have passed laws further regulating OxyContin. For example, in 2003, state legislators in Pennsylvania amended their state law to make OxyContin a Schedule I drug rather than a Schedule II drug. West Virginia has listed all drugs containing oxycodone as Schedule I drugs. Physicians in these states are still allowed to prescribe the drug to patients with severe pain.

Some experts believe that these laws have made or will make physicians unlikely or unwilling to prescribe OxyContin. Some pharmacies have refused to sell OxyContin and have posted signs that they do not stock the drug in an attempt to decrease their risk of robberies.

Withdrawal from OxyContin

Symptoms of withdrawal from OxyContin addiction include bone and muscle pain, diarrhea, vomiting, involuntary leg movements, cold flashes, restlessness, and insomnia. Some patients have sought a rapid detoxification from OxyContin, although studies have not shown whether quickly detoxifying from OxyContin under medical supervision will enable addicted patients to stay off of the drug.

A rapid detoxification may remove the physical dependence on the drug. However, if users remain psychologically dependent on the drug, they may need further help.

See also DETOXIFICATION; NARCOTICS; OPIATES; PAIN; PAINKILLING MEDICATIONS; PAIN MANAGEMENT; PAIN MANAGEMENT CENTERS; PRESCRIPTION DRUG ABUSE; TREATMENT CONTRACT/MEDICATIONS.

General Accounting Office Report to Congressional Requesters. "Prescription Drugs: OxyContin Abuse and Diversion and Efforts to Address the Problem," GAO-04-110. Washington, D.C.: United States General Accounting Office, December 2003.

National Drug Intelligence Center. *National Drug Threat Assessment 2003.* U.S. Department of Justice (DOJ) Product No. 2003-Q0317-001. Washington, D.C.: DOJ, January 2003.

pain Discomfort that ranges from mild to severe. Some people become addicted to opioids or other prescription medications that they first take because of their chronic pain conditions, such as back pain, arthritis, and other illnesses. Many experts believe, however, that an addiction with such a beginning is not a common occurrence. Instead, most addictions to opioids and other such medications stem from the pursuit of a EUPHORIA that an illicit use induces among patients who are not in pain. This euphoria is usually not found to result among patients who are in severe pain who use opioids.

Whether some patients should continue to receive opioids on a long-term basis for their severe chronic pain is a controversial issue. Many physicians fear that the patient will become addicted to the drug, while others believe that pain relief is the most important concern. In addition, undertreatment of pain can lead to great suffering and even to suicide and violence. Further studies of the long-term effects of narcotics on patients with cancer pain and severe chronic pain are urgently needed so that physicians and policy makers can create plans that are fair and reasonable to patients in severe pain while at the same time are protective of individuals who are at risk for becoming addicted to prescription drugs.

See also NARCOTICS; OPIATES; OXYCONTIN; PAIN-KILLING MEDICATIONS; PAIN MANAGEMENT; PRESCRIPTION DRUG ABUSE.

painkilling medications Drugs that decrease the brain's ability to perceive pain or that decrease the abnormal body process that leads to pain. Drugs such as aspirin and other nonsteroidal anti-inflammatory drugs decrease inflammatory processes at the site of the pain while decreasing the brain's

reporting of pain. Opiate pain relievers block brain response to pain through activating specific brain receptor sites devoted to pain perception.

Some painkilling medications can be addictive, particularly narcotics such as METHADONE and OXYCONTIN. Some experts believe that when patients in severe pain are managed properly, addiction from narcotics is a low risk. This is a controversial issue.

Some individuals addicted to painkilling drugs present to doctors and emergency rooms pretending to be in severe pain in order to obtain addictive medications. Trained emergency room physicians can generally distinguish individuals who are faking pain from those who are truly ill.

See also NARCOTICS; PAIN; PAIN MANAGEMENT; PAIN MANAGEMENT CENTERS; PRESCRIPTION DRUG ABUSE; TRAMADOL.

pain management Treatment provided by physicians for patients with severe chronic pain problems, such as cancer, back pain, arthritis, sickle cell anemia, stroke, and many other medical problems that generate pain. The use of prescription medications such as NARCOTICS, including drugs such as OXYCONTIN and METHADONE, are often indicated for patients with severe unremitting pain, although many patients are fearful of becoming addicted to these drugs. Although this is a valid concern, experts report that when physicians are trained and knowledgeable about narcotics, are careful with dosages, and do not overtreat or undertreat their patients, problems with addiction are rare. One caveat, however, is that most studies on patients with chronic pain who are taking opiates are of patients who have used the drug for less than a year, and thus the long-term effects of opiates are unclear.

If doctors overtreat their chronic pain patients, prescribing an excessive dose of medication, patients receive too much medication and risk the development of serious side effects that are associated with narcotics, such as a rapid tolerance or a dependence on the drug. It is possible for a patient who is treated in a pain management clinic to receive an inappropriately high dosage of narcotics such that the patient becomes dependent on narcotics. This situation comes under the oversight of organizations such as the Drug Enforcement Administration as well as other federal, state, and local law enforcement organizations.

In contrast, if the doctor undertreats patients' problems with pain, then patients may seek further pain remedies and risk dangerous medication interactions from the effects of multiple drugs. Undertreated patients who seek further medications may be mistakenly perceived as drug seekers or even as drug addicts by some physicians, when in fact they are pseudoaddicts.

Some physicians believe that it is far more likely that patients are undertreated for pain than it is that they would be overtreated. Studies have shown that some elderly patients in nursing homes have received little or no medication beyond over-the-counter drugs for advanced cancer pain due to physician fear of legal consequences. The fear of causing addiction has led some physicians into an overreaction and a failure to prescribe narcotics when they are clearly needed.

Balancing the Need to Treat Pain with the Desire to Prevent Addiction

According to some experts, policy makers must balance the need to treat patients with pain with the desire to protect patients from the risk of addiction and drug abuse.

According to a position statement from the task force of the College on Problems of Drug Dependence, published in a 2003 issue of *Drug and Alcohol Dependence*, "When formulating policy decision about prescription opioid nonmedical use and abuse, a careful and balanced approach is needed, so that the risk management strategies developed to prevent and reduce diversion of prescription opioids do not deter physicians from prescribing high-efficacy opioids when those drugs are indicated."

In addition, the authors also stated, "Pain is still undertreated in this country and to reduce availability of opioids in an attempt to stem diversion to illicit sources would further exacerbate a problem already affecting many pain patients—inadequate pain relief." They further stated, "Recommended steps to take include further epidemiological research, laboratory testing of prescription opioids to determine abuse liability, and clinical trials to determine the efficacy of different approaches to the prevention and treatment of prescription opioid abuse."

Pain management clinics must keep careful records of their patients. Many doctors also require patients to sign contracts that patients will obtain narcotic painkillers only from their pain management physician, although the enforceability of these contracts is questionable. Doctors may also request periodic and random drug screening of their patients if they are concerned about excessive drug use or about patients combining their medications with alcohol or other drugs. Despite such tests, however, there is only so much screening that the physician can accomplish within the constraints of his or her office.

Pharmacists may report physicians to law enforcement personnel if they feel physicians are writing an unusually high number of narcotic prescriptions or the dosages seem unreasonably high.

Pain management clinics are also at risk for burglary because some individuals believe that clinics maintain a large amount of narcotics. Because of this and other risks, most clinics maintain very little or no inventory of narcotic pain relievers.

Noncompliance with Opioid Therapy

Sometimes patients fail to comply with their prescribed narcotic regimens for various reasons. They may not wish to take the drugs because of the side effects (narcotics are very constipating). In addition, they may not wish to take opioids because of the social stigma associated with taking methadone, morphine, OxyContin, and other drugs.

In contrast, some patients may take excessive doses of the drug. They may believe that taking large doses of the drug will relieve them of all their pain, generally an unreasonable expectation. They may also be addicted to the drug.

Some examples of such noncompliance, which may be an indication of addiction, were provided by Dr. Jane Ballantyne and Dr. Jianren Mao in their 2003 article for the *New England Journal of Medicine*. They included such behaviors as reporting to their physician that they have lost medications or prescriptions on multiple occasions, tampering with prescriptions, frequently going to the emergency room to seek medication, missing follow-up appointments with the doctor, and asking for dosage increases too often. Such patients may receive a toxicology screening and have findings not in concert with the drugs they are supposed to be taking.

More Studies Are Needed

Further studies of the long-term use of opioids for nonmalignant chronic pain are needed to answer many questions that physicians and patients have about addiction as well as side effects and potential problems. Clinical studies would be difficult to manage, however, because of the nature of the patients. Giving a placebo to patients in extreme pain would be unethical. One possible solution would be to randomize some patients to rehabilitation therapy or to nonnarcotic medications, but a lack of funding has precluded such studies as of this writing.

See also CANCER; CARISOPRODOL; MORPHINE; OXY-CONTIN; PAIN; PAINKILLING MEDICATIONS; PAIN MANAGEMENT CENTERS; PRESCRIPTION DRUG ABUSE; TRAMADOL.

Ballantyne, Jane C., M.D. and Jianren Mao, M.D. "Opioid Therapy for Chronic Pain," *New England Journal of Medicine* 349, no. 20 (November 13, 2003): 1,943–1,953.

Mitka, Mike. "Experts Debate Widening Use of Opioid Drugs for Chronic Nonmalignant Pain," *Journal of the American Medical Association* 289, no. 18 (May 14, 2003): 2,347–2,348.

Zacny, James, et al. "College on Problems of Drug Dependence Taskforce on Prescription Opioid Non-Medical Use and Abuse: Position Statement," *Drug and Alcohol Dependence* 69, no. 3 (2003): 215–232.

pain management centers Facilities that specialize in treating patients with severe chronic pain that is caused by CANCER, spinal disorders, arthritis, and a wide variety of other serious, pain-inducing medical problems. These centers may be staffed by physicians with special training in pain management, although generally any licensed physician may open a pain clinic. In a multidisciplinary pain center, the facility may be comprised of anesthesiologists, psychiatrists, neurologists, physiatrists (physicians who are trained in physical medicine, also known as sports medicine), psychologists, and other experts.

Physicians at most pain management centers prescribe medications, including narcotics, when they are determined necessary to alleviate intractable pain. Pain management centers may also offer physical therapy and lawful steroid injections. The doctors should have a thorough knowledge of drug interactions and the side effects of narcotics as well as an understanding of issues of cross-tolerance and withdrawal. Sometimes doctors become concerned about patients becoming addicted to drugs, although most studies indicate that few patients with chronic pain develop such addictions unless they have a prior history of a problem with addictions.

The Committee on Accreditation of Rehabilitation Facilities offers a certification program for inpatient and outpatient pain centers. The American Academy of Pain Management provides certification for chronic pain treatment centers.

See also MORPHINE; NARCOTICS; OPIATES; PAIN; PAIN MANAGEMENT; TREATMENT CONTRACT/MEDICATIONS.

Hendler, Nelson, M.D. "Pain Clinics," in *Pain Management Secrets: Questions and Answers Reveal the Secrets to Successful Pain Management,* 2nd ed. Ronald Kanner, M.D., ed. Philadelphia, Pa.: Hanley & Belfus, Inc., 2003.

pancreatitis, alcoholic A severe and possibly life-threatening inflammation of the pancreas, often caused by long-term ALCOHOLISM. Alcoholic pancreatitis is most common among men in their 40s who are alcoholics.

The patient with pancreatitis suffers from profound abdominal pain and may also experience nausea and vomiting. Patients with alcoholic pancreatitis need to be treated in a hospital because of the seriousness of this condition, which can lead to death in the worst case. Patients require intravenous fluids and painkilling medications until they are stabilized.

Diagnosis and Treatment

Patients with pancreatitis often present to the hospital emergency room, complaining of extreme pain. In the case of chronic pancreatitis, a plain X-ray may show some calcification of the pancreas. A computerized tomography scan can also show the severity of the pancreatitis. An ultrasound is usually also performed to rule out the presence of gallstones, which can cause symptoms similar to pancreatitis or may cause pancreatitis itself.

The diagnosis of pancreatitis can be confirmed with blood tests, specifically tests for the pancreatic enzymes lipase and amylase.

Patients with alcoholic pancreatitis are urged to stop drinking alcohol immediately because continued drinking will lead to further increasingly painful bouts with pancreatitis and finally to pancreatic failure.

See also ALCOHOLIC HEALTH PROBLEMS.

Minocha, Anil, M.D., and Christine Adamec. *The Encyclopedia of Digestive Diseases and Disorders.* New York: Facts On File, Inc., 2004.

PCP (phencyclidine)   A hallucinogenic drug that was initially developed as an anesthetic to be used during surgical procedures in the 1950s. PCP was removed from the market for human use in 1965 because patients became too delusional and agitated when the anesthetic wore off. Veterinarians continued to use the drug as a tranquilizer until about 1978, when legal manufacture of the drug ceased in the United States. Today, there is no legal production of PCP, according to the DRUG ENFORCEMENT ADMINISTRATION.

PCP is currently a Schedule II drug under the CONTROLLED SUBSTANCES ACT in the United States. PCP is manufactured illegally in clandestine laboratories in a liquid or powder form, and it is smoked, snorted, or taken orally.

Studies have shown that an estimated 3 percent of high school students have ever used PCP in the United States in 2002 and about 3 percent of the population ages 12 and older have used PCP at least once. The National Household Survey on Drug Abuse has estimated that about 6 million people in the United States ages 12 and older have used PCP at least once in their lives.

The drug has such negative effects in contrast to other drugs of abuse that understanding its appeal is difficult. However, its addictive qualities may draw users to using PCP again and again. Some users report that the drug makes them feel powerful, while others say it has a numbing effect on their brains.

Effects of PCP

After ingestion, the drug takes effect rapidly, usually within minutes, and the effects of PCP may last for days. Physical changes caused by the drug may include an increased blood pressure and heart rate, and the user's body temperature may become so elevated that the person suffers from hyperthermia. Severe muscle contractions may also occur, and these muscle contractions may become so extreme that the individual suffers from bone fractures. High doses of PCP can lead to convulsions, coma, and death.

PCP induces strong auditory and visual HALLUCINATIONS in users and may induce a PSYCHOTIC BREAK. They may experience paranoia and delusions and thus their symptoms may be difficult to distinguish from severe mental illness, such as paranoid SCHIZOPHRENIA.

The drug also induces dissociative feelings of detachment and distortions of body images, as other hallucinogenic drugs may also cause. PCP has led to acts of violence and suicide. People in a hospital or detention setting who take this drug are a danger to themselves and to others.

Adolescents who take PCP may find that the drug impedes their growth and development. It can also impede the learning process. Over the long term, users of PCP may develop permanent problems with thinking and with speech as well as with depression. These problems may continue for as long as a year after the person discontinues using PCP.

In contrast to other hallucinogens, the continued use of PCP can lead to addiction, and physical withdrawal symptoms may also occur when the drug is stopped. Chronic users may suffer from memory loss and depression after they stop taking PCP.

See also ECSTASY; LSD; METHAMPHETAMINE; MUSHROOMS/PSILOCYBIN; TEENAGE AND YOUTH DRUG ABUSE.

National Institute on Drug Abuse. "PCP (Phencyclidine)," *NIDA Info Facts.* Bethesda, Md.: National Institutes of Health, September 2003. Available online. URL: http://www.nida.nih.gov/Infofax/pcp.html. Accessed April 2005.

peer pressure   Urging from individuals that a person regards as his or her equal to perform acts that the individual might not choose to do on his or her own. For example, teenage peers may urge an adolescent to engage in SMOKING or drinking, including BINGE DRINKING, or to perform other addictive behaviors so that the person will be considered as one of the group. Unfortunately, the addictive behavior often remains well after the individual has grown up and may have lost all interest in his or her former adolescent friends.

See also CODEPENDENCY; ENABLERS.

peyote   A Mexican cactus that contains mescaline, a potent hallucinogen (which causes HALLUCINATIONS). Peyote has been used in some tribal religious ceremonies. Peyote is not a popular drug of abuse in the United States, but it is used by some young adults. According to the National Household Survey on Drug Abuse in 2001, less than 1 percent of youths ages 12–17 reported ever using peyote. A peyote button, the mushroomlike crown of the peyote plant, is a powerful cathartic, causing excessive vomiting.

physicians and health care professionals and addiction   Physicians, dentists, pharmacists, nurses, and other health care professionals generally regarded as role models in society but who, like anyone else, may develop an addiction to illegal drugs, prescribed medications, or alcohol.

No one knows how many health care professionals have addictive behaviors. It is generally believed that in many cases, addicted health professionals are not reported to medical licensing boards. Some experts believe that the extreme stress faced by doctors and other health care professionals may increase the risk of developing a SUBSTANCE ABUSE problem. Others say that insufficient data is available to know why some health care workers become addicted while others in the same type of environment do not develop such a problem.

According to Dr. Abraham Verghese in his article for the *New England Journal of Medicine*, most impaired health care professionals use alcohol. He says that anesthesiologists are overrepresented in substance abuse programs. This may be at least in part due to their ready access to addicting drugs. Dr. Verghese also says that emergency room physicians who abuse drugs are more likely to choose cocaine, while impaired psychiatrists are more likely to choose mood-altering drugs. Some examples of mood-altering drugs are stimulants, antidepressants, and tranquilizers.

Fortunately, according to Dr. Verghese, impaired physicians who undergo rehabilitation for their addiction are often successful. He says, "The incentive is great: physicians cannot pursue their livelihood without a license, and any drug use will put that license in jeopardy."

This ability of physicians to recover has been backed up by studies. For example, according to a 2001 issue of the *Journal of the American Medical Association*, the University of Florida studied a random selection of 24 physicians in the Florida Physician Recovery Network who received treatment for alcohol or drug addiction in 1995. The purpose of the study was to determine if the doctors were employed and drug-free five years later after treatment. The research showed that 22 of the 24 physicians were successfully rehabilitated, based on evaluations from mental health professionals, work records, and random weekly (or more frequent) urinalysis testing for drugs. This is a stunning success rate compared with the 30–35 percent success rate of other individuals who have completed drug and alcohol treatment.

The Scope of the Problem

It is generally believed that only a few doctors and other health care professionals become addicted to alcohol or drugs, but that those individuals represent a significant problem to patients and other doctors. In one study of physicians who were disciplined by a state medical board in California, reported in the *Journal of the American Medical Association* in 1998, the researchers found that 375 doctors were disciplined for 465 offenses from October 1995 to April 1997. About 15 percent of all licensed physicians practice in California, and thus the California data provides useful and broad information.

The most common reasons for disciplinary action against physicians in this study were negligence or incompetence (34 percent) followed by abuse of alcohol or other drugs (14 percent). According to the researchers, about 10,000 complaints are made about doctors every year to the Medical Board of California, but most of these (about 80 percent) are dismissed as invalid.

Indications of Impairment in Health Care Professionals

Experts say that impaired doctors may be more readily noticed in busy hospitals and clinics as opposed to more suburban or rural areas. In general, alcohol-impaired doctors are likely to report in sick frequently or may fail to appear at all. They begin to isolate themselves from others more than in the past and attempt to work alone whenever possible. They may become drunk at parties or other public functions. The odor of alcohol on the breath may be present. The doctor's work performance may be noticeably poorer than in the past.

In contrast to alcoholic doctors, drug-addicted health care professionals are more likely to spend extra time around the hospital or clinic, where they may have easy access to addictive drugs, such as narcotics. They may make a habit of coming in early and staying late and may volunteer to work extra shifts. They may volunteer to be in charge of the keys to the cabinet where controlled medications are kept.

Drug-addicted health care professionals may exhibit marked mood swings, from euphoria to irritability, over a short period of time. They may constantly make trips to the bathroom, where they can use drugs. They may request other doctors to write narcotic prescriptions for them or for their family and patient prescriptions may be written with inappropriately high dosages. Their record keeping for narcotics is often sloppy and inadequate, and there may be shortages of narcotics in the medicine supply cabinet.

As with other addicts, a health care professional who has a drug addiction may also have physical signs, such as dilated pupils and needle marks on the arms. The individual's personal hygiene may deteriorate, and a once-neat individual may look dirty and unkempt. The drug-impaired individual also tends to make more mistakes than in the past and refuses to accept responsibility for them.

Denial Is Common

Many physicians with a drug or alcohol problem do not believe that they are addicted. Denial is common because physicians believe that they are smart people and in control. Because they self-prescribe, they may believe their prescriptions are appropriate and necessary. Like other addicts in denial, they believe that they can stop using the drug or alcohol whenever they choose to do so. In addition, because health care professionals, especially physicians, are trained to be self-sufficient and to rely on their own decisions, which they make quickly and confidently, they may feel discouraged from seeking help or admitting to any personal weakness.

In the book *Drug-Impaired Professionals* by Robert Holman Coombs, which was based on interviews with 91 addicted professionals (whose confidentiality was preserved), such as physicians, medical students, dentists, pharmacists, nurses, and pilots, a physician was quoted as saying, "I didn't think it could happen to me because I'm too smart and I have all this knowledge. I'm unique, a doctor, a cut or two above the average citizen. When I found out I was addicted, I was devastated. It sneaked up on me and had me by the throat before I even had an inkling that I had a problem."

Some individuals realize that what they are doing is illegal and potentially harmful. However, they believe that this behavior is all right because they believe it does not affect their professional life. This is another form of denial. In a case cited in *Drug-Impaired Professionals,* an addicted person talked about when he was a resident and an anesthesiologist resident had died of drug abuse. The department chair called everyone to a special meeting and said that he knew that some of the residents were using drugs. The department head was quoted as saying, "You might think that what you do socially has nothing to do with what you do here. Well, let me tell you something. I confronted a resident in the not-so-distant past with information I had regarding his use of recreational drugs and he told me, 'What I do on my own time is my business.' He was one of my best residents. He's dead now, and I'm here to tell you that if you are using drugs 'on your own time' *it isn't only your business!* I learned the hard way that it is *my* business, and any of you who are using recreational drugs must stop. If you need help, get it. If you don't know where to get help, ask me and I will tell you. I promise you that if you come to me for help, I will not throw you out of the program. I also promise you that if you continue to use drugs, I will throw you out. It's your choice. You know who you are. I don't want any more dead residents."

Addicted Individuals May Fear the Consequences of Revealing Their Addiction

Addicted health care professionals know that when the addiction is identified by others, the penalties can be very severe, such as suspension from the job or even outright loss of professional licensing. Although they may be able to retain their professional license as a condition of or subsequent to undergoing rehabilitative treatment in many states, the addicted professional may still fear the permanent loss of the license and an entire professional career.

Family Members, Friends, and Colleagues Often Cover for the Addict

In many cases, family members and friends will assist the addicted person in covering up the addiction because they do not want the addict or the addict's family to suffer the consequences that public disclosure would cause. Family members may call in to the office and say that the health care professional is "sick" when he or she is actually suffering from the effects of drugs, alcohol, or withdrawal from drugs or alcohol.

The professional's own staff may cover for the addicted person. They may fear reprisals such as getting fired or being sued if they do not cover for the addict. They may fear the professional will lose his or her livelihood, which in turn could also cause staff members to lose their jobs.

Sometimes professionals cover for each other, believing that doctors, nurses, and other health care professionals need to stick up for each other. They do not want to ruin the reputation of a colleague and may fear being treated as a whistleblower if they did so. They may also fear legal retaliation from the addicted person, particularly if they have made an error about the addiction. According to malpractice attorney Lee J. Johnson of Mount Kisco, New York, this is not a valid fear. Johnson told *Medical Economics* in a 2002 article,

"In most states, there's immunity for good faith reporting."

State Programs

Some states offer special programs for health care professionals who have become substance abusers, allowing them to retain their professional licenses if they successfully complete particular rehabilitative programs. For example, in 1994, Minnesota passed a law that created a diversion program for impaired physicians and others that would allow licensing boards to monitor their treatment confidentially. Prior to the passage of the law, most health care professionals faced disciplinary actions that were reported in public records.

The new law allowed for confidentiality as long as the health care professional complied with the program. This program is designed for addicted professionals only. However, some individuals are not eligible for this program. Those health care professionals who improperly gave narcotics to others, who had failed a similar program in Minnesota or another state in the past, who were accused of sexual misconduct, or who would "create a serious risk of harm to the public" if they continued to practice were not included. Other categories were also excluded from participating in this diversion program.

Other Professionals with Addictions

It should also be noted that health care professionals are not the only types of professionals who may develop addictive behaviors. Airline pilots, attorneys, ship captains, and many other professionals who are trusted by the public sometimes develop serious substance abuse problems.

See also DIVERSION PROGRAMS; ENABLERS.

American Medical Association. "Treatment Helps Addicted Physicians," *Journal of the American Medical Association* 286, no. 24 (December 26, 2001): 3,071.

Coombs, Robert Holman. *Drug-Impaired Professionals.* Cambridge, Mass.: Harvard University Press, 1997.

Harbison, Kent G. "New Law Avoids Unnecessary Punishment of Impaired Physicians," http://www.fredlaw.com/articles/health/heal_9409_kghmm.html. Accessed on December 20, 2003.

Morrison, James, M.D. and Peter Wickersham. "Physicians Disciplined by a State Medical Board," *Journal of the American Medical Association* 279, no. 23 (June 17, 1998): 1,889–1,893.

Terry, Ken. "Impaired Physicians Speak No Evil? (Reporting an Impaired Colleague)," Available online. URL: http:www.findarticles.com/cf_dls/m3229/19_79/932 12856/print.jhtml. Accessed on December 20, 2003.

Verghese, Abraham, M.D. "Physicians and Addiction," *New England Journal of Medicine* 346, no. 20 (May 16, 2002): 1,510–1,511.

pica An unusual eating disorder, which may be an addictive behavior, in which the individual habitually consumes nonfood items, such as paper, clay, or other items. It may be caused by anemia or by a mental illness and should be treated by a physician within the appropriate specialty.

posttraumatic stress disorder (PTSD) A form of anxiety disorder and a delayed or chronic reaction to one or more severe traumatic events that occurred in the past, even many years in the past. Individuals who suffer from PTSD may have a greater risk of developing substance abuse and other addictive behaviors in an unconscious attempt to resolve their emotional pain. They may also suffer from DEPRESSION and/or ANXIETY DISORDERS.

According to the Substance Abuse and Mental Health Administration, of the entire population exposed to a traumatic event, about 7 percent may develop PTSD. Of those who have been assaulted, about 54 percent develop PTSD. In general, women have a greater risk for developing the disorder.

According to Rachel Yehuda in her 2002 article on PTSD for the *New England Journal of Medicine*, the individual with PTSD has been exposed to an event to which he or she responded with shock, horror, fear, or helplessness. Individuals with PTSD actively avoid reminders of the event, including staying away from the people and places that may remind them of it. Physicians may be reluctant to probe individuals about disturbing events that have occurred to them. However, if a patient has otherwise unexplained symptoms, such as shortness of breath, heart palpitations, and insomnia, these symptoms may indicate the presence of PTSD and the physician should consider this possibility. If the diagnosis seems likely, the patient should be referred to a mental health professional.

Patients may be treated with therapy and education. Some therapists use exposure therapy, helping patients confront painful memories, while others use cognitive-behavioral therapy, teaching patients to challenge irrational beliefs. Patients with PTSD may also be treated with ANTIDEPRESSANTS.

See also BIPOLAR DISORDER; DUAL DIAGNOSIS; MENTAL ILLNESS/PSYCHIATRIC PROBLEMS; PSYCHIATRIC MEDICATIONS; PSYCHIATRISTS.

Yehuda, Rachel. "Post-Traumatic Stress Disorder," *New England Journal of Medicine* 346, no. 2 (January 10, 2002): 108–114.

pregnancy The time during which a fetus is carried and nurtured by a woman. Pregnant women who use drugs or who are addicted to drugs, alcohol, and/or tobacco and who continue their pregnancies risk harming their babies. They run a greater risk of delivering a low-birth-weight baby, and the baby also has a greater risk of physical and developmental problems.

Some studies indicate that pregnant women who abuse drugs and/or alcohol are more likely to have been reared by parents who were also drug or alcohol abusers. As with other addicts, they may also have underlying psychiatric disorders, such as DEPRESSION or antisocial personality disorder.

According to data from the federal Drug and Alcohol Services Information System, the percentage of pregnant women receiving SUBSTANCE ABUSE treatment for cocaine (27 percent) is higher than that for nonpregnant women using cocaine (20 percent). In contrast, the percentage of women receiving treatment for alcohol is much lower among pregnant women (24 percent) than nonpregnant women (38 percent). (See figure on page 199.)

A slightly higher percentage of pregnant women than nonpregnant women receive substance abuse treatment for marijuana use. The reasons for these discrepancies are open to interpretation. Pregnant women may be more likely to be tested for drugs because of the pregnancy, and thus, when they are tested, cocaine or marijuana use is detected. In contrast, nonpregnant women are generally tested only if they run afoul of the law.

As seen in the figure on page 199, women who are pregnant are less likely than nonpregnant women to be in treatment. This may be because they are less likely to drink or because they are less likely to seek treatment for their continued drinking problem because they are fearful of the consequences of discovery. They may also be fearful of seeking prenatal care because their substance abuse may be discovered, resulting in their referral to mandated treatment.

Many women who are pregnant are also fearful of seeking treatment for their drug or alcohol addiction because they may be afraid that their children who are already in the family will be taken away from their custody and placed into foster care. They may also fear that their newborn baby will be taken away upon its birth. As a result, frequently the only way that pregnant women will enter treatment is if it mandated by government authorities. The courts may require drug or alcohol treatment as a precondition to avoid incarceration or as part of a sentence. State social services workers may require treatment as a condition for retaining or regaining custody of a child. They may threaten legal termination of parental rights if the woman does not comply.

Many treatment programs for drug or alcohol dependence are primarily based on the needs of males rather than on the unique needs of pregnant women, who require ongoing medical care as well as treatment. In addition, pregnant women may need help with minor children under their care. Specialized treatment programs for drug-addicted pregnant women have been developed in many states.

Drug Use

According to the National Survey on Drug Use and Health as reported in a 2004 issue of *The NSDUH Report,* about 3 percent of pregnant women ages 15–44 years used an illegal drug in the past month, compared with 9 percent of nonpregnant women in this age group. Younger women were more likely to abuse drugs. Pregnant women ages 15–25 years were more likely to use illegal drugs than women ages 26–44 years old.

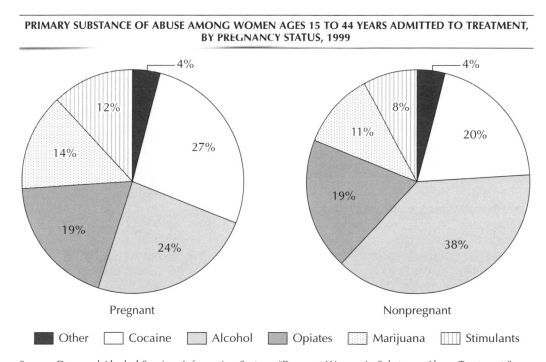

PRIMARY SUBSTANCE OF ABUSE AMONG WOMEN AGES 15 TO 44 YEARS ADMITTED TO TREATMENT, BY PREGNANCY STATUS, 1999

Pregnant

Nonpregnant

■ Other □ Cocaine ▨ Alcohol ▨ Opiates ⬚ Marijuana ▥ Stimulants

Source: Drug and Alcohol Services Information System, "Pregnant Women in Substance Abuse Treatment," *The DASIS Report,* Office of Applied Studies, Substance Abuse and Mental Health Services Administration (SAMHSA). Rockville, Md.: SAMHSA, May 17, 2002.

Some drugs are particularly problematic for pregnant women. For example, studies reported in the *New England Journal of Medicine* in 1999 have shown that cocaine use can increase the risk of a spontaneous abortion in pregnant women, as can tobacco use.

Alcohol Use

The National Survey on Drug Use and Health research revealed that 9 percent of pregnant women reported drinking any alcohol in the past month. (About 45 percent of nonpregnant women reported any alcohol use.) Less than 1 percent reported heavy alcohol use, compared with about 5 percent for nonpregnant women.

As with drug use, the rate of alcohol use was higher among younger pregnant women, ages 15–25 (5 percent) than among pregnant women ages 26–44 years old (2 percent). Alcohol use increases the risk of the infant being born with FETAL ALCOHOL SYNDROME, a condition with profound developmental effects and that usually includes mental retardation as well as many physical problems.

Cigarette Use

The National Survey on Drug Use and Health data revealed that about 17 percent of pregnant women reported smoking. Younger women, ages 15–25, had a higher rate of smoking than pregnant women ages 26–44 years. Smoking results in a significantly increased risk for delivering a low-birth-weight baby. As can be seen from the table below, in 2001, about 7 percent of nonsmokers had babies with low birth weight, compared with nearly 12 percent of mothers who were smokers. Tobacco is a problematic drug in terms of both the prevalence of its use and its dangerousness to the fetus.

Pregnant women who wish to quit smoking should discuss the issue with their doctors. They should not use nicotine replacement options unless the doctor recommends them, nor should they take drugs such as bupropion (Zyban) that are used to treat nonpregnant individuals wishing to stop smoking.

Because of the additional stress of pregnancy, it may be very difficult for women to stop smoking. This difficulty may be compounded if they also have a dependence on alcohol or drugs and/or are experiencing family problems.

Treatment for Addictions

Treating pregnant women who are addicted to substances and/or to cigarettes can be difficult. Physicians want women to stop using illegal drugs or harmful substances but they do not want to harm the fetus with the DETOXIFICATION process. This seems illogical because continued drug exposure is generally more dangerous than detoxifying from drugs.

According to information reported in a 2002 issue of *The DASIS Report,* studies of pregnant women ages 15–44 years, based on nationwide treatment statistics, revealed that they were less likely to be admitted to detoxification programs than nonpregnant women and were more likely to be admitted to outpatient programs. Of pregnant women who were admitted to treatment for opiate addiction, they were more likely to be admitted to methadone maintenance programs than were nonpregnant women. Yet withdrawal from heroin can be performed more quickly and the fetus can withdraw from the drug in utero rather than being subjected to a lengthy withdrawal from the much-longer-acting methadone.

One study of 244 pregnant women with substance abuse problems in North Carolina was

	1995	1996	1997	1998	1999	2000	2001
LOW-BIRTH-WEIGHT LIVE BIRTHS (LESS THAN 2,500 G), PERCENT OF LIVE BIRTHS ACCORDING TO MOTHER'S SMOKING STATUS, 1995–2001							
Cigarette smokers	12.18	12.13	12.06	12.01	12.06	11.88	11.90
Nonsmokers	6.79	6.91	7.07	7.18	7.21	7.19	7.32

Source: Fried, V. M., et al. *Chartbook on Trends in the Health of Americans. Health, United States, 2003.* Hyattsville, Md.: National Center for Health Statistics, 2003.

reported in the *American Journal of Drug and Alcohol Abuse*. Of these women, 192 (79 percent) were African American and 52 (21 percent) were non-Hispanic white. Their ages ranged from 20–41 years and all were eligible for Medicaid (a medical program for very low-income individuals who fit categorical requirements, such as being pregnant or disabled). Most did not receive any prenatal care until the second or third trimester; only 27 percent received care in the first trimester.

Of the 244 women, 236 (97 percent) were referred for outpatient treatment and 61 percent complied. About half the women were also referred for inpatient treatment (56 percent), and about 59 percent of them complied with the treatment.

The researchers found that women who complied with their referrals to outpatient treatment were significantly more likely to have received substance abuse treatment in the past. (Many of the women who complied, 45 percent, had undergone prior substance abuse treatment versus 28 percent of the women who failed to comply with outpatient treatment.) Their reputation has already been diminished and the secret of their substance abuse is out, and so these women may think that they have more to gain and less to lose by undergoing treatment. The researchers also found that women who complied with treatment were significantly more likely to have partners who themselves had also experienced prior substance abuse treatment.

With regard to compliance with inpatient treatment referrals, women who complied were also significantly more likely to have received prior substance abuse treatment, although their partners' prior substance abuse record was not significantly related.

The authors said, "Women who have never been in substance abuse treatment might be afraid that seeking help would cause them to be labeled as a drug user and then shunned by friends and/or family members, causing them to leave treatment early or to forego it. Women who have experienced treatment, however, may realize that it might be necessary to forge new drug-free relationships that could only be achieved through successful completion of a treatment program."

In another study, this time of women recruited from 15 residential substance abuse treatment programs for pregnant and parenting women in northern California, the researchers studied 36 women, including 12 who were pregnant at the time of the study and 24 women who had had a child the previous year. Two-thirds of the women had entered a substance abuse treatment program during their pregnancy, and the average age of entry to the program was 17 weeks gestation. Thirteen of the women had been referred to substance abuse treatment by child social services authorities as a condition of obtaining custody of a child who was already in foster care, or the women were ordered by a court to obtain treatment. The majority of the women (28 women) were African American, followed by 8 white women, 7 Latina women, and 1 Native American woman.

The researchers found that the majority of the women (78 percent) were fearful and worried about losing custody of their infants as well as of being arrested, prosecuted, and incarcerated for their use of drugs during their pregnancies. Some of the women stated that they had not sought prenatal care because they had feared they would suffer punitive consequences.

The researchers also identified other barriers to seeking treatment, such as the limits on the age and number of children that addicted women could bring with them to treatment. Many women experienced difficulty finding someone to care for their children during treatment. Women who were opiate dependent reported finding difficulty being accepted into a program, especially women who were in methadone treatment programs, because they were regarded by treatment providers as individuals with problems that were too complex to treat.

Pregnancy itself was perceived as a barrier to obtaining treatment for addictions. Clients in the study reported that treatment programs excluded them or, if they were accepted, did not provide transportation to receive prenatal care.

Clark, Kathryn Anderson, et al. "Treatment Compliance among Prenatal Care Patients with Substance Abuse Problems," Available online. URL: http://www.findarticles.com/cf_dls/m0978/1_27/75119727/print.jhtml Downloaded on February 27, 2004.

Drug and Alcohol Services Information System. "Pregnant Women in Substance Abuse Treatment," *The

DASIS Report, Office of Applied Studies, Substance Abuse and Mental Health Services Administration (SAMHSA). Rockville, Md.: SAMHSA, May 17, 2002.

Fried, V. M., et al. *Chartbook on Trends in the Health of Americans. Health, United States, 2003.* Hyattsville, Md.: National Center for Health Statistics, 2003.

Jessup, Martha A., et al. "Extrinsic Barriers to Substance Abuse Treatment Among Pregnant Drug Dependent Women," *Journal of Drug Issues* 2 (Spring 2003): 285–304.

National Survey on Drug Use and Health (NSDUH). "Pregnancy and Substance Use," *The NSDUH Report.* Rockville, Md.: Office of Applied Studies, Substance Abuse and Mental Health Services Administration, January 2, 2004.

Ness, Roberta B., M.D., et al. "Cocaine and Tobacco Use and the Risk of Spontaneous Abortion," *New England Journal of Medicine* 340, no. 5 (February 4, 1999): 333–339.

prescription drug abuse   The nonmedical use of a prescribed medication, whether it is used by someone other than the person for whom the drug was prescribed or a patient has been using his or her own prescribed drugs to excess. In some cases, prescription drugs are obtained through forged prescriptions or they are stolen from other individuals or pharmacies, hospitals, and other locations. Some people consult with two or more physicians, obtaining the same prescription from each doctor and purposely withholding the fact that they have already obtained this prescription from other doctors. In some cases, family members give other family members their prescribed medications, which, although it may be well-intended, is another form of prescription drug abuse. It is also an illegal act.

Pain medicines are the most commonly abused form of prescription drugs, especially narcotics. However other forms of prescription drugs are also abused, such as stimulants, diet pills, and psychiatric medications, such as sedatives and anti-anxiety drugs.

Prescription drug abuse may occur because individuals wish to achieve a euphoric high, lose weight, stay awake, alleviate pain, or control their distressing symptoms of withdrawal from the drug.

It can be extremely dangerous and even fatal to use another's prescription medications, whether on purpose or by accident. Using one's own prescription drugs to excess is also clearly dangerous and may be fatal. Of course, it is also dangerous to use prescription drugs obtained through illegal acts, such as through forged prescriptions or theft.

Most Commonly Abused Prescription Painkiller Drugs

Of the prescription painkiller drugs abused in 2002, most were scheduled drugs, according to the National Survey on Drug Use and Health. (See figure on page 203.) Darvocet, DARVON, and Tylenol with codeine were the most abused drugs. Nearly 19 million Americans ages 12 and older had used these particular drugs nonmedically in their lifetimes, followed by 13.1 million people who had abused Vicodin, Lortab, and Lorcet.

Emergency Department Visits Due to Prescription Drug Abuse

Prescription drug abuse is a problem seen in emergency departments in hospitals throughout the United States. According to the Drug Abuse Warning Network (DAWN), narcotic analgesics were involved in an estimated 14 percent of all drug abuse-related emergency department visits in 2001

PERCENTAGES OF PERSONS AGES 12 AND OLDER REPORTING LIFETIME AND PAST YEAR NONMEDICAL PAIN DRUG USE

Total	Lifetime Nonmedical Pain Reliever Use Chararacteristics	Past Year Dependence or Abuse
	Percentage	Percentage
Age		
12–17	11.2	1.0
18–25	22.1	1.4
26 and older	11.1	0.5
Gender		
Male	14.3	0.7
Female	11.0	0.6
Race/ethnicity		
White	13.6	0.7
African American	9.7	0.4
Asian	7.0	0.1
Hispanic	11.0	0.9

Source: Office of Applied Studies, Substance Abuse and Mental Health Services Administration (SAMHSA). "Nonmedical Use of Prescription Pain Relievers," *The NSDUH Report.* Rockville, Md.: SAMHSA, May 21, 2004.

ESTIMATED NUMBER (IN MILLIONS) OF LIFETIME NONMEDICAL USE OF SELECTED PAIN RELIEVERS AMONG PERSONS AGES 12 OR OLDER: 2002

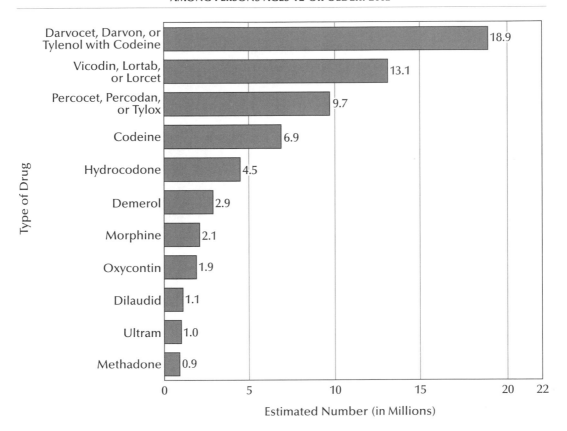

Source: Office of Applied Studies, Substance Abuse and Mental Health Services Administration (SAMHSA). "Nonmedical Use of Prescription Pain Relievers," *The NSDUH Report.* Rockville, Md.: SAMHSA, May 21, 2004.

in the United States. In a third of the cases, the narcotic was not named. In the cases where the drug was named, hydrocodone led, with 21,567 mentions, followed by oxycodone, with 18,409 mentions. The average age of patients treated for narcotic analgesic abuse in the emergency department was 37 years.

The numbers of analgesic-related emergency department visits have increased nationwide from 1994 to 2001, from 41,687 to 90,232, although the reasons for these increases remain unclear. (See figure on page 204.)

According to *The DAWN Report* for January 2003, "Most of the increases in narcotic analgesic mentions occurred toward the end of the 1990s. Total mentions increased 44 percent from 1999 to 2001, apparently driven by increases in oxycodone (186%), methadone (98%) and hydrocodone (41%). From 2000 to 2001, statistically significant increases were observed for oxycodone (70%) and methadone (37%). Although unspecified narcotic analgesics (NOS) increased 288 percent from 1994 to 2001 and 24 percent from 2000 to 2001, it is not possible to determine which, if any, specific drugs are driving the overall increase in that category."

In considering gender and prescription drug abuse in emergency department admissions for drugs, the most commonly abused narcotic by males in 2001 was oxycodone and the most commonly abused narcotic by females was hydrocodone.

TRENDS IN NARCOTIC ANALGESIC-RELATED EMERGENCY DEPARTMENT VISITS: 1994–2001

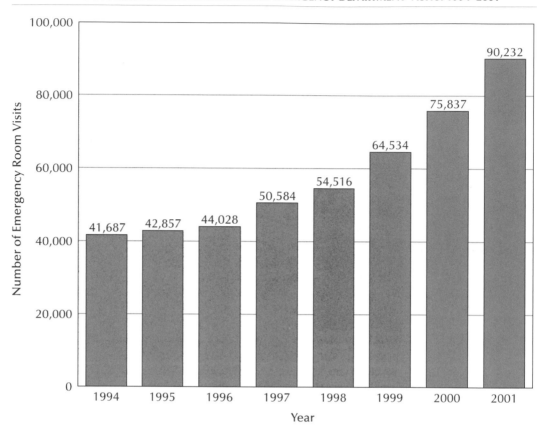

Source: Office of Applied Studies, Substance Abuse and Mental Health Services Administration (SAMHSA). "Narcotic Analgesics: In Brief," *The Dawn Report.* Rockville, Md.: SAMHSA, January 2003.

In looking at the race and ethnicity of narcotic abusers in the emergency rooms in the United States in 2001, most (62,937 patients) were white, followed by 9,986 African-American patients, and 8,329 Hispanic patients. In more than 8,000 cases, the patient's race and ethnicity were unknown.

When the motives for abusing the drugs could be determined, the most common motive was a dependence/addiction (44 percent) to the drug in order to function. The next most common motive was suicide, and 27 percent of the emergency department patients took narcotics alone or with other drugs or alcohol in order to end their lives. A small number, 15 percent, said they took drugs because of the psychological effects of the narcotics or for other reasons.

Abused Tranquilizers

Tranquilizers (antianxiety medications) have fallen from popularity as drugs of abuse, although they became increasingly popular again in the 1990s, as with other drugs. The most frequently abused tranquilizers are in the class of BENZODIAZEPINES. According to the overview of the key findings of *Monitoring the Future: National Results on Adolescent Drug Use* in 2002, Valium and Xanax were the most commonly abused drugs of this type by high school students.

Illegal Methods of Obtaining Prescription Drugs

As mentioned, adults may obtain drugs for prescription drug abuse through pharmacy theft, prescription fraud, or doctor shopping (visiting various doctors to obtain prescriptions for the same drug). In contrast, adolescents are more likely to obtain prescription drugs from their friends. They may receive drugs from other teenagers who have legitimate prescriptions. They may also steal medications from their family members or from their school dispensaries.

See also CARISOPRODOL; MORPHINE; NARCOTICS; OPIATES; OXYCONTIN; PAINKILLING MEDICATIONS; PAIN MANAGEMENT; PROPOXYPHENE; SCHEDULED DRUGS; TRAMADOL.

Johnston, Lloyd D., Patrick O'Malley, and Jerald G. Bachman. *Monitoring the Future: National Results on Adolescent Drug Use. Overview of Key Findings, 2002.* Bethesda, Md.: National Institute on Drug Abuse, U.S. Department of Health and Human Services, National Institutes of Health, 2003.

Office of Applied Studies, Substance Abuse and Mental Health Services Administration (SAMHSA). "Narcotic Analgesics: In Brief," *The Dawn Report.* Rockville, Md.: SAMHSA, January 2003.

Office of Applied Studies, Substance Abuse and Mental Health Services Administration. "Nonmedical Use of Prescription Pain Relievers," *The NSDUH Report* May 21, 2004.

propoxyphene (Darvon) A central nervous system depressant medication combined with aspirin. Darvon is a mild opioid that is structurally related to methadone and is used as a painkilling medication. When combined with acetaminophen rather than aspirin, the brand name is Darvocet. Propoxyphene in any form is a Schedule IV drug under the CONTROLLED SUBSTANCES ACT because it has some addictive potential. The drug can be taken orally or injected.

Effects of Propoxyphene

In addition to pain relief, the drug may induce EUPHORIA in some people. It may also cause stomach upset, nausea, and vomiting as well as constipation, fatigue, and blurred vision. The drug may lower both blood pressure and heart rate. High doses of propoxyphene can lead to coma, seizures, and accidental death. The combined use of propoxyphene and alcohol can be substantially more dangerous than the use of either substance alone. Some experts believe that this combination is even more dangerous than the benzodiazepine/alcohol interaction.

The long-term use of the drug can cause gastrointestinal damage such as stomach bleeding. It may also damage the kidneys and the liver. Physicians and patients should carefully monitor the use of this drug.

Patients should be sure to tell their doctors about other medications they take because some medications have serious interactions with propoxyphene. For example, warfarin (Coumadin) is a blood thinner. When combined with propoxyphene, the two drugs could lead to a dangerous bleeding problem.

See also OPIATES; SCHEDULED DRUGS.

prostitution Receiving money, drugs, or other commodities in exchange for sexual favors. Most prostitutes exhibit addictive behaviors to alcohol, illegal drugs, and cigarettes. They spend a great deal of time in jail. If they have children, prostitutes usually lose custody of them.

Some women may prostitute themselves out of desperation in order to obtain illegal drugs. For others, the act of prostitution occurs first and the drug abuse occurs later. Prostitution is illegal everywhere in the United States except in some parts of Nevada. If prostitutes are under the age of 18 years old, individuals who use their services can be prosecuted for statutory rape or child sexual abuse.

Studies

A study reported in a 1999 issue of *Psychiatric Services* analyzed data on 1,142 female jail detainees in Chicago between 1991 and 1993 to determine the primary pathways of the women into prostitution. (About a third, 34.1 percent, of the women had prostituted themselves.)

The researchers found three distinct pathways to prostitution. First, early adolescent runaways often became prostitutes. Women who had run away were more likely (44.7 percent) to have ever prostituted themselves than nonrunaways (29.7 percent). They were also more likely to prostitute themselves routinely (35.6 percent) than nonrunaways (21.5 percent).

Childhood sexual abuse was another major factor among women who became prostitutes. The researchers said this factor doubled the risk for entering into prostitution and remaining as a prostitute. More than a third of the sample was abused as children, and the average age at the time of first abuse was 10.6 years. It is also true that the sexual abuse was the reason why some women ran away as children.

Women who had been abused as children had a 44.2 percent rate of ever prostituting, versus 28.5 percent for those with no history of child sexual abuse. They also had a higher rate of routine prostitution, or 34.6 percent, versus 20.6 percent for nonabused detainees.

The researchers also found that illegal drug use was a significantly greater factor leading toward prostitution than others. However, it was not as powerful a factor as running away or child sexual abuse.

Because of these different pathways into prostitution, the researchers argued that different approaches were needed to help different populations of people. They said, "First, early recovery of children who run away is necessary to reduce entry to prostitution. Services must address children's basic survival needs by providing a stable emotional and environmental support system."

They added, "Second, the impact of childhood sexual abuse on entry into prostitution appears to persist over the life course. Victims of childhood sexual abuse need mental health services to help them come to terms with their victimization and restore a sense of mastery and control over their lives. The need for this help—and the potential impact on a victim's ability to make positive choices—does not diminish as women age."

"Third, although preventing or treating drug abuse may not be the most powerful deterrent to entry into prostitution, intervention is still vital. Addict-prostitutes tend to be heavy users and report that narcotic use increases with further involvement into prostitution. Although entrance into prostitution before addiction may be due to effects of sexual abuse, entering prostitution after developing an addiction may be an economic necessity."

In another study of a small sample of prostitutes (43 women), all of whom worked the streets to sell their sexual favors, the authors sought to identify basic factors about women who are prostitutes. This research was published in a 2000 issue of the *Journal of Sex Research*.

Less than half of the prostitutes were controlled by a pimp, and the rest reportedly were free agents. The women were an average of 33 years old, and they included 20 whites, 18 African Americans, and 5 Native Americans. Fourteen of the women were in prison. Their average education level was 9.3 years. The average age at entry into prostitution was 19.4 years.

Of the 43 women, 41 were drug abusers. Sixteen began abusing drugs before they entered a life of prostitution and 17 after they started prostituting. Eight said drug abuse was "concurrent" with prostitution. CRACK COCAINE was the most popular drug among the women, and other substances that were commonly used included MARIJUANA, ALCOHOL, and HEROIN.

The authors said, "Sexual abuse is repeatedly identified in the extant literature as a correlate to later prostitution. These data concur; sexual abuse consistently emerged in the participants' life histories." The researchers found that 63 percent of the women had been sexually molested as children.

Literal or imagined abandonment was another common theme among the women. Said the authors, "Parental alcoholism, drug abuse, mental instability, and severe domestic violence resulted in feelings of emotional (or symbolic) abandonment, as well. Symbolic abandonment also comprised instances when sexual abuse was reported but ignored."

Running away was another common theme among the women in this study, and 17 of the women had run away in early adolescence. One woman had traveled with carnivals, others had run off with boyfriends, and others hitched rides with strangers.

The researchers reported that condom use among the prostitutes was intermittent, and some women failed to require any condom use at all. The women reportedly did not care if they became pregnant or if they contracted a sexually transmitted disease or the human immunodeficiency virus. Five of the women had become pregnant by clients. Of the 43 women, 38 had borne children but only five of the children lived with the women. Most were in foster care, and some had been adopted. Others lived with other family members.

See also CHILD ABUSE AND NEGLECT; CRIME; SEX ADDICTS ANONYMOUS; SEXUAL ADDICTION; VIOLENCE.

Dalla, Rochelle L. "Exposing the 'Pretty Woman' Myth: A Qualitative Examination of the Lives of Female Streetwalking Prostitutes," *Journal of Sex Research* (November 2000). Available online. URL: http://articles.findarticles.com/p/articles/mi_m2372/is_4_37/ai_72272308/print Accessed June 14, 2004.

McClanahan, Susan F., et al. "Pathways into Prostitution among Female Jail Detainees and Their Implications for Mental Health Services," *Psychiatric Services* 50, no. 12 (December 1999): 1,606–1,613.

psychiatric medications Drugs that are used to treat psychiatric problems, such as ANXIETY DISORDERS, DEPRESSION, BIPOLAR DISORDER, OBSESSIVE-COMPULSIVE DISORDER and SCHIZOPHRENIA.

ANTIDEPRESSANTS are drugs given to treat individuals with depression. Antianxiety drugs (also called anxiolytics) are given to treat patients with anxiety disorders. Antipsychotic medications are given to patients with psychotic disorders who cannot reason for themselves and who appear to a mental health professional to be a threat to themselves or to other individuals because of HALLUCINATIONS and/or delusions (false beliefs). Stimulant medications and related drugs are given to patients with ATTENTION DEFICIT HYPERACTIVITY DISORDER (ADHD) to help them control their symptoms of distractibility, disorganization, and impulsivity as well as the hyperactivity that many individuals with ADHD have. Some patients need more than one psychiatric medication.

In general, people cannot be forced to take psychiatric medications against their will unless they are temporarily or permanently incarcerated or they are in an emergency situation in which their lives or another person's lives are threatened.

Some psychiatric medications are abused by individuals who do not have such illnesses. For example, sometimes people without ADHD seek to convince adolescents diagnosed with ADHD to share their prescribed stimulant medication with others. To do so would be illegal. Drugs such as methylphenidate (Ritalin) and other stimulants can induce a euphoric high among individuals who do not have ADHD.

BENZODIAZEPINES, used to treat anxiety disorders, are also sometimes used by people who do not have anxiety disorder and are engaging in PRESCRIPTION DRUG ABUSE.

psychiatric problems Serious or severe mental or emotional problems, including ANXIETY DISORDERS, BIPOLAR DISORDER, DEPRESSION, OBSESSIVE-COMPULSIVE DISORDER, SCHIZOPHRENIA, and many other psychiatric diagnoses. Individuals with addictive behaviors have a significantly greater risk of having a psychiatric disorder than people who are not addicts.

See also DUAL DIAGNOSIS; IMPULSE CONTROL DISORDERS; IMPULSIVITY; MOOD STABILIZERS; PSYCHIATRIC MEDICATIONS; PSYCHIATRISTS.

Petrakis, Ismene L., M.D., et al. "Comorbidity of Alcoholism and Psychiatric Disorders: An Overview," *Alcohol Research & Health* 26, no. 2 (2002): 81–89.

psychiatrists Medical doctors who are experts in mental health issues and medications. Psychiatrists assist people with addictive behaviors as well as moderate or serious psychiatric disorders, such as ATTENTION DEFICIT HYPERACTIVITY DISORDER, DEPRESSION, ANXIETY DISORDERS, BIPOLAR DISORDER, EATING DISORDERS, OBSESSIVE-COMPULSIVE DISORDER, and SCHIZOPHRENIA.

Psychiatrists may treat individuals with medications, and some psychiatrists also treat patients with talk therapy. Some psychiatrists refer patients to psychologists or social workers for psychotherapy while the psychiatrist manages the medications.

See also DUAL DIAGNOSIS.

psychotic break A severe psychiatric illness in which the person loses touch with reality and may become a danger to himself or herself or to others. Some hallucinogenic substances, such as lysergic acid diethylamide, phencyclidine, METHAMPHETAMINE, and ECSTASY (methylenedioxymethamphetamine) can cause a temporary or permanent psychotic break. An alcoholic undergoing WITH-DRAWAL and in the midst of DELIRIUM TREMENS may also suffer a psychotic break. A person who has undergone a psychotic break is in urgent need of psychiatric hospitalization. He or she may recover in a few weeks or months with treatment or may remain ill for an extended period. It can be very difficult for doctors to predict the prognosis.

See also AMPHETAMINE PSYCHOSIS; COCAINE; DUAL DIAGNOSIS; LSD; PCP.

recovery The process by which an addicted person successfully overcomes addictive behavior, whether through therapy, medications, and/or other means. Experts report that many people seeking recovery from their addictive behaviors have one or more RELAPSES as they move toward overcoming the problem and toward health.

See also DETOXIFICATION; REHABILITATION.

rehabilitation The process by which a person overcomes an addiction. Often rehabilitation (or rehab) is achieved in an institutional setting, although addicted individuals may also seek recovery as outpatients, depending on the type of addictive behavior that they seek to overcome. In general, long-term alcohol or drug abuse usually requires treatment in a residential treatment facility for an individual to experience a recovery.

See also DETOXIFICATION; RECOVERY; RELAPSES; TREATMENT.

relapses A return to performing addictive behaviors after a period of refraining from them. Many experts believe that relapses are common and to be expected with many addictive behaviors, although it is hoped that individuals have few or no relapses. People may relapse for many different reasons, such as associating with others who exhibit the addictive behavior (such as an ex-smoker spending time with heavy smokers or a reformed drinker who associates with others who encourage him or her to drink). Severe stress may lead to a relapse because the individual may feel a need to exhibit the addictive behavior in order to relieve the emotional stress.

Rohypnol (flunitrazepam) A central nervous system depressant that is classified as a Schedule IV drug under the CONTROLLED SUBSTANCES ACT. Rohypnol can induce amnesia and has been known to be used as a DATE RAPE DRUG. However, because of concern about this use, in 1997, the manufacturer reformulated the drug so that if it is mixed with a liquid, the fluid becomes blue. Despite this change in the formulation, some sexual predators have overcome this precautionary step by placing the drug into blue drinks or in dark containers, thus keeping it possible for unwitting victims to be drugged.

Rohypnol can also be injected. The drug has also been used illegally by drug abusers to counteract the stimulating effects of COCAINE or METHAMPHETAMINES.

Most abusers of Rohypnol are young and between the ages of 13 and 30 years old. An estimated 2 percent of all high school seniors have used the drug, according to studies by the University of Michigan.

Effects of the Drug
Rohypnol generally causes sedation, dizziness, memory impairment, and confusion, although it can cause aggression in some users. The effects of the drug are quickly felt within about 15 minutes and may last as long as 12 hours or more.

See also CLUB DRUGS.

S

scheduled drugs Term used by the DRUG ENFORCEMENT ADMINISTRATION (DEA) to denote drugs that have been designated as having varying potential for abuse or addiction, based on regulations set in the CONTROLLED SUBSTANCES ACT, a federal law. NARCOTICS, MARIJUANA, some sedatives, and many other specific drugs are scheduled drugs.

Although not required to do so, many doctors photocopy prescriptions they have written for scheduled drugs for their own records before they give the prescription to the patient. This provides the doctor with a copy of the original prescription in the event that the patient attempts to tamper with the prescription regarding the dose or the number of pills ordered. Some doctors will give the prescription only to the patient directly or to a person they know, such as a spouse, because they are concerned about potential drug abuse by other individuals, such as other family members.

Schedule I drugs are considered to have the greatest potential for abuse, and they are also drugs that are illegal in the United States. Schedule II drugs may be legally prescribed, but they do have a high potential for abuse. Some levels of scheduled drugs require stricter controls. For example, doctors must write out a prescription for a Schedule II medication rather than calling one in to the pharmacy, and they may only write the prescription for one month with no refills. They are also required to keep careful office records.

Lower levels of scheduled drugs, such as Schedule III and IV medications, can be called in to the pharmacy. Refills may be ordered by the doctor.

HEROIN is a Schedule I drug. Possessing or selling heroin is illegal in the United States. Marijuana is also a Schedule I drug because the DEA does not acknowledge any medical use for it. ECSTASY (methylenedioxymethamphetamine) is another Schedule I drug, as is lysergic acid diethylamide. Some other examples of Schedule I drugs include mescaline, PEYOTE, and psilocybin.

Drugs that are classified as Schedule II drugs are considered to have a high potential for abuse, but they do have a currently accepted medical use in the United States, under strict control. Some examples of Schedule II drugs are MORPHINE, COCAINE, METHADONE, and various forms of oxycodone (OXYCONTIN, Percocet, Tylox, Roxicodone, and Roxicet).

Schedule III drugs have a lower potential for abuse than drugs in both Schedule I and Schedule II categories, and they also have a currently accepted medical use in the United States. ANABOLIC STEROIDS are examples of Schedule III drugs, as are some BARBITURATES such as butalbital and secobarbital. KETAMINE is a Schedule III drug. (It is also sometimes illegally used as a DATE RAPE DRUG.)

Schedule IV drugs have a lower potential for abuse than Schedules I through III, and they have a currently accepted medical use in the United States. Some examples of drugs that are classified as Schedule IV are antianxiety drugs or sedatives such as alprazolam (Xanax), chlordiazepoxide (Librium), clonazepam (Clonopin, Klonopin), diazepam (Valium), and zalepion (Sonata).

Schedule V drugs have the lowest potential for abuse among the scheduled drugs. They have a medical use in the United States. Over-the-counter cough preparations that contain codeine are classified as Schedule V drugs, as are some antidiarrheal medications, such as dephenoxylate (Lomotil and Logen).

See also ADDICTION; BENZODIAZEPINES; COUGH SYRUP; CRACK COCAINE; LSD; MUSHROOMS/PSILOCYBIN; OPIATES.

schizophrenia A psychotic disorder that is characterized by disordered thinking, delusions, and auditory and/or visual HALLUCINATIONS. Some individuals also experience other sensory hallucinations, such as feeling touches when no one is touching them (tactile hallucinations). People with schizophrenia may also exhibit paranoia, believing that others are actively plotting against them, and convincing them otherwise is impossible because of their strong sense of certainty.

Schizophrenia is often confused by the public with multiple personality disorder (also known as dissociative identity disorder). However, the person with schizophrenia does not have multiple personalities. Instead, he or she is confused, disoriented, and has difficulty differentiating between reality and delusions.

Schizophrenia occurs in about 1–2 percent of the population worldwide. It appears to have a genetic basis, although some cases may be triggered by drug abuse, particularly from the use of drugs such as lysergic acid diethylamide or COCAINE. Some people who abuse large amounts of amphetamines over weeks or longer may develop AMPHETAMINE PSYCHOSIS, which may resemble schizophrenia, although it is not the same problem. For this reason, physicians should screen individuals exhibiting psychotic symptoms by DRUG TESTING methods. The illness occurs in both males and females and generally presents in early adulthood, although rarely schizophrenia can have its onset in adolescence or earlier.

Behavior of People with Schizophrenia

Undiagnosed individuals with schizophrenia, or diagnosed patients with schizophrenia who have refused to take their medication or in whom the medication is not controlling their symptoms, may exhibit a variety of symptoms. They may talk to themselves or to unseen individuals, or they may exhibit fear for no apparent reason because of the paranoid ideas that they hold. They may speak in a confused and illogical manner. Some patients with schizophrenia may seem to be intoxicated or under the influence of drugs even when they have not used any alcohol or drugs.

Substance Abuse Issues

Many people with schizophrenia also exhibit addictive behaviors. An estimated 50 percent or greater have SUBSTANCE ABUSE problems, with alcohol being the major problem. One theory is that people with schizophrenia abuse drugs in an attempt to self-medicate the troubling symptoms stemming from the illness or from the side effects caused by medications used to treat the illness. This may be a valid view. However, some patients who attempt to self-medicate may possibly suffer from anxiety disorders, depression, or other psychiatric illnesses. In addition, often alcohol abuse occurs before the onset of schizophrenic symptoms rather than afterward, so it does not appear to be a response to the disease.

One study reported in a 2001 issue of the *American Journal of Psychiatry* seems to refute this belief that patients use drugs or alcohol to self-medicate. Instead, some patients may use drugs or alcohol because they are impulsive and sensation seeking. The researchers studied the medical records of 76 hospitalized patients with schizophrenia or schizoaffective disorder (a form of schizophrenia that includes a mood disorder, such as depression) and 24 outpatients with these same diagnoses. Of these subjects, 27 had a lifetime abuse of or dependence on alcohol and 27 had the same with cannabis (MARIJUANA). Seventeen subjects abused more than one substance.

The researchers sought to discover if patients with schizophrenia and schizoaffective disorder who abused substances or became addicted to them had high levels of impulsivity and sensation seeking, as do nonpsychotic individuals who are substance abusers. The researchers confirmed that they did. Said the researchers, "Our results indicate that schizophrenic patients with a lifetime comorbidity of substance abuse or dependence are more impulsive and seek more intense sensations than schizophrenic patients without abuse or dependence."

In another study, reported in the *American Journal of Drug and Alcohol Abuse* in 2000, researcher Cheryl D. Swofford reported on her findings that provided predictive data for patients with schizophrenia who were likely to relapse. In this study, there were 262 patients, of whom 56 percent were male, 80 percent were African American, 19 percent were Caucasian, and 1 percent were listed as other. The average patient age was 42 years, and the average number of hospitalizations was five. A majority, 55 percent, of all the patients had used alcohol or drugs in the past.

The researchers compared the substance-abusing patients with the nonsubstance abusers and found distinctive differences. Said Swofford, "There was a strong relationship between substance use with younger age at first psychiatric hospitalization and number of both lifetime hospitalizations and hospitalizations in the past 2 years. There was also a higher rate of poor treatment adherence, as measured by missed appointments."

Treatment of Schizophrenia

Antipsychotic medications have enabled many patients with schizophrenia to cope with their most troubling symptoms. In the past, many patients failed to take their medications because of the severe side effects caused by the drugs, such as lethargy, poor physical coordination, and forgetfulness. Over the long term, some patients developed tardive dyskinesia, a severe and permanent muscle condition, causing contortions of the face, tongue thrusting, and lip smacking, and that resulted in distress and embarrassment to patients. Newer medications, such as clozapine (Clozaril) and especially ariprazole (Abilify), suppress psychotic symptoms without causing the severe side effects of the older antipsychotic drugs.

Because of the severe side effects of the older antipsychotics, they were so unappealing to patients with schizophrenia that most patients stopped taking them within several months. Some of these patients may have resorted to using alcohol and drugs to attempt to control their symptoms. It is too soon to know, but within the next decade, researchers will be able to determine if patients with schizophrenia are better stabilized on the newer antipsychotic medications and also if these patients have a lower rate of substance abuse than patients in the past who had only the older antipsychotic medications upon which to rely.

Treating Schizophrenia and Substance Abuse

Patients with both schizophrenia and substance abuse need both problems treated, and this can be difficult. Many patients with schizophrenia do not accept that there is anything wrong with them. In addition, many facilities center on treating either mental illness or substance abuse and not both

problems. According to Drake and Mueser in their 2002 article for *Alcohol Research & Health*, the best approach is stage-wise treatment and a multidisciplinary approach. The authors say that patients with schizophrenia and substance abuse generally go through four stages of recovery, which are as follows:

1. Engagement or building a trusting relationship with treatment providers

2. Persuasion and developing the motivation to manage the illnesses and seek recovery

3. Active treatment; in this stage, the patient works on developing skills and the supports needed to manage the illness and the recovery

4. Relapse prevention, including developing strategies to seek to avoid and minimize the effects of relapses

Contrary to past hopeless views about schizophrenia as the "cancer of psychiatry," today, with treatment and medication, many individuals with schizophrenia can develop effective coping skills and live in society; often holding jobs or attending classes. Patients with schizophrenia who are also drug addicts or alcoholics urgently need treatment. With community support and appropriate treatment, many individuals with schizophrenia can overcome drug and alcohol dependence.

See also DUAL DIAGNOSIS; HOMELESSNESS; LSD.

Condren, Rita M., John O'Connor, and Roy Browne. "Prevalence and Patterns of Substance Misuse in Schizophrenia: A Catchment Area Case-Control Study," *Psychiatric Bulletin* 25, no. 1 (2001): 17–20.

Dervaux, Alain, M.D., et al. "Is Substance Abuse in Schizophrenia Related to Impulsivity, Sensation Seeking, or Anhedonia?" *American Journal of Psychiatry* 158, no. 3 (2001): 492–494.

Drake, Robert E., M.D., and Kim T. Mueser. "Co-Occurring Alcohol Use Disorder and Schizophrenia," *Alcohol Research & Health* 26, no. 2 (2002): 99–102.

Swofford, Cheryl D. "Double Jeopardy: Schizophrenia and Substance Use," *American Journal of Drug and Alcohol Abuse* (August 2000). Available online. URL: http://www.findarticles.com/p/articles/mi_m0978/is_3_26/ai_65803039/print. Accessed on September 1, 2004.

secondhand smoke Smoke that is generated by cigarettes, cigars, or pipes that other individuals are smoking. It is also known as environmental tobacco smoke. According to the American Cancer Society, 35,000–40,000 people who are not smokers die of heart disease because of exposure to secondhand smoke.

According to the Environmental Protection Agency (EPA) in the United States, secondhand smoke contains more than 4,000 substances, and at least 40 of them are carcinogenic (cancer causing). The EPA has classified secondhand smoke as a known cause of LUNG CANCER in humans that causes about 3,000 lung cancer deaths in nonsmokers every year. The EPA also estimates that there are between 7,500–15,000 hospitalizations of infants and children under the age of 18 months each year for respiratory tract infections that are caused by secondhand smoke. Children with asthma who live with smokers must cope with a greater number of attacks that are more severe.

There are two forms of secondhand smoke. Sidestream smoke is from the lighted cigarette, cigar, or pipe. Mainstream smoke is exhaled by the person who is smoking. When either form of smoke is inhaled by nonsmokers, it is called passive smoking or involuntary smoking.

Recommendations for Smokers

For their own health and the health of others, all smokers should stop smoking. Until then, people who smoke should smoke outside their home or workplace so that others will not be exposed to secondhand smoke. Parents should make sure that they tell babysitters and family members they disapprove of smoking and should not allow smoking around their children. If a family member or other person smokes inside the house despite requests for no smoking, windows should be opened and exhaust fans turned on.

See also NICOTINE REPLACEMENT THERAPY; SMOKING AND HEALTH PROBLEMS; SMOKING CESSATION; SMOKING, CIGARETTE.

For further information, contact the following organizations:

Office on Smoking and Health/Centers for Disease Control and Prevention
Center for Chronic Disease Prevention and Health Promotion

Mail Stop K-50
4770 Buford Highway
Atlanta, GA 30341
(800) CDC-1311 or (404) 488-5705

National Cancer Institute
Building 41, Room 10A24
9000 Rockville Pike
Bethesda, MD 20892
(800) 4-CANCER (toll-free)

National Heart, Lung, and Blood Institute
Information Center
4733 Bethesda Avenue
Suite 530
Bethesda, MD 20814
(301) 951-3260

Sex Addicts Anonymous A self-help organization loosely modeled on the TWELVE STEPS principle developed by ALCOHOLICS ANONYMOUS and designed for individuals who have determined that they are sex addicts and wish to become sexually healthy. Some individuals may have been arrested for their behavior. Many feel ashamed and out of control.

The organization has over 500 meetings worldwide, including telephone conference meetings and online meetings. Sex Addicts Anonymous also publishes a newsletter, "Plain Brown Rapper," which can be downloaded from their Web site.

See also SEXUAL ADDICTION.

For further information, contact the organization at:

ISO of SAA
P.O. Box 70949
Houston, TX 77270
(713) 869-4902
(800) 477-8191 (toll-free from the United States or Canada: Monday through Friday, 10 A.M. to 6 P.M., Central Time)
http://www.sexaa.org

sexual addiction A compulsion to obsess about or to engage in sexual acts on a very frequent basis, despite the risks involved to the health and safety of the individual (such as the risk of contracting a sexually transmitted disease) or others or whether the act is legal or not. Sexual addiction has also been called sexual dependency and sexual compulsivity. Psychologist Patrick Carnes was the first mental health professional to identify sexual addiction. His research indicated that most sex addicts (80 percent) are male.

According to Dr. Carnes in his book *Don't Call It Love: Recovery from Sexual Addiction,* there are 10 signs that indicate a sexual addiction, including:

1. A pattern of out-of-control behavior
2. Severe consequences due to sexual behavior
3. Inability to stop despite adverse consequences
4. Persistent pursuit of self-destructive or high-risk behavior
5. Ongoing desire or effort to limit sexual behavior
6. Sexual obsession and fantasy as a primary coping strategy
7. Increasing amounts of sexual experience because the current level of activity is no longer sufficient
8. Severe mood changes around sexual activity
9. Inordinate amounts of time spent in obtaining sex, being sexual, or recovering from sexual experiences
10. Neglect of important social, occupational, or recreational activities because of sexual behavior

Manifestations of Sexual Addiction

Some sex addicts engage in constantly reading pornographic books or viewing pornographic material on the Internet, while others participate in compulsive sex acts with others. Some sex addicts may induce or force minors to engage in sexual acts with them; this is pedophilia and is illegal in the United States and most other countries. The main feature of a sexual addiction is that sexual activity becomes the driving force and the focus of the individual's life, similar to the focus of alcohol for the alcoholic or gambling for the compulsive gambler.

Driven by Guilt, Shame, and Powerlessness

Many people assume that sex addicts have a much greater enjoyment of sex than others, but there is no evidence that this is true. In fact, in general, sexual addicts may enjoy sex less than most people because of the driven and compulsive nature of their behavior. They may enjoy the sex act, but they do not enjoy the guilt and shame that precedes it or that follows, nor do they enjoy the powerlessness that constantly pervades their lives.

Because they feel that they must engage in sexual acts, some sex addicts will hire prostitutes, have anonymous affairs, sexually abuse children, compulsively masturbate, and engage in many other behaviors that they do not approve of and yet are drawn to repeat, again and again. Most psychiatrists believe that many sex addicts were sexually abused as children and are compelled to reenact scenes that they were a part of as children.

Other Addictive Behaviors

Sex addicts have an increased risk of SUBSTANCE ABUSE. In her 1993 article on cocaine abuse in the *Annals of Internal Medicine,* Dr. Elizabeth Warner described sex addiction among cocaine abusers. Said Warner, "Compulsive sexuality, defined by excessive preoccupation, loss of control, and continuation of sexual practices despite adverse effects has been associated with cocaine use. Sometimes referred to as 'sexual addiction,' compulsive sexuality may be related to the higher incidence of sexually transmitted diseases in cocaine users. As a form of barter, sexual activities may be performed in exchange for cocaine."

Many sex addicts may have problems with abuse of other drugs in addition to COCAINE, as well as with eating disorders, COMPULSIVE SHOPPING, and compulsive GAMBLING.

Other Emotional Problems

People with sexual addictions may have other problems as well. For example, sexual obsessions may occur in patients with BIPOLAR DISORDER as well as substance abuse and personality disorders. They may also have an underlying problem with DEPRESSION.

Treatment

Patients with sex addiction generally need therapy with an experienced psychotherapist. Many patients have experienced many losses because of their addiction, such as the loss of a spouse or partner, loss of custody of their children, and unplanned pregnancies. Counseling can help them cope with these losses and learn to change their behavior so future losses can be limited. Patients cannot be expected to give up sex, but they can learn healthier ways of sexual interaction.

Patients with sex addiction may also benefit from self-help groups such as SEX ADDICTS ANONYMOUS. If there is an underlying psychiatric problem, medication may help. For example, if the individual has bipolar disorder, he or she may benefit by treatment with a mood stabilizer, or if he or she has depression, an antidepressant may help the patient cope better.

For further information on sexual addiction, contact the following organizations:

National Council on Sexual Addiction and
  Compulsivity
P.O. Box 725544
Atlanta, GA 31139
(770) 541-9912
http://www.ncsad.org

Sex Addicts Anonymous
ISO of SAA
P.O. Box 70949
Houston, TX 77270
(713) 869-4902
(800) 477-8191 (toll-free from the United States or
  Canada: Monday through Friday, 10 A.M. to
  6 P.M., Central Time)
http://www.sexaa.org

Carnes, Patrick. *Don't Call It Love: Recovery from Sexual Addiction.* New York: Bantam Books, 1991.
Warner, Elizabeth A. "Cocaine Abuser," *Annals of Internal Medicine* 119, no. 3 (August 1993): 226–235.

sex, unplanned   Usually refers to unanticipated sexual acts that are also unsafe in that they do not involve the use of contraceptives or condoms. People who are under the influence of alcohol or illegal drugs are more likely to engage in unplanned sex than others, and consequently, they are also more likely to contract sexually transmitted diseases and to create unplanned pregnancies. Individuals with some psychiatric disorders, such as BIPOLAR DISORDER, have an increased risk of engaging in unplanned sex acts.

See also ATTENTION DEFICIT HYPERACTIVITY DISORDER; IMPULSE CONTROL DISORDER; IMPULSIVITY; PROSTITUTION.

shopping addiction   See COMPULSIVE SHOPPING.

smokeless tobacco   Tobacco that is chewed or sniffed rather than smoked. The four key types of smokeless tobacco products are dry snuff, moist snuff, plug/twist, and loose leaf chewing "spit" tobacco. According to the Federal Trade Commission, about 64 million pounds of moist snuff was sold in 2001, which was greater than the combined sales of all the other forms of smokeless tobacco. In all, an estimated 113 million pounds of smokeless tobacco products were sold in 2001, generating over $2 billion in sales.

About 9.6 million people in the United States use smokeless tobacco products, and the overwhelming majority are males. As with cigarette smoking, many users are initiated into the use of smokeless tobacco by their peers during adolescence. Of the few females who regularly use smokeless tobacco, many are reportedly embarrassed or ashamed of their use. However, the nicotine in smokeless tobacco is as addicting to females as it is to males.

College students may use or try smokeless tobacco. In one study reported in a 2000 issue of the *Journal of the American Medical Association,* of about 14,000 college students, about 9 percent of the males reported currently using smokeless tobacco and 14 percent had used it in the past year. (Less than 1 percent of females were current users and only 1.3 percent had used smokeless tobacco in the past year.) The researchers found that students in rural areas or small towns were more likely to be smokeless tobacco users, as were intercollegiate athletes.

Younger individuals, especially adolescents, often believe that smokeless tobacco is less addicting and thus healthier than smoked tobacco. This common belief is erroneous. Some people have used smokeless tobacco to help them stop smoking; however, they are simply trading one form of nicotine delivery for another form. In fact, some experts have stated that smokeless tobacco may contain a higher level of nicotine than cigarettes.

Some forms of tobacco are flavored, apparently to appeal to younger palates and increase the appeal of trying the product. If chewed, the tobacco is either swallowed or spit out.

State-by-State Differences

Broad variations occur among states in the percentage of people who use smokeless tobacco. For example, only 2.6 percent of Arizona adult males use smokeless tobacco, compared with a high of 18.4 percent of the men in West Virginia. Usage rates are low among women, according to this federal data, ranging from zero or near-zero in many states to a high of 1.7 percent in Georgia. (See the table below for a comparison of many states and the percentage of residents who used smokeless tobacco in 1997.)

Health Issues

Using smokeless tobacco can cause ORAL CANCER in the mouth and throat. It increases the risk of developing this cancer by an estimated 50 times, according to the American Cancer Society. The cancer is most commonly found in the cheek, gums, and inner lips. Use of smokeless tobacco may cause esophageal cancer. It can cause bleeding gums and sores, and it stains the teeth a yellowish brown color. Smokeless tobacco also causes chronic bad breath. The constant spitting that smokeless tobacco users must perform often disgusts onlookers.

Ending the Addiction

NICOTINE REPLACEMENT THERAPY may work for individuals who are addicted to smokeless tobacco. Some patients may improve with bupropion (ZYBAN). Studies are mixed on the success rates of smoking cessation therapies for smokeless tobacco, and further research is needed.

See also NICOTINE; SMOKING AND HEALTH PROBLEMS; SMOKING CESSATION; SMOKING, CIGARETTE; TEENAGE AND YOUTH SMOKING; TOBACCO.

Federal Trade Commission. *Federal Trade Commission Smokeless Tobacco Report for the Years 2000 and 2001.* Available online. URL: http://www.ftc.gov/os/2003/08/2k2k1smokeless.pdf. Accessed on March 16, 2004.

Rigotti, Nancy A., M.D., Jae Eun Lee, and Henry Wechsler. "U.S. College Students' Use of Tobacco Products: Results of a National Survey," *Journal of the American Medical Association* 284, no. 6 (August 9, 2000): 699–705.

smoking and health problems Medical problems that are directly or indirectly caused by the inhalation of tobacco products, including cigarettes, pipes, and cigars. Most research, though, centers around health problems that stem from cigarette smoking. Researchers have extensively studied cigarette smoking because of the large numbers of people who smoke cigarettes in contrast to those who use other tobacco products. However, smoking cigars and pipe tobacco also lead to the development of diseases such as CANCER and bronchitis. The use of SMOKELESS TOBACCO has many health risks as well, including ORAL CANCER.

Cigarette Smoking and Health Problems

According to the 2004 report, *The Health Consequences of Smoking: A Report of the Surgeon General,* smoking cigarettes is harmful to nearly every organ in the body, while quitting smoking has both immediate and long-term health benefits. An estimated 440,000 people die each year from smoking-related illnesses in the United States. Smokers are more likely to miss work than nonsmokers, and they incur more medical costs. They are admitted to hospitals more frequently and for longer periods of time than nonsmokers.

PERCENTAGE OF CURRENT SMOKELESS TOBACCO USE AMONG ADULTS, BY STATE AND SEX, UNITED STATES, 1997

State	Men %	Women %	Total %
Alabama	9.9	1.4	5.4
Alaska	9.2	1.6	5.5
Arizona	2.6	0.3	1.4
Georgia	6.4	1.7	4.0
Indiana	6.8	0.0	3.2
Kansas	10.3	0.2	5.1
Kentucky	12.2	0.6	6.1
Louisiana	7.6	0.3	3.7
Montana	10.5	0.2	5.3
Ohio	5.1	0.0	2.4
Oklahoma	7.7	0.3	3.8
Pennsylvania	7.4	0.4	3.8
South Carolina	4.8	1.0	2.8
Virginia	6.1	0.1	3.0
Washington	5.6	0.2	2.9
West Virginia	18.4	0.2	8.8
Wyoming	14.7	0.7	7.6

Source: Centers for Disease Control and Prevention. "State-Specific Prevalence Among Adults of Current Cigarette Smoking and Smokeless Tobacco Use and Per Capita Tax-Paid Sales of Cigarettes—United States, 1997," *Morbidity and Mortality Weekly Report* 47, no. 43 (November 6, 1998): 924.

Cancer and cigarette smoking   Most causes of LUNG CANCER (about 90 percent) are caused by smoking, as are the broad majority of cases of oral cancer. Lung cancer is a very serious disease and often a fatal one. Unfortunately, the disease is often not diagnosed until it is in an advanced stage. Smoking is also associated with bladder cancer and esophageal cancer. In 2004, the Surgeon General further expanded the list of cancers caused by smoking to include cervical cancer, kidney cancer, pancreatic cancer, and stomach cancer as well as acute myeloid leukemia.

Respiratory problems and cigarette smoking Smoking increases the risk of bronchitis and pneumonia. Chronic bronchitis and EMPHYSEMA are extremely common in smokers. (See the table on page 219.)

Pregnancy complications with cigarette smoking According to the Surgeon General's report and other sources, only about 18–25 percent of all women who smoke before pregnancy stop smoking when they become pregnant, despite the many health risks to their infants and to themselves.

Smoking cigarettes significantly increases the risk of complications, premature deliveries, fetal deaths, and stillbirths. The infants of mothers who smoke during pregnancy have a greater risk of being low-birth-weight babies. In fact, low birth weight is a leading cause of infant deaths in the United States, and more than 300,000 low-birth-weight newborns die each year in the United States. Pregnant smokers generally eat more than pregnant nonsmokers but their babies weigh less. However, this weight difference in the babies is less if pregnant smokers stop smoking early in their pregnancy.

Smoking is directly linked to sudden infant death syndrome (SIDS). The infants born to mothers who smoke have twice the risk of developing SIDS. Babies whose mothers smoked both before and after their birth have three to four times the risk of dying from SIDS.

When women smoke during their pregnancy, they reduce their babies' lung capacity.

Mothers who breast-feed and also smoke deliver nicotine to their babies in their breast milk.

Cardiovascular problems with cigarette smoking Smoking cigarettes is associated with cardiovascular problems, such as stroke and coronary artery disease. Coronary artery disease is the number one cause of death in the United States. Cigarette smoking is a major cause of stroke, which is the third leading cause of death in the United States. Smoking cigarettes is associated with sudden cardiac death in both men and women. Vascular diseases of all kinds are markedly more prevalent among smokers.

Smoking among seniors   Older people who smoke greatly increase their risks for serious health problems. For example, elderly smokers have two to three times the risk of developing cataracts of the eye than do nonsmokers. Smoking also reduces bone density and is related to an increased risk for hip fractures in both men and women.

Smoking causes EMPHYSEMA, a breathing disorder that limits daily activities and that is most prevalent among older men and women. It increases the risk of abdominal aortic aneurysm. Of course, smoking causes cancer, stroke, and heart disease in older individuals as well as younger people. Stopping smoking reduces the risk for developing cancer, stroke, and heart disease in elderly people.

Other health problems with cigarette smoking Cigarette smoking may also affect fertility. In 2004, the Surgeon General's report concluded, "The evidence is sufficient to infer a causal relationship between smoking and reduced fertility in women." According to the Surgeon General's report, smoking also causes dental diseases, such as periodontitis (serious gum disease).

The report also states that smokers have a lower survival rate after surgery than nonsmokers because of delayed wound healing and reduced wound response as well as damage to the body's host defenses. Smokers have a generally greater risk for postoperative complications, including infections, pneumonia, and respiratory complications.

There may be a link between erectile dysfunction (impotence) and smoking. However, the Surgeon General's study established only an increased risk rather than a causal link and suggested further studies are needed.

Children and adolescents who smoke   Children and adolescents who smoke experience chronic coughing and wheezing. Many become addicted to nicotine and develop a lifelong smoking habit that is difficult to break. According to the Surgeon General, teenage smokers are less physically fit than their peers and they have more respiratory illnesses. In general, the younger the person is when he or she starts smoking, the more difficult it is to quit smoking later in life.

Problems for children of cigarette smokers The children and the other family members of smokers are at risk for developing respiratory diseases such as bronchitis, serious ear infections, and frequent colds due to their exposure to SECONDHAND SMOKE.

Some of the Major Ways that Smoking Harms the Body

According to the Surgeon General's report, smoking harms the body in the following key ways:

- Nicotine reaches the brain 10 seconds after smoke is inhaled. It has been found in every part of the body, including breast milk.

- Toxic ingredients in cigarette smoke travel throughout the body, causing damage in several different ways.

- Carbon monoxide binds to hemoglobin in the red blood cells, preventing the affected cells from carrying a full load of oxygen.

- Carcinogens (cancer-causing agents) in tobacco smoke damage the genes that control cell growth, causing cells to grow abnormally or reproduce too rapidly.

- The carcinogen benzo[a]pyrene, a chemical compound in tobacco smoke, binds to cells in the airways and major organs of smokers.

- Smoking can cause oxidative stress that mutates DNA, promotes atherosclerosis, and also leads to chronic lung injury. Oxidative stress is believed to be behind the aging process and the development of cancer and cardiovascular disease.

- Smoking lowers levels of antioxidants in the body. Antioxidants repair damaged cells.

- Smoking is linked to higher levels of chronic inflammation in the body.

Quitting Smoking Rapidly Brings Benefits

To avoid the health-related risks that are associated with tobacco, people should stop smoking cigarettes or using smokeless tobacco or any other form of tobacco. Often they may also need to avoid a close association with others who smoke because of the CRAVING that may be generated to smoke by the smoking of others. Some individuals who wish to quit smoking benefit by joining self-help groups, such as NICOTINE ANONYMOUS. Many people use NICOTINE REPLACEMENT THERAPY.

See also CARCINOGENS; DEATH; NICOTINE; SMOKING CESSATION; SMOKING, CIGARETTE; TEENAGE AND YOUTH AND SMOKING; ZYBAN.

U.S. Department of Health and Human Services. *The Health Consequences of Smoking: A Report of the Surgeon General.* Atlanta, Ga.: U.S. Department of Health and

NUMBER AND PERCENTAGE OF CIGARETTE SMOKING-ATTRIBUTABLE HEALTH CONDITIONS AMONG CURRENT AND FORMER SMOKERS, BY CONDITION, UNITED STATES, 2000

Condition	Current Smokers		Former Smokers		Overall	
	Number	%	Number	%	Number	%
Chronic Bronchitis	2,633,000	49	1,872,000	26	4,505,000	35
Emphysema	1,273,000	24	1,743,000	24	3,016,000	24
Heart Attack	719,000	13	1,755,000	34	2,474,000	19
All Cancers except lung cancer	358,000	7	1,154,000	16	1,512,000	12
Stroke	384,000	7	637,000	9	1,021,000	8
Lung cancer	46,000	1	138,000	2	184,000	1
Total	5,412,000	100	7,299,000	100	12,711,000	100

Source: Centers for Disease Control and Prevention. "Cigarette Smoking-Attributable Morbidity—United States, 2000" *Morbidity and Mortality Weekly Report* 52, 35 (September 5, 2003): 843.

Human Services, Centers for Disease Control and Prevention, National Center for Chronic Disease Prevention and Health Promotion, Office on Smoking and Health, 2004.

smoking cessation Ending a smoking habit. Because of the addictive nature of NICOTINE, it can be very difficult for many people to stop smoking. However, effective treatments and therapies can assist them in achieving this goal. It is also important to stop smoking in order to regain good health and significantly limit the risk of developing oral and lung cancer as well as the risk of developing other serious diseases such as stroke and emphysema. In addition, smoking cessation will end the transmission of secondhand smoke to family members and others who could otherwise develop health problems as a result of this exposure.

Smoking Cessation Pharmacotherapy

Pharmacotherapy for smoking cessation includes prescribed medications such as bupropion (ZYBAN), to treat nicotine addiction. Some drugs, such as nortriptyline and clonidine, have been found to help patients stop smoking, but they have not been approved for this use by the Food and Drug Administration.

Nicotine Replacement Therapy

NICOTINE REPLACEMENT THERAPY also helps many individuals to stop smoking. Nicotine replacement therapy comes in the form of skin patches, nasal spray, gum, and a vapor inhaler. The plan is to replace the nicotine that was smoked with another form of nicotine that is steadily reduced over time. The individual should not also smoke when using nicotine replacement therapy. If the individual continues to smoke as many cigarettes as before as well as use nicotine replacement, he or she could receive toxic levels of nicotine that could be dangerous or even fatal.

Some studies indicate that the gum with 4 mg of nicotine appears to be the most effective form of nicotine replacement therapy for heavy smokers (those who smoke at least 25 cigarettes per day). The skin patch and the gum are sold as over-the-counter drugs, but the nasal spray and inhalers are available only as prescribed drugs.

Therapy and Other Methods

Some people quit smoking by receiving assistance in the form of counseling, psychotherapy, and/or hypnosis. Many people buy books, videotapes, and audiotapes to help themselves stop smoking.

Hotlines for Quitting Smoking

Some individuals have found relief by participating in an active telephone quitline or in support group meetings for people who wish to stop smoking.

The National Cancer Institute in the United States offers a smoking quitline that is available to answer individual questions about quitting smoking from Monday through Friday from 9 A.M. to 4:30 P.M. This toll-free line is: 1-877-44U-QUIT. The TTY line is 1-800-332-8615. For further information on state and federal quitline access phone numbers, go to the Department of Health and Human Services Web site at: http://www.smokefree.gov.

Efficacy of Smoking Cessation Methods

In general, bupropion appears to be the most effective and longest lasting method for smoking cessation of all methods. In one study, reported in a 1999 issue of the *New England Journal of Medicine,* researchers reported their findings on the abstinence rates after one year for four groups of former smokers, including patients in a sustained-release bupropion group, those in a nicotine patch group, those in a group using a combination of both bupropion and the nicotine patch, and patients in a fourth placebo (no medicine) group. The bupropion-only group received nine weeks of bupropion (150 mg per day for the first three days and then 150 mg twice a day thereafter).

After one year, the researchers found that the abstinence rates from smoking were 15.6 percent for the placebo group, 16.4 percent for the nicotine patch group, 30.3 percent for the bupropion group, and 35.5 percent for the bupropion and nicotine patch group.

The researchers also noted that no significant weight gain differences occurred between the treatment groups. (Many people who quit smoking, especially females, worry about gaining weight or even becoming obese. However, most people who stop smoking gain only a few pounds.)

Physician Training Can Help Patients Stop Smoking

Studies have also shown that when primary care physicians are more knowledgeable about smoking cessation, they are also more effective at helping their patients to quit smoking. This was demonstrated in a study that was published in a 2002 issue of the *Annals of Internal Medicine.*

In this study, 35 medical residents were given counseling skills training on helping patients stop smoking. The residents were trained in both smoking cessation and dyslipidemia so that they would not know which effect was being studied by the researchers. They were told that cardiovascular problems were being addressed. Some patients were in the smoking cessation intervention group with the residents, while others were in the control group on dyslipidemia.

The residents were taught to identify which of three stages the smokers were in. For example, if they were in the precontemplation stage (with no intention to stop smoking), the residents were trained to talk about the advantages of no longer smoking and to challenge the patients' wrong beliefs about smoking. If smokers were in the contemplation stage (thinking about stopping smoking sometime in the next six months but not within the next 30 days), the residents were trained to use different strategies, such as discussing barriers to cessation and solutions. For patients who were ready to stop smoking (which was called the preparation stage), the residents were trained to provide support, and they were given suggested behavioral hints and information on nicotine replacement therapy for their patients.

One year later, the patients were evaluated. Researchers found that the training program had been effective and abstinence from smoking was significantly higher in the intervention group (13 percent) than among the smokers in the control group (5 percent). The researchers believed that the program was effective because participants spent more than half the time in active learning rather than didactic learning.

In other words, rather than being told by the doctor once or twice, "Smoking is bad and causes cancer. You should stop smoking," instead, the doctors individualized the responses to patients and their particular situation. The doctors provided them with active suggestions on not only why they should stop smoking but how they could stop as well as assuring them that stopping was a goal that they could achieve.

Said the researchers, "We conclude that a physician training program in smoking cessation based on active learning of counseling skills with standardized patients is effective."

Suggestions on Smoking Cessation

In their booklet *Clearing the Air: Quit Smoking Today,* the National Cancer Institute offers many helpful hints for people who wish to stop smoking. These hints include START, which stands for:

S = Set a quit date.
T = Tell family, friends, and coworkers that you plan to quit smoking.
A = Anticipate and plan ahead for the challenges that you will face while quitting.
R = Remove cigarettes and other tobacco products from your home, car, and work.
T = Talk to your doctor about getting help to quit.

Smokers should also think about reasons why they wish to stop smoking. In addition to improving health, they can save money and set a better example for their children. Women may wish to quit smoking to avoid getting wrinkles on their faces. Many people regard nonsmokers as more self-disciplined than smokers. Smokers who wish to quit smoking may wish to list their reasons for quitting on a piece of paper where they can periodically review it.

Smokers also need to discover their personal triggers that may cause them to smoke, such as finishing a meal or talking on the phone. Once triggers are identified, they can be replaced. For example, the smoker could eat in a nonsmoking section of a restaurant if finishing a meal is usually followed by smoking. At home, the person could move the dining table so that the visual cues are different. It is important to remember that the urge to smoke lasts about three to five minutes and it can be overcome. After several days, the urges start to abate.

The initial period of withdrawing from smoking can be a difficult time for the smoker, who may feel irritable and moody. This is normal and to be expected, as the toxic effects of the nicotine leave the body. Within several days, however, the body begins to recover and become healthy again.

Cornuz, Jacques, M.D. "Efficacy of Resident Training in Smoking Cessation: A Randomized, Controlled Trial of a Program Based on Application of Behavioral Theory and Practice with Standardized Patients," *Annals of Internal Medicine* 136, no. 6 (March 19, 2002): 429–437.

Jorenby, Douglas E., et al. "A Controlled Trial of Sustained-Release Bupropion, A Nicotine Patch, or Both for Smoking Cessation," *New England Journal of Medicine* 340, no. 9 (March 4, 1999): 685–691.

National Cancer Institute. "Clearing the Air: Quit Smoking Today," NIH Publication No. 03-1647. Bethesda, Md.: U.S. Department of Health and Human Services, National Institutes of Health, April 2003.

Rigotti, Nancy A., M.D. "Treatment of Tobacco Use and Dependence," *New England Journal of Medicine* 346, no. 7 (February 14, 2002): 506–512.

Zhu, Shu-Hong, et al. "Evidence of Real-World Effectiveness of a Telephone Quitline for Smokers," *New England Journal of Medicine* 347, no. 14 (October 3, 2002): 1,087–1,093.

smoking, cigarette   Ingestion of tobacco products through cigarettes. Smoking is an addiction that many people acquire as a teenager or young adult, often because of PEER PRESSURE and a desire to seem older or sophisticated. The individual then develops a nicotine addiction that is usually difficult to break. Smoking causes many serious health problems over both the short term and the long term of an individual's life.

Although smoking cigars and pipe tobacco as well as using chewing tobacco or snuff are also unhealthy, most research centers around cigarette smoking. All users of tobacco products have an increased risk of developing ORAL CANCER compared with nonsmokers.

According to state-by-state research performed by the Centers for Disease Control and Prevention (CDC) and reported in a 2002 issue of *Morbidity and Mortality Weekly Review*, in 2001, about 22.5 percent of American adults smoked cigarettes. This statistic is likely about the same as of this writing in 2005.

Deaths Caused by Smoking

Smoking causes many people to lose their lives. In 2002, the CDC estimated the annual number of lives lost from various diseases and the yearlong numbers of the total that could be attributed to smoking based on data available from 1995–99. The researchers found that more than 440,000 people died per year from ailments related to cigarette smoking. In addition, the CDC also calculated the number of years of life that were lost due to smoking, and they found that an estimated 5.6 million total years were lost because of the smoking habit. (See table on page 223.)

In this chart, the column on total deaths shows the total number of people who died per year from an illness. Then the next column shows the estimated number of men who died from smoking-attributable mortality (SAM), followed by a column with the years of potential lives lost (YPLL). The column on males are followed by data on females, and the estimated number of women who died from smoking-attributable mortality and the years of potential life lost. Thus, with oral cancer, 5,180 men died of the disease, but the experts estimated that 3,873 of these deaths were attributable to smoking, and 64,022 years of potential life were lost. In the case of women, 2,645 died of oral cancer, and of these, 1,264 cases were attributable to smoking, causing 21,499 years of potential life lost.

Demographics of Cigarette Smoking

Research has revealed some broad differences between smokers and nonsmokers in terms of their geographic area, race and ethnicity, and education.

State-by-state differences   Research by the CDC on cigarette smoking among people from different states in the United States in 2001 revealed that there were broad variations of the percentages of smokers among states and territories. The areas with the highest percentages of smokers were Kentucky (30.9 percent), Guam (31.2 percent), and Oklahoma (28.7 percent). The areas with the lowest percentages of smokers were the Virgin Islands (9.6 percent), Puerto Rico (12.5 percent), and Utah (13.2 percent).

Lifetime smoking status   In a report published in 2003, the National Center for Health Statistics provided detailed data comparing the lifetime smoking status of three groups of individuals: those who had never smoked, former smokers, and current smokers. (See table on page 224.) Many different conclusions may be drawn from

ANNUAL DEATHS DUE TO SMOKING-ATTRIBUTABLE MORTALITY (SAM) AND YEARS OF POTENTIAL LIFE LOST (YPLL), BY CAUSE OF DEATH AND SEX, UNITED STATES, DATA FROM 1995–1999

Disease Category	Male			Female		
Cancers	Total Deaths	SAM (Smoking-Attributable Mortality)	YPLL (Years of Potential Lives Lost)	Total Deaths	SAM	YPLL
Lip, oral cavity, pharynx	5,180	3,873	64,022	2,645	1,264	21,499
Esophagus	8,627	6,280	94,359	2,778	1,613	25,686
Pancreas	13,429	3,065	46,112	14,339	3,415	52,481
Larynx	3,031	2,525	37,823	816	602	10,793
Trachea, lung, bronchus	91,295	80,571	1,106,117	61,593	44,242	763,669
Cervix uteri	—	—	—	3,772	1,053	13,290
Urinary bladder	7,778	3,699	40,208	3,772	1,053	13,290
Kidney, other urinary	7,066	2,799	41,867	4,537	236	4,172
Total	136,406	102,812	1,430,507	94,618	52,949	905,194
Cardiovascular disease						
Hypertension	17,575	3,320	51,291	25,182	2,740	36,286
Ischemic heart disease						
Ages 35–64 years	52,977	22,059	514,926	19,381	7,069	185,580
Ages 65 and older	191,172	29,312	252,380	217,962	25,536	219,813
Other heart diseases	98,088	18,822	243,327	117,645	10,546	127,756
Cerebrovascular diseases						
Ages 35–64 years	9,726	3,898	93,903	8,103	3,586	101,493
Ages 65 years and older	51,369	4,697	37,751	88,452	5,284	47,581
Atherosclerosis	6,008	1,644	14,877	10,050	883	7,925
Aortic aneurysm	9,971	6,489	76,568	6,201	3,135	39,655
Other arterial diseases	4,718	665	8,535	6,183	940	12,359
Total	441,602	90,906	1,293,559	499,159	57,699	778,447
Respiratory diseases						
Pneumonia, influenza	38,295	8,802	84,878	47,420	6,774	71,255
Bronchitis, emphysema	10,935	9,944	109,011	9,585	7,752	107,365
Chronic airways obstruction	42,765	34,919	353,137	39,727	29,816	379,052
Total	42,765	34,919	353,137	39,727	29,816	379,052
Perinatal conditions						
Short gestation/low birth weight	2,198	227	16,685	1,768	175	13,871
Respiratory distress syndrome	931	85	6,273	639	24	1,925
Other respiratory—newborn	912	84	6,147	645	33	2,646
Sudden infant death syndrome	1,766	202	14,805	1,197	175	13,872
Total	5,808	599	43,910	4,249	408	32,314
Burn deaths	—	589	17,270	—	377	10,486
Secondhand smoke deaths						
Lung cancer	—	1,110	—	—	1,890	—
Ischemic heart disease	—	14,407	—	—	20,646	—
Overall total	—	264,067	3,332,272	—	178,311	2,284,113

Source: Centers for Disease Control and Prevention. "Annual Smoking-Attributable Mortality, Years of Potential Life Lost, and Economic Costs—United States, 1995–1999," *Morbidity and Mortality Weekly Report* 51, 14 (April 12, 2002): 302.

PERCENT DISTRIBUTION OF LIFETIME SMOKING STATUS FOR ADULTS 18 YEARS OF AGE AND OLDER, BY SELECTED CHARACTERISTICS: UNITED STATES, 1997–1998, BOTH MEN AND WOMEN

		Lifetime Cigarette Smoking Status		
	Total	Never Smoker	Former Smoker	Current Smoker
Age				
18–24 years	100.0	64.0	7.7	28.3
25–44 years	100.0	56.1	15.8	28.0
45–64 years	100.0	44.6	30.7	24.7
65–74 years	100.0	43.2	41.7	15.0
75 years and older	100.0	56.6	36.5	6.8
Race/ethnicity				
Hispanic	100.0	63.1	18.0	18.9
White/non-Hispanic	100.0	49.5	25.1	25.4
African American, non-Hispanic	100.0	58.7	15.8	25.5
Asian/Pacific Islander, non-Hispanic	100.0	70.1	15.8	14.1
Education				
Less than high school graduate	100.0	45.6	20.1	34.4
GED diploma	100.0	31.3	24.4	44.3
High school graduate	100.0	49.4	22.4	28.2
Some college, no degree	100.0	50.5	25.2	24.3
Associates' degree	100.0	52.1	25.2	22.7
Bachelor's degree	100.0	61.8	25.5	12.7
Master's, doctorate, medical degree	100.0	68.4	23.3	8.4
Poverty status *				
Below poverty level	100.0	49.7	16.6	33.6
Poverty–1.99 times poverty level	100.0	48.5	20.4	31.1
2.00–3.99 times poverty level	100.0	50.6	23.6	25.8
4.00 times poverty level or more	100.0	54.1	27.4	18.5

* Poverty status was based on family income and family size using the U.S. Census Bureau poverty thresholds for 1996 and 1997.
Source: Schoenborn, Charlotte A., Jackline L. Vickerie, and Patricia Barnes, *Cigarette Smoking Behavior of Adults: United States, 1997–98,* Advance data from Vital and Health Statistics Series, no. 331, Centers for Disease Control and Prevention, February 7, 2003.

this data. For example, among individuals ages 75 and older, 56.6 percent had never smoked. Only 6.8 percent continued to smoke. Never smoking or stopping smoking may have been a reason for this group's longevity.

Race and ethnicity   There are clear differences with regard to other characteristics that the CDC has found between smokers and nonsmokers. For example, when considering race and ethnicity, whites and African Americans are the most likely to be smokers, in about the same percentages. Asians and Pacific Islanders who were non-Hispanic are the least likely to be current smokers (14.1 percent), followed by Hispanics (18.9 percent).

Poverty   With regard to poverty, people below the poverty line were the most likely to be current smokers (33.6 percent of this group). With increasing income came a decreasing percentage of current smokers, such that those whose income was equal to or greater than four times the poverty level had almost half the percentage of current smokers (18.5 percent).

Education   Education is clearly a factor among people who smoke, and more education usually means a decreased likelihood to smoke. Those with less than a high school diploma were more likely to be current smokers (34.4 percent) than most other groups. Interestingly, those with a general equivalency diploma had the highest percentage of current smokers (44.3 percent). The percentages fell with increased education, from high school graduates (28.2 percent were current smokers) to individuals with a Master's degree, doctorate, or medical degree (8.4 percent were current smokers).

Mental illness Mentally ill individuals have a higher rate of smoking than people without mental illness. For example, in a study of data from over 4,000 people ages 15–54 years, reported in a 2000 issue of the *Journal of the American Medical Association,* the researchers found that among patients with BIPOLAR DISORDER, DEPRESSION, SCHIZOPHRENIA, and panic disorder, significantly higher rates of smoking occurred among these patients than among individuals without diagnosed mental disorders. The smoking rates for patients with mental illness were 41 percent compared with 22.5 percent for patients with no mental illness. Many mentally ill patients did stop smoking, however.

It is possible that some mentally ill people smoked heavily in the past because older antipsychotic medications were powerful dopamine agonists and caused many side effects. Nicotine is a dopamine agonist and seems to ameliorate some of the side effects of these drugs.

Treatment for Smoking Cessation

A small number of smokers have reported that they decided to quit, stopped smoking, and that they have never smoked again. However, many more smokers have reported that they tried to quit but found it extremely difficult to do so. There is no reason to doubt the sincerity of their efforts, and the underlying problem is the intensity of the addiction. Why some people are able to stop smoking suddenly and why most people struggle to do so remains a mystery for most therapists.

One popular treatment for smoking cessation is NICOTINE REPLACEMENT THERAPY, a form of therapy that allows the individual to receive a small amount of nicotine through a skin patch, nasal spray, gum, or other method of delivery. The goal is to decrease the amount of nicotine that is used steadily. It can be very dangerous for individuals to use any form of nicotine replacement therapy and to continue to smoke, because the combined levels of nicotine can reach toxic levels and be harmful, even to long-term smokers used to high doses of nicotine.

Some individuals use medications to help them stop smoking, such as bupropion (ZYBAN), a drug that is also sometimes used as an ANTIDEPRESSANT (Wellbutrin). Other individuals attend no-smoking group sessions or have individual counseling. Some people have claimed that acupuncture or hypnosis has helped them quit smoking. Studies indicate that a combination of therapies may be useful, such as using nicotine replacement therapy and taking Zyban.

See also CANCER; CARCINOGENS; EMPHYSEMA; LUNG CANCER; NICOTINE; SMOKING AND HEALTH PROBLEMS; SMOKING CESSATION.

Centers for Disease Control and Prevention. "State-Specific Prevalence of Selected Chronic Disease-Related Characteristics—Behavioral Risk Factor Surveillance System, 2001," *Morbidity and Mortality Weekly Report* 52, no. SS-8 (August 22, 2003): 1–80.

Lasser, Karen, M.D., et al. "Smoking and Mental Illness: A Population-Based Prevalence Study," *Journal of the American Medical Association* 284, no. 20 (November 22–29, 2000): 2,606–2,610.

Schoenborn, Charlotte A., Jackline L. Vickerie, and Patricia Barnes. "Cigarette Smoking Behavior of Adults: United States, 1997–98," no. 331, Centers for Disease Control and Prevention, February 7, 2003.

substance abuse The recurrent use of alcohol and/or legal or illegal drugs that result in an individual failing to perform important work, school, and family obligations and thus suffering consequences. As defined by the *Diagnostic and Statistical Manual of Mental Disorders, Text Revision*, a publication produced by the American Psychiatric Association, substances of abuse, in addition to alcohol, include AMPHETAMINES, MARIJUANA, COCAINE, hallucinogenic drugs, INHALANTS, opioids, phencyclidine, sedatives, hypnotics or anxiolytics (antianxiety drugs), and polysubstance (multiple drugs) as well as the general category of "other" substances.

Substance abuse is not as severe as an addiction to substances. With substance dependence (also known as addiction), an individual has built up a tolerance to alcohol or a drug, needing greater quantities to achieve the same effect. In addition, if the person with substance dependence stops using the addictive substance, then he or she will experience withdrawal symptoms.

Although substance abuse is not as severe as substance dependence, it may lead to serious consequences such as losing a job, getting suspended or expelled from school, or being divorced by a spouse. Substance abuse may also lead to the commission of crimes, including crimes of VIOLENCE such as CHILD ABUSE, DATE/ACQUAINTANCE RAPE, and rape.

Some individuals use the term *substance abuse* to encompass both or either substance abuse and substance dependence. Thus, whenever possible, it is best to ascertain whether abuse or addiction is meant.

See also OPIATES; PCP.

American Psychiatric Association. *Diagnostic and Statistical Manual of Mental Disorders. Fourth Edition. Text Revision, DSM-IV-TR.* Washington, D.C.: American Psychiatric Association, 2000.

suicide   The voluntary attempt or successful ending of one's own life. A successful suicide is also called a completed suicide. Some people whose life is centered around addictive behaviors turn to suicide, especially those who have problems with ALCOHOLISM or who are addicted to substances such as COCAINE or other drugs that impair their judgment. In addition, many people who attempt or complete suicide have psychiatric disorders, such as DEPRESSION or BIPOLAR DISORDER. Individuals with both a substance use disorder and a serious psychiatric problem such as depression and who are not under ongoing treatment with a mental health professional are at risk for suicide.

Sometimes knowing if a death was a suicide or an accident is difficult. For example, if a person has taken an overdose of drugs or has used both drugs and alcohol, the combination may have been taken purposely to end life or it may have been an unintentional and ACCIDENTAL OVERDOSE. If the individual has not left a note or expressed a suicide wish to others, ascertaining the intention of the individual may be difficult or impossible.

A Leading Cause of Death Among Young People

In the United States, 70.6 percent of all the deaths of youths and young adults between the ages of 10–24 years result from only four causes: motor vehicle crashes (31.4 percent), other unintentional injuries (12 percent), homicide (15.3 percent), and suicide

(11.9 percent). Thus suicide is a leading cause of death and one that should be considered seriously in any young person who threatens suicide.

Alcoholism and Suicide

The authors of *The Encyclopedia of Understanding Alcohol and Other Drugs,* volume I, say that suicide is a problem among many people who are addicted to alcohol. They said, "Alcoholics of both genders are at particularly high risk of committing suicide. Although estimates of the level of risk vary, at least one study reported it to be 30 times greater than the risk of suicide among the general population." According to the authors, in up to 80 percent of completed suicides, the victim was drinking at the time of the suicide.

Impact of Childhood Abuse

Adults can carry the emotional scars of childhood abuse, and sometimes these psychological scars ultimately lead to an increased risk for suicide. In a large study of over 17,000 adults, about 4 percent had ever attempted suicide. The researchers sought linkages between suicide and household dysfunction, childhood abuse, and substance abuse, and they reported their findings in a 2001 issue of the *Journal of the American Medical Association.*

According to the researchers, "The prevalence of self-reported alcoholism, illicit drug use, and depressed affect was 6.5%, 16.5%, and 28.4%, respectively." Thus, depression (depressed affect) was the largest factor in suicide attempts, followed by illicit drug use and self-reported alcoholism.

The researchers found that the prevalence of suicide attempts among adults who had suffered from adverse childhood events was high. For example, if the individual had experienced no emotional abuse during childhood, the suicide prevalence was 2.5 percent. (Chronic emotional abuse includes such behavior as constantly screaming at a child and/or belittling the child in front of others. Emotional abuse can be very harmful even when no physical abuse occurs.) If emotional abuse did occur in childhood, the suicide prevalence among adults was 14.3 percent.

Some of the adults in the study had been sexually abused as children. The researchers found that if there was no sexual abuse in childhood, the prevalence for suicide in the adults was 2.4 percent. If sexual abuse did occur in childhood, however, the rate of suicide was nearly quadrupled to 9.1 percent among the adults.

Seeing a parent beaten during childhood can have a lifelong effect on individuals. The researchers found that if no domestic violence occurred in the home during childhood, the prevalence for suicide was 3.1 percent among the adults. If a battered mother was in the home during childhood, the prevalence for suicide tripled to 9.0 percent.

These statistics are significant because it is also known that a large proportion of childhood abuse is linked to the use of alcohol and/or drugs by the abusers. Thus substance abuse was likely an issue in at least some adults who were abused as children and who later committed suicide.

First Week of the Month is Riskiest

Some researchers have looked at other aspects of suicide, such as when the deaths occurred. In one unique study of deaths including suicides, homicides, accidents, and other causes of death, the researchers found that the risk for death was highest in the first week of the month and it was also associated with substance abuse. In their study results published in a 1999 issue of the *New England Journal of Medicine*, the researchers studied computerized death certificates in the United States for the period 1973–88. To assess a possible role of alcohol or drugs, they also looked at the secondary causes of death from 1983–88, the years for when that information was available.

The researchers found that the increased deaths in the first week of the month were particularly strong in the cases of deaths from homicides, suicides, accidents, and deaths that involved substance abuse. They speculated that the greater number of deaths in the first week might be related to many people who were receiving their government benefits checks at the beginning of the month, providing the funds that became available to buy the drugs or alcohol that then led to suicide.

Adolescents and Suicide

Among adolescents, any suicide talk should be taken seriously, no matter how well-adjusted the individual may appear to others. Teenagers and children can and do attempt suicide, and sometimes they die. According to the Centers for Disease Control and Prevention (CDC), about 14 percent of high school students in the United States have made a suicide plan, with girls (10.0 percent) much more likely to attempt suicide than boys (4.9 percent). In about 2.4 percent of high school students, a suicide attempt required medical attention. The rates of plans and attempts varied from state to state. (See table on page 228.)

Suicide attempts among high school students also vary by race, according to the CDC. Hispanic females have the greatest risk of attempting suicide (15.9 percent), followed by white females (10.3 percent), and white males have the lowest risk (5.3 percent). When considering grades 9 through 12, female students in grade 9 had the greatest risk for attempting suicide (13.2 percent) as well as the greatest risk for requiring medical attention after a suicide attempt (3.8 percent).

Dr. Iris Borowsky and colleagues reported on their suicide attempt findings among children and adolescents in a 2001 issue of *Pediatrics*. They studied the data from the National Longitudinal Study of Adolescent Health of more than 13,000 students. They found that key suicide risk factors for children and adolescents in the United States were a previous attempted suicide or the use of alcohol, marijuana, or other illicit drugs. Other risk factors for suicide were exhibiting violence, being a victim of violence, or having school problems. However, prior suicide attempts were the greatest indicator of a subsequent completed suicide.

The researchers found that 3.6 percent of the sample group had attempted suicide. These suicide attempts were more prevalent among white girls (5.6 percent) and Hispanic girls (5.5 percent) and were the least prevalent among white boys (1.9 percent) and African-American boys (1.6 percent). There were also some gender differences in risk factors. For example, carrying weapons was a suicide risk factor for both African-American and white boys but only for African-American girls and not white girls. The repeating of a grade in school was a suicide risk factor for Hispanic girls only.

The researchers also found protective factors against suicide attempts, such as family connectedness and emotional well-being.

Adolescents with Psychiatric Disorders and Substance Abuse Problems

Adolescents with psychiatric problems who abuse drugs and/or alcohol have an increased risk for

PERCENTAGE OF HIGH SCHOOL STUDENTS WHO SERIOUSLY CONSIDERED ATTEMPTING SUICIDE, WHO MADE A SUICIDE PLAN, AND WHO ATTEMPTED SUICIDE, BY SEX, SELECTED U.S. SITES. YOUTH RISK BEHAVIOR SURVEY, 2001

State	Felt Sad or Hopeless			Seriously Considered Attempting Suicide			Made a Suicide Plan			Attempted Suicide		
	Female	Male	Total	Female	Male	Total	Female	Male	Total	Female	Male	Total
Alabama	33.6	21.8	27.6	17.6	13.2	15.6	14.3	9.6	12.0	10.2	5.2	7.8
Arkansas	37.4	22.3	29.7	23.9	15.4	19.6	17.8	10.7	14.2	11.6	5.9	8.8
Delaware	32.3	21.3	27.0	19.6	12.9	16.3	13.9	10.3	12.1	8.9	5.3	7.1
Florida	34.7	21.8	28.2	19.4	11.4	15.4	13.3	9.2	11.3	10.0	6.6	8.4
Idaho	33.1	19.7	26.4	20.1	13.4	16.7	15.9	12.2	14.1	10.5	5.5	8.1
Maine	34.1	19.6	26.7	24.9	12.5	18.6	20.3	12.8	16.5	11.6	6.7	9.2
Massachusetts	35.0	22.7	28.8	25.3	15.0	20.1	18.3	12.2	15.2	12.2	6.9	9.6
Michigan	32.9	21.8	27.3	23.1	13.1	18.1	18.2	11.4	14.8	11.7	8.4	10.2
Mississippi	33.1	24.8	29.1	17.4	11.6	14.6	14.1	9.0	11.7	8.5	3.8	6.3
Missouri	33.3	24.1	28.5	23.0	15.6	19.2	18.4	10.5	14.3	11.0	5.9	8.4
Montana	33.8	19.6	26.6	24.4	14.4	19.4	20.0	12.8	16.3	13.3	7.4	10.4
Nevada	35.5	24.2	29.7	25.5	14.0	19.6	20.9	12.2	16.4	13.2	8.3	10.8
New Jersey	35.9	25.3	30.7	19.7	14.8	17.3	12.7	13.4	13.0	8.2	8.7	8.4
North Carolina	38.0	20.8	29.3	21.8	14.3	18.1	n/a	n/a	n/a	n/a	n/a	n/a
North Dakota	31.6	20.1	25.9	22.0	15.7	19.0	17.5	10.0	13.9	9.0	5.7	7.5
Rhode Island	30.9	20.5	25.7	19.5	13.7	16.5	15.6	9.2	12.4	10.3	5.9	8.1
South Dakota	30.2	16.3	23.1	23.9	14.8	19.3	21.0	14.6	17.7	14.7	11.4	13.1
Texas	36.3	22.5	29.3	23.2	12.5	17.7	16.1	10.9	13.4	12.7	5.3	9.0
Utah	31.3	23.3	27.2	22.4	16.4	19.4	15.8	12.2	14.5	11.9	6.3	9.2
Vermont	n/a	n/a	n/a	n/a	n/a	n/a	16.8	10.2	13.4	9.5	4.1	6.8
Wisconsin	35.7	18.1	26.7	25.4	14.6	19.9	n/a	n/a	n/a	11.3	5.8	8.6
Wyoming	33.1	20.0	26.2	22.6	14.6	18.5	16.5	12.1	14.2	10.0	4.9	7.4

Source: Grunbaum, Jo Anne, et al. "Youth Risk Behavior Surveillance—United States, 2001," *Morbidity and Mortality Weekly Report* 51, no. SS-4 (June 28, 2002): 32.

attempted suicide. Research on this topic is described in a 2004 article in *Drug and Alcohol Dependence*. The researchers found that adolescent males with ATTENTION DEFICIT HYPERACTIVITY DISORDER who abused drugs and/or alcohol were at risk for attempting suicide, as were females with mood disorders and substance abuse. The researchers also found that the increased suicide risk began early: age 12.5 for males and age 11 years for females.

In their study, which included 503 adolescents, ages 12.2–19.0 years, the researchers found that 17 percent had attempted suicide. In looking at gender alone, 29.8 percent of the females and 9.2 percent of the males had one or more suicide attempt. Depression greatly increased the risk for a suicide attempt. For example, among females who were diagnosed with major depression, 91.1 percent had attempted

depression; while among males, the percentage was lower but it was still very high (79.3 percent).

The researchers advised that clinicians should carefully monitor adolescents with substance abuse problems for their suicide risk. They should also be aware of gender differences in the risk for suicide.

The researchers also found that the abuse of some types of substances increased the risks for a suicide attempt. They said, "Males with hallucinogen use disorders, inhalant use disorders, and sedative-hypnotic use disorders had a higher risk for attempting suicide and females with substance disorders other than cannabis [marijuana] use disorder had higher odds for attempting suicide than non-suicide attempting adolescents."

In another study, Dr. Alec Roy studied the characteristics among 84 cocaine-dependent patients who had attempted suicide and 130 patients who had never attempted suicide. He found patterns of behavior among the suicidal patients. He reported his findings in a 2001 issue of the *American Journal of Psychiatry.*

According to Dr. Roy, suicidal patients were more likely to be females with a family history of suicidal behavior. In addition, they reported more childhood trauma and were more introverted and hostile than those patients who did not attempt suicide.

The Elderly and Suicide

Older Americans are at risk for suicide, often caused by depression, alcoholism, PRESCRIPTION DRUG ABUSE, or a combination of causes. In fact, in the United States, people over the age of 65 years have the highest suicide rate of all age groups and older men are especially at risk for suicide. Older people who are widowed or divorced have a high risk of suicide. Of adults over age 65, men represent 83 percent of all suicides. The highest suicide rate of 64.9 deaths per 100,000 people is found among white males, ages 85 and older. The national rate for all ages is 10.6 suicides per 100,000 people.

Older people may also commit homicide-suicide; that is, they kill another person (usually a spouse) and then kill themselves. Nearly all elderly perpetrators of homicide-suicides are male.

Dealing with Suicide Attempts

Any person of any age who talks about suicide or who has attempted suicide is in urgent need of psychiatric assistance. The person may be suffering from depression or another mental illness in conjunction with a substance abuse problem. Because subsequent attempts at suicide are often successful, it is particularly important that family members and the individual see a first, failed attempt as a chance to identify the underlying problem and treat it. A combination of antidepressants or other psychiatric medications along with counseling may considerably alleviate suicidal ideation and attempts in many individuals.

In the most extreme cases, when a physician believes that an individual is a threat to himself or herself, an individual may be involuntarily committed to a psychiatric hospital for a short period, depending on state laws. Physicians will seek to stabilize the person and then will work on identifying the prevailing problems that have apparently led to the suicide attempt or threatened suicide. Medication and therapy can be very effective for many patients. Patients with both substance abuse problems and psychiatric problems will need to receive treatment for both problems.

See also ANXIETY DISORDERS; CHILD ABUSE AND NEGLECT; DUAL DIAGNOSIS.

Borowsky, Iris Wagman, M.D., Marjorie Ireland, and Michael D. Resnick. "Adolescent Suicide Attempts: Risks and Protectors," *Pediatrics* 107, no. 3 (March 2001): 485–493.

Dube, Shanta R., et al. "Childhood Abuse, Household Dysfunction, and the Risk of Attempted Suicide Through the Life Span: Findings from the Adverse Childhood Experiences Study," *Journal of the American Medical Association* 286, no. 24 (December 26, 2001): 3,089–3,096.

Kandel, Joseph, M.D., and Christine Adamec. *The Encyclopedia of Senior Health and Well-Being.* New York: Facts On File, Inc., 2003.

Kelly, Thomas M., Jack R. Cornelius, and Duncan B. Clark. "Psychiatric Disorders and Attempted Suicide Among Adolescents with Substance Use Disorders," *Drug and Alcohol Dependence* 73, no. 1 (2004): 87–97.

Phillips, David P., Nicholas Christenfeld, and Natalie M. Ryan. "An Increase in the Number of Deaths in the United States in the First Week of the Month: An Association with Substance Abuse and Other Causes of Death," *New England Journal of Medicine* 341, no. 2 (July 8, 1999): 93–98.

Roy, Alec, M.D. "Characteristics of Cocaine-Dependent Patients Who Attempt Suicide," *American Journal of Psychiatry* 158, no. 8 (August 2001): 1,215–1,219.

teenage and youth drinking Consumption of alcohol by adolescents as young as 12 and as old as 18 years old. Chronic alcohol consumption among youths is a serious problem in the United States. According to the NATIONAL INSTITUTE ON ALCOHOL ABUSE AND ALCOHOLISM (NIAAA), underage alcohol use is more likely to kill young people than the use of all illegal drugs combined. In addition, youths who are heavy drinkers have a serious risk of suffering from ALCOHOLISM as adults. Studies have also shown that alcohol abuse is associated with an increased risk for attempted and completed SUICIDE among adolescents.

Health Effects on the Brain

Some researchers are concerned about the effect of heavy drinking on the adolescent brain. Some studies have shown measurably smaller sizes in a part of the brain of alcoholic adolescents. The hippocampus, which is important for learning and memory, was significantly smaller in the alcoholic teenagers, according to a 2003 report in *Alcohol Alert.*

Alcohol and High-Risk Behaviors

Alcohol abuse among adolescents is associated with many other problems, such as DRIVING WHILE INTOXICATED/DRIVING UNDER THE INFLUENCE of alcohol. This is extremely dangerous behavior since the fatal crash rate involving young alcohol-involved drivers between the ages of 16 and 20 years old is more than double the rate for alcohol-involved drivers ages 21 and older, according to the NIAAA.

Alcohol is also associated with an increased risk for unsafe sex. Teenagers are more likely to engage in sex and less likely to use condoms when they are under the influence of alcohol than when they are not. The consequences can be very serious and may include unwanted pregnancy. Teenagers engaging in unsafe sex also risk contracting a sexually transmitted disease, including the human immunodeficiency virus as well as herpes, gonorrhea, syphilis, and many other diseases that can be transmitted sexually. It should also be noted that sexually transmitted diseases can be contracted through oral sex as well as through intercourse. Oral sex protects only against pregnancy, not against diseases.

Sexual assault occurs more commonly when alcohol is involved, whether the alcohol is used by the victim, the offender, or both of them.

Some parents attempt to control teenage alcohol use by allowing their teenagers to drink at home at private parties. This is illegal behavior and could cause the parent to be charged with the criminal offense of providing alcohol to a minor.

Extent of the Problem

Surveys such as the national annual *Monitoring the Future* survey in the United States reveal how prevalent drinking is among high school students. Based on the results released for 2002, 49 percent of high school seniors admitted drinking an alcoholic beverage a month before the survey, 35 percent of 10th graders said they had been drinking in the month before the survey, and 20 percent of eighth graders had been drinking.

It is worth noting that, according to this survey, the trends of lifetime use among adolescents apparently are down compared with previous years. For example, when looking at any use of alcohol, the percentages have been steadily dropping each year. (See table on page 232.) In 2001, the percentage for eighth graders was 50.5, and it fell to 47.0 percent in 2002. The percentage of students who reported being drunk has also steadily fallen, although the rates for students who are seniors in high school are still very high. They have fallen from 63.9 percent in 2001 to 61.6 percent in 2002.

Some students, however, are using alcohol on a daily basis. The Monitoring the Future data revealed that about 3.5 percent of high school seniors are using alcohol daily, which probably indicates that they are alcoholics. (See table on page 233.) As can be seen from the chart, less than 1 percent (0.7 percent) of eighth graders reported drinking daily in 2002.

BINGE DRINKING, or drinking five or more drinks in a row in the past two weeks, is a serious problem for many high school students. (See table on page 233.) In 2002, 28.6 percent of high school seniors admitted to binge drinking, as did 22.4 percent of 10th graders and 12.4 percent of eighth graders. Binge drinking can lead to ALCOHOL POISONING and death. It can also lead to car crashes and the other dangerous consequences associated with excessive alcohol use. The rates of binge drinking dropped at all grade levels from 2001–02, but they are still far too high. Certainly it is a dangerous proposition when nearly a third of high school seniors and a quarter of high school sophomores in the United States are engaging in binge drinking.

Psychiatric Problems Contributing to Heavy Drinking in Adolescents

Many youths and adolescents apparently turn to alcohol because of serious underlying psychiatric problems. DEPRESSION is a key problem for many youths. Sometimes the depression predates the alcohol abuse. At other times, however, the depression may be triggered by alcohol abuse.

Other adolescents may suffer from ANXIETY DISORDERS, and they may attempt to use alcohol to self-medicate their symptoms. This seems to be especially true of female adolescents. Some studies indicate that adolescents with undiagnosed ATTENTION DEFICIT HYPERACTIVITY DISORDER (ADHD) may use alcohol as a means to overcome the discomfort that their symptoms of impulsivity, inattention, and hyperactivity cause them.

Some experts, however, disagree that adolescents with ADHD are more likely to abuse alcohol than youths without ADHD. For example, Dr. Biederman and his colleagues have found that the presence of BIPOLAR DISORDER and conduct disorder are much more predictive of alcohol abuse than is ADHD among adolescents.

Drinking Problems in Adolescence Are Highly Predictive of Alcoholism in Adulthood

In a study of substance abuse among 35-year-old adults, researchers sought to find if their substance abuse that occurred when they were in high school was later predictive of alcohol abuse behavior present as adults. They found out that it was predictive. (This research was reported in a 2004 issue of the American Journal of Public Health.)

The researchers used data from the annual Monitoring the Future survey and queried adults who had been surveyed in the past, contacting over 2,000 individuals. According to the researchers,

TRENDS IN LIFETIME PREVALENCE OF USE OF ALCOHOL IN THE UNITED STATES, FOR EIGHTH, 10TH, AND 12TH GRADERS, BY PERCENT												
	1991	1992	1993	1994	1995	1996	1997	1998	1999	2000	2001	2002
Any use												
8th grade	70.1	69.3	55.7	55.8	54.5	55.3	53.8	52.5	52.1	51.7	50.5	47.0
10th grade	83.8	82.3	71.6	71.1	70.5	71.8	72.0	69.8	70.6	71.4	70.1	66.9
12th grade	88.0	87.5	80.0	80.4	80.7	79.2	81.7	81.4	80.0	80.3	79.7	78.4
Been drunk												
8th grade	26.7	26.8	26.4	25.9	25.3	26.8	25.2	24.8	24.8	25.1	23.4	21.3
10th grade	50.0	47.7	47.9	47.2	46.9	48.5	49.4	46.7	48.9	49.3	48.2	44.0
12th grade	65.4	63.4	62.5	62.9	63.2	61.8	64.2	62.4	62.3	62.3	63.9	61.6

Source: Johnston, Lloyd D., O'Malley, Patrick, and Bachman, Jerald. *Monitoring the Future: National Results on Adolescent Drug Use. Overview of Key Findings, 2002.* NIH Publication No. 03-5374, Bethesda, Md.: National Institute on Drug Abuse, U.S. Department of Health and Human Service, National Institutes of Health, 2003.

TRENDS IN 30-DAY PREVALENCE OF DAILY USE OF ALCOHOL IN THE UNITED STATES FOR EIGHTH, 10TH, AND 12TH GRADERS, BY PERCENT

	1991	1992	1993	1994	1995	1996	1997	1998	1999	2000	2001	2002
Any daily use												
8th grade	0.5	0.6	1.0	1.0	0.7	1.0	0.8	0.9	1.0	0.8	0.9	0.7
10th grade	1.3	1.2	1.8	1.7	1.7	1.6	1.7	1.9	1.9	1.8	1.9	1.8
12th grade	3.6	3.4	3.4	2.9	3.5	3.7	3.9	3.9	3.4	2.9	3.6	3.5
Been drunk daily												
8th grade	0.1	0.1	0.2	0.3	0.2	0.2	0.2	0.3	0.4	0.3	0.2	0.3
10th grade	0.2	0.3	0.4	0.4	0.6	0.4	0.6	0.6	0.7	0.5	0.6	0.5
12th grade	0.9	0.8	0.9	1.2	1.3	1.6	2.0	1.5	1.9	1.7	1.4	1.2
5+ drinks in a row in last 2 weeks												
8th grade	12.9	13.4	13.5	14.5	14.5	15.6	14.5	13.7	15.2	14.1	13.2	12.4
10th grade	22.9	21.1	23.0	23.6	24.0	24.8	25.1	24.3	25.6	26.2	24.9	22.4
12th grade	29.8	27.9	27.5	28.2	29.8	30.2	31.3	31.5	30.8	30.0	29.7	28.6

Source: Johnston, Lloyd D., O'Malley, Patrick, and Bachman, Jerald. *Monitoring the Future: National Results on Adolescent Drug Use. Overview of Key Findings, 2002.* NIH Publication No. 03-5374, Bethesda, Md.: National Institute on Drug Abuse, U.S. Department of Health and Human Service, National Institutes of Health, 2003.

"When compared with those who did not drink heavily as high school seniors, participants who drank heavily had 3 times the odds of drinking heavily at age 35 years."

Other researchers have looked at the long-term picture as well. In their research, Phyllis Ellickson and colleagues considered public health problems associated with drinking in grades seven and 12 and how it affected young adults at age 23. They reported on their findings in a 2003 issue of *Pediatrics.*

The researchers reviewed data from a longitudinal survey of 6,527 students recruited from 30 schools in California and Oregon in 1985 when they were in grade seven and then again in 1990 when they were in grade 12. They were reassessed in 1995 when they were age 23.

The researchers found that the students who were drinkers in the seventh grade were more likely to have problems at the age of 23 years. For example, about 8 percent of the juvenile nondrinkers had been arrested for predatory violence as adults, compared with 16 percent of the juvenile drinkers. When considering all arrests, about 16 percent of the people who were nondrinkers as juveniles had ever been arrested as adults, compared with 32 percent of those who drank in the seventh grade.

Other negative effects were seen as well. For example, about 17 percent of the nondrinkers in seventh grade became alcoholics when they were 23 years old, compared with 40.5 percent of the students who drank when they were in seventh grade. About 3 percent of the nondrinkers in seventh grade had multiple drug problems as adults, compared with 9.3 percent of the seventh grade drinkers as adults. The adults who drank as young people were also more likely to miss work for no good reason and to get fired from their jobs.

The researchers also found that even those who experimented with alcohol in the seventh grade a few times often suffered long-term effects, such as a higher incidence of alcoholism, drug abuse, predatory violence, drunk driving, and the other measures. Thus even brief but excessive use of alcohol can create significant life problems.

This research lends credence to the old saying that the "child is the father to the man" and that adolescent behavior can have lifelong consequences.

Adolescent Drinking Problems Can be Predicted by Parental Substance Abuse

Teenagers are also affected by the substance abuse behavior of their parents. In part, this may be due to a genetic predisposition to alcohol abuse. However, it may also be caused by observed and learned/modeled behavior.

Researchers Joseph Biederman and his colleagues believed that patterns of alcohol and drug abuse in young people could be predicted by the substance abuse patterns of their parents. They reported on their findings in a 2000 issue of *Pediatrics.*

The researchers controlled for the effects of socioeconomic status, the presence of attention deficit hyperactivity disorder, and other possible risk factors. They found that parental substance abuse was predictive of adolescent substance abuse.

The researchers said, "Controlling for duration of exposure, we also found that adolescence was a critical developmental period for exposure to parental SUDS [substance use disorders]. These results especially highlight adolescence as a critical period for the deleterious effects of exposure to parental SUDS."

They also added, "There are 2 main values of this information: education and referral. Substance-abusing parents need to know that they are placing their children at high risk for substance abuse and that they should seek treatment for the disorder not only for their sake but also for the well-being of their children. Even if referral to a mental health professional does not stop the parents' addiction, it could be useful in modifying the parenting styles and modeling behaviors that may lead to substance use in high-risk children."

Religious Beliefs Mitigate Against Drinking

Researchers have found some factors appear to have a protective effect against youths using alcohol. One such factor is the presence of religious beliefs. As part of the research for the National Survey on Drug Use and Health, researchers asked youths ages 12–17 about whether religious beliefs were important in their lives, if their religious beliefs influenced their decisions, and how often they attended religious services.

The researchers found that about 78 percent said their religious beliefs were very important in their lives. A majority, 69 percent, said that their religious beliefs influenced how they made decisions. About 33 percent of the youths reported attending religious services 25 times or more in the past year.

Of the youths who reported that their religious beliefs were very important to them, about 15 percent reported using alcohol in the past month, compared with 27 percent of the less-religious group. When considering the adolescents who said their religious beliefs influenced how they made decisions, about 14 percent of this group said they used alcohol in the past month, compared with 27 percent of the youths in the less-religious group. Of the youths who had attended 25 or more religious services in the past year, about 13 percent said they had used alcohol in the past year, compared with 20 percent of the less-religious group.

Although religious beliefs did not prevent all drinking, it dramatically reduced the percentage of individuals who used alcohol and thus had a positive and protective effect.

Treatment of Alcohol Disorders

Because the image of the stereotypical alcoholic is so far from that of a young adolescent, adults can have difficulty accepting that teenagers can be alcoholics and that when they are addicted to alcohol, they need treatment. However, a person may develop an alcohol disorder at any age.

Unfortunately, many adolescent alcoholics do not receive treatment. According to one report, "Alcohol Use by Persons Under the Legal Drinking Age of 21," about 3 million people ages 12–20 met the criteria for alcohol dependence (alcoholism) or alcohol abuse in the past 12 months in 2001, based on the numbers of problems they had experienced. However, only about 400,000 people in that same age group received alcohol treatment. Thus many underage drinkers were and probably still are not receiving the treatment that they need.

It is also true that many adult alcoholics do not receive treatment. For example, according to the *2002 National Survey on Drug Use and Health,* 1.5 million people of all ages received treatment for their alcohol use in 2002. However, an estimated 17.1 million people needed treatment. The reasons for their nontreatment are unknown.

In a study of facilities that do provide treatment for adolescents, reported in a 2003 issue of the *DASIS Report,* the researchers looked at the National Survey of Substance Abuse Treatment Services, an annual survey of all treatment facilities in the United States, public and private, which offer substance abuse treatment. This data revealed that in 2002, there were 13,843 facilities and 897 (7 percent) concentrated on clients under the age of 18 years old.

Of the adolescent facilities, 73 percent of the clients received treatment for alcohol and drug abuse and only 8 percent received treatment exclusively for alcohol problems. Most facilities (68 percent) provided outpatient care. The services that the clients received were individual therapy (97 percent), group therapy (94 percent), substance abuse assessment (90 percent), discharge planning (86 percent), and drug/alcohol urine screening (80 percent).

See also COLLEGE STUDENTS; DATE/ACQUAINTANCE RAPE; DRINKING GAMES; TEENAGE AND YOUTH DRUG ABUSE; TEENAGE AND YOUTH GAMBLING; TEENAGE AND YOUTH SMOKING.

Biederman, Joseph, M.D., et al. "Patterns of Alcohol and Drug Use in Adolescents Can Be Predicted by Parental Substance Use Disorders," *Pediatrics* 106, no. 4 (October 2000): 792–797.

Deas, Deborah M.D., and Suzanne Thomas. "Comorbid Psychiatric Factors Contributing to Adolescent Alcohol and Other Drug Use," *Alcohol Research & Health* 26, no. 2 (2002): 116–121.

Ellickson, Phyllis, Joan S. Tucker, and David J. Klein. "Ten-Year Prospective Study of Public Health Problems Associated with Early Drinking," *Pediatrics* 111, no. 5 (May 2003): 949–955.

Johnston, Lloyd D., Patrick O'Malley, and Jerald Bachman. *Monitoring the Future: National Results on Adolescent Drug Use. Overview of Key Findings, 2002.* NIH Publication No. 03-5374, National Institute on Drug Abuse, U.S. Department of Health and Human Service, National Institutes of Health, 2003.

Li, Ting-Kai, M.D. "Underage Drinking: A Major Public Health Challenge," *Alcohol Alert* 59, no. 59 (April 2003): 1–4.

Merline, Alicia, et al. "Substance Use Among Adults 35 Years of Age: Prevalence, Adulthood Predictors, and Impact of Adolescent Substance," *American Journal of Public Health* 94, no. 1 (January 2004): 96–102.

National Institute on Alcohol Abuse and Alcoholism. "Underage Drinking: A Major Public Health Challenge," *Alcohol Alert* 59 (April 2003): 1–4.

National Survey on Drug Use and Health. "Religious Beliefs and Substance Use Among Youths," *The NSDUH Report* (January 30, 2004): 1–3.

Office of Applied Studies. "Alcohol Use by Persons Under the Legal Drinking Age of 21," *The NHSDA Report* (May 9, 2003): 1–5.

teenage and youth drug abuse Adolescents ages 12–17 and their illegal use of substances, such as COCAINE, ECSTASY (methylenedioxymethamphetamine/MDMA), METHAMPHETAMINE, MARIJUANA, and other drugs.

Based on the findings from the 2002 National Survey on Drug Use and Health in the United States, the survey showed that 11.6 percent of youths ages 12–17 had used illicit drugs at some time. Of this group, an estimated 8.2 percent had used marijuana and 4.0 percent had illegally used prescription-type drugs. The survey also showed that one in six youths had been offered drugs for sale by someone in the past month and that those who were approached by others and offered drugs had almost a six times greater risk (36.2 percent) of using a drug than those who were not approached (6.7 percent) by drug sellers.

Most youths do not abuse drugs on a regular basis nor are they addicted to drugs. However, even a one-time use of an illegal drug can lead to significant harm and even death. For example, the first time an INHALANT is used can lead to a severe toxic reaction. In addition, the abuse of drugs such as MDMA or cocaine have caused many young patients to require EMERGENCY TREATMENT in hospital emergency rooms for hyperthermia (excessively high body temperature) or cardiac arrhythmias. If death does not ensue, lifelong brain damage or other serious health problems may occur instead.

Often many different substances are combined as drugs of abuse, greatly increasing the risk of harm to the individual's health. There is no Food and Drug Administration control or other governmental oversight over substances that are used illegally, which is a fact that is sometimes forgotten by those people who act irresponsibly. The individual may have little or no idea what substance he or she is ingesting. Many adolescents also combine drug use with alcohol abuse, which further escalates the risk of harm.

It should also be noted that drug abuse, particularly with drugs such as cocaine and inhalants, have been linked to an increased risk for SUICIDE among adolescents who have psychiatric disorders, as discussed in a 2003 issue of *Drug and Alcohol Dependence*.

Reasons for Drug Abuse

In general, among those who are not addicts, illicit drugs are often used for the purposes of obtaining a EUPHORIA or getting high. Among adolescents, however, PEER PRESSURE may initially be a far more compelling reason to abuse drugs than the desire to get high. Another reason for drug abuse may be that pills may seem like a quick fix solution to the often seemingly overwhelming problems of adolescence. This may explain the increasing problem of PRESCRIPTION DRUG ABUSE among adolescents. According to the 2002 National Survey on Drug Use and Health, the lifetime rate of prescription drug abuse among youths ages 12–17 years old who were taking nonmedical pain relievers increased from 9.6 percent in 2001 to 11.2 percent in 2002. (The rate was only 1.2 percent in 1989, and it has steadily increased upward ever since then.)

Another reason for drug abuse may be that adolescents may be modeling their own parents' behavior. Adolescents and youths whose parents abuse or are addicted to drugs are at high risk for developing SUBSTANCE ABUSE problems, according to many clinical studies.

How Youths Obtain Drugs

Youths often purchase illegal drugs from each other. According to the 2002 National Survey on Drug Use and Health, marijuana users were asked where they obtained the drug from. Most users (79 percent) who bought their marijuana said they obtained it from a friend. More than half (55.9 percent) said they purchased the drug inside a home, apartment, or dormitory. Almost 9 percent of youths said they bought their marijuana inside a school building. Schools are designated as DRUG-FREE ZONES, which are areas where penalties are automatically much higher for drug sales.

Some youths abuse prescription drugs that they illegally purchase or are given from others or that they steal, such as prescription painkillers. There have also been some reports of adolescents who have illegally ordered prescription narcotics from over the Internet, using their parents' credit cards without their knowledge. In some cases, they have

reportedly died from abusing these drugs. The drugs may be ordered from other countries as far away from the United States as Thailand or India. This is a matter of concern to law enforcement agencies, such as the DRUG ENFORCEMENT ADMINISTRATION.

Drugs of Abuse Can Be Very Harmful

Some drugs have a profound effect on the body and can rapidly cause addiction or impair the body in such a way that the individual behaves out of character. For example, cocaine can induce violent rages, aggressive behavior, and paranoia. Some drugs, such as lysergic acid diethylamide (LSD) and gamma-hydroybutyrate, can induce HALLUCINATIONS. Other drugs reduce normal inhibitions, such that youths may engage in unsafe sex with others, increasing the risk of unplanned pregnancies and the transmission of sexually transmitted diseases. The addition of alcohol further increases the unpredictability of the drug's effects on the body.

In addition to the ill effects that drugs can cause on people of all ages, they can cause additional harm to the developing body of the adolescent, causing a delay in puberty and causing menstrual problems in females.

Demographics of Drug Use

Knowing which groups of adolescents are most at risk for drug abuse can help educators and policy makers better help such groups. The 2002 National Survey on Drug Use and Health provides this type of demographic information. It does not, however, offer reasons or explanations for the data. For example, the rate of drug abuse is extremely high among American Indians/Alaska Natives and extremely low among Asians, although why this finding is true is unknown.

Racial data The rate of drug abuse for all youths in the survey was 11.6 percent. Illicit drug use was highest among American Indians/Alaska Natives youths ages 12–17 years old (20.9 percent). The rate for other races/ethnicities were as follows: whites 12.6 percent; blacks or African Americans 10.0 percent; two or more races 12.5 percent; and Hispanic or Latin 10.7 percent. The rate was lowest among Asian youths (4.8 percent).

Age and drug of choice among youths The drug of choice depended on the age of the youth. According to the 2002 National Survey on Drug

Use and Health, the types of drugs abused by 12 and 13 year olds in 2002 were as follows: 1.7 percent used prescription-type drugs nonmedically, 1.4 percent used marijuana, and 1.4 percent used inhalants.

Among 14- and 15-year-old teenagers, the most popular drug was marijuana (7.6 percent), followed by prescription-type drugs used nonmedically (4.0 percent) and inhalants (1.6 percent). Among teenagers ages 16 and 17 years old, marijuana was the most popular drug (15.7 percent), followed by prescription-type drugs used nonmedically (6.2 percent), hallucinogens (1.9 percent), and cocaine (1.3 percent). Less than 1 percent of 16 and 17 year olds used inhalants.

Gender differences in drug abuse among youths
The 2002 National Survey on Drug Use and Health (and all other surveys) revealed that in general, males are more likely than females to abuse drugs. Males are also more likely than females to abuse alcohol.

Among youths ages 12–17 years old, the illicit drug use rate was 12.3 percent for boys and 10.9 percent for girls. Boys had a higher rate of marijuana abuse (9.1 percent) than girls (7.2 percent). However, girls had a higher rate of psychotherapeutic drug abuse (4.3 percent) than boys (3.6 percent). Psychotherapeutic drugs include drugs such as prescription pain relievers, tranquilizers, stimulants, and sedatives. It also includes methamphetamine. It does not include any over-the-counter drugs.

Gender differences in treatment   According to the 2002 National Survey on Drug Use and Health, among persons age 12 and older in 2002, males were more likely to receive treatment for an illicit drug problem or alcohol problem in the past year (2.1 percent) than females (0.9 percent). The reason for this disparity is unknown.

Drug Use Is Linked to Emotional Problems

According to the 2002 National Survey on Drug Use and Health, in 2002, an estimated 4.8 million youths ages 12–17 received treatment or counseling for emotional or behavioral problems that occurred in the year prior to the interview. The reasons most cited by the youths for their latest treatment session was they "felt depressed" (49.5 percent), "thought about killing self or tried to kill self" (19.5 percent), and "felt very afraid or tense" (19.5 percent).

The rate of mental health treatment among adolescents who used illegal drugs was higher (26.7 percent) than among those who did not use them (17.2 percent). Some research indicates that depressed people are more likely to take drugs, while other research indicates that taking illicit drugs may trigger DEPRESSION. Psychiatrists continue to debate this issue of cause and effect with regard to depression and drug and alcohol abuse.

Monitoring the Future Data on Drug Use by Adolescents

Information on drug, alcohol, and tobacco use is also provided from annual survey data taken each year from students in the eighth, 10th, and 12th grades nationwide in the United States in the Monitoring the Future survey data. Data from 1991–2002 show some trends in ups and downs of drug usages. Considering several different categories of drugs is instructive in order to provide a basis for comparison and contrast, not only to each other now but also to compare drug use now with drug use in the past. (See table on page 238.)

Use of any illicit drug   As can be seen from the table, the percentages of illicit drug use when all drugs are considered have dropped from 2001–02 in all grades. Eighth graders' illicit drug use was down from 26.8–24.5 percent. Tenth graders' drug use was also down, from 45.6–44.6 percent. Twelfth graders' use was down from 53.9–53.0 percent. These were all positive signs; however, the abuse rates are still high. For example, when considering 12th graders alone, the chart shows that from 1991–96, seniors had lower levels of drug use in all of those years compared with 2002.

MDMA (Ecstasy) use   The abuse of MDMA was down among all three grades from 2001–02 and use was down in lifetime use, annual use, and 30-day use. This drug had been climbing in popularity since 1998. According to the authors of the Monitoring the Future study, "Disapproval of ecstasy use rose sharply in all three grades in 2002, indicating that peer norms against use of this drug were strengthening."

Cocaine use   Among eighth graders, 3.6 percent who were surveyed said they had ever used cocaine, and 6.1 percent of 10th graders and 7.8

LIFETIME PREVALENCE OF USE OF VARIOUS DRUGS FOR EIGHTH, 10TH, AND 12TH GRADERS IN THE UNITED STATES, BY PERCENT

	1991	1992	1993	1994	1995	1996	1997	1998	1999	2000	2001	2002
Any illicit drug												
8th grade	18.7	20.6	22.5	25.7	28.5	31.2	29.4	29.0	28.3	26.8	26.8	24.5
10th grade	30.6	29.8	32.8	37.4	40.9	45.4	47.3	44.9	46.2	45.6	45.6	44.6
12th grade	44.1	40.7	42.9	45.6	48.4	50.8	54.3	54.1	54.7	54.0	53.9	53.0
MDMA (Ecstasy)												
8th grade	—	—	—	—	—	3.4	3.2	2.7	2.7	4.3	5.2	4.3
10th grade	—	—	—	—	—	5.6	5.7	5.1	6.0	7.3	8.0	6.6
12th grade	—	—	—	—	—	6.1	6.9	5.8	8.0	11.0	11.7	10.5
Cocaine												
8th grade	2.3	2.9	2.9	3.6	4.2	4.5	4.4	4.6	4.7	4.5	4.3	3.6
10th grade	4.1	3.3	3.6	4.3	5.0	6.5	7.1	7.2	7.7	6.9	5.7	6.1
12th grade	7.8	6.1	6.1	5.9	6.0	7.1	8.7	9.3	9.8	8.6	8.2	7.8
Crack cocaine												
8th grade	1.3	1.6	1.7	2.4	2.7	2.9	2.7	3.2	3.1	3.1	3.0	2.5
10th grade	1.7	1.5	1.8	2.1	2.8	3.3	3.6	3.9	4.0	3.7	3.1	3.6
12th grade	3.1	2.6	2.6	3.0	3.0	3.3	3.9	4.4	4.6	3.9	3.7	3.8
Amphetamines												
8th grade	10.5	10.8	11.8	12.3	13.1	13.5	12.3	11.3	10.7	9.9	10.2	8.7
10th grade	13.2	13.1	14.9	15.1	17.4	17.7	17.0	16.0	15.7	15.7	16.0	14.9
12th grade	15.4	13.9	15.1	15.7	15.3	15.3	16.5	16.4	16.3	15.6	16.2	16.8
Heroin												
8th grade	1.2	1.4	1.4	2.0	2.3	2.4	2.1	2.3	2.3	1.9	1.7	1.6
10th grade	1.2	1.2	1.3	1.5	1.7	2.1	2.1	2.3	2.3	2.2	1.7	1.8
12th grade	0.9	1.2	1.1	1.2	1.6	1.8	2.1	2.0	2.0	2.4	1.8	1.7
Marijuana												
8th grade	10.2	11.2	12.6	16.7	19.9	23.1	22.6	22.2	22.0	20.3	20.4	19.2
10th grade	23.4	21.4	24.4	30.4	34.1	39.8	42.3	39.6	40.9	40.3	40.1	38.7
12th grade	36.7	32.6	35.3	38.2	41.7	44.9	49.6	49.1	49.7	48.8	49.0	47.8
Inhalants												
8th grade	17.6	17.4	19.4	19.9	21.6	21.2	21.0	20.5	19.7	17.9	17.1	15.2
10th grade	6.1	6.4	6.8	8.1	9.3	10.5	10.5	9.8	9.7	8.9	8.9	7.8
12th grade	17.6	16.6	17.4	17.7	17.4	16.6	16.1	15.2	15.4	14.2	13.0	11.7
Tranquilizers (such as Xanax)												
8th grade	3.8	4.1	4.4	4.6	4.5	5.3	4.8	4.6	4.4	4.4	5.0	4.3
10th grade	5.8	5.9	5.7	5.4	6.0	7.1	7.3	7.8	7.9	8.0	9.2	8.8
12th grade	7.2	6.0	6.4	6.6	7.1	7.2	7.8	8.5	9.3	8.9	10.3	11.4
Anabolic steroids												
8th grade	1.9	1.7	1.6	2.0	2.0	1.8	1.8	2.0	2.7	3.0	2.8	2.5
10th grade	1.8	1.7	1.7	1.8	2.0	1.8	2.0	2.0	2.7	3.5	3.5	3.5
12th grade	2.1	2.1	2.0	2.4	2.3	1.9	2.4	2.7	2.9	2.5	3.7	4.0

Source: Johnston, Lloyd D., Patrick O'Malley, and Jerald Bachman. *Monitoring the Future: National Results on Adolescent Drug Use. Overview of Key Findings, 2002.* NIH Publication No. 03-5374. Bethesda, Md.: National Institute on Drug Abuse, U.S. Department of Health and Human Service, National Institutes of Health, 2003.

percent of high school seniors had ever used this drug. The use of crack cocaine was much lower among all groups: 2.5 percent of eighth graders, 3.6 percent of 10th graders, and 3.8 percent of 12th graders used crack in 2002.

Amphetamine use As the table on page 238 reveals, amphetamine levels are slightly up in 12th grade, from 16.2 percent in 2001 to 16.8 percent in 2002. Levels were down in grades eight and 10.

Heroin use Few adolescents are heroin users. As can be seen from the table on page 238, though, there are small numbers. In the eighth grade, 1.6 percent use heroin. In grade 10, the rate is 1.8 percent. The percent is lower in grade 12 (1.7 percent). Although it is not known why, it may be speculated that some heroin addicts probably do not continue to the 12th grade and have dropped out of school by that point.

Marijuana use Marijuana use was also about the same in 2002 as in 2001. Nearly half (47.8 percent) of high school seniors were using the drug in 2002, while numbers were lower in 10th grade (38.7 percent) and eighth grade (19.2 percent). About 6 percent of 12th graders are using marijuana or hashish on a daily basis. This is triple the rate of daily users in 1991. (See table below.)

Inhalant use Inhalant use shows a downward trend from 2001–02 in all grades. (See table on page 238.) As can be seen from the table, the percentage of eighth graders, the biggest users of inhalants, using inhalants dropped from 17.1 percent in 2001 to 15.2 percent in 2002. The percentage of 10th grade users dropped from 8.9 percent in 2001 to 7.8 percent in 2002. The lifetime prevalence among 12th graders dropped from 13.0 percent in 2001 to 11.7 percent in 2002.

Although most children and adolescents in the United States do not abuse inhalants such as GLUE, paint, and other household products, huffing, or inhaling products for their intoxicating effects, is an abuse problem. It is a serious problem because even one use can lead to brain damage or death. Some youths develop an abusive or addictive use of inhalants. Most states in the United States have passed laws making it illegal to use household and commercial products as inhalants. Some states have enacted laws restricting retail sales to minors of common household products that can be inhaled, such as glue.

Tranquilizer use In the category of tranquilizer use, including such antianxiety drug as alprazolam (Xanax), abuse was up among 12th graders, from 10.3 percent in 2001 to 11.4 percent in 2002. This is also the highest rate over the 1991–2002 period. The rates for both eighth graders and 10th graders were down from 2001–02.

Steroid use Drug use of anabolic steroids among 10th graders was flat in 2002 but slightly up among 12th graders. At 4 percent among 12th graders, it is at its highest level over the period 1991–2002 and nearly double the 2.1 percent rate of 1991.

Youths and Hallucinogens

Drugs that are hallucinogens, such as Ecstasy (MDMA), LSD, phencyclidine (PCP), and related drugs, can cause depression, anxiety, delusions (false beliefs), panic, and even psychosis. An estimated 1.4 million youths ages 12–17 years old had used a hallucinogenic drug at least once in their lives, according to federal data released in 2001. (See table below.) The most commonly used hallucinogens

TRENDS IN 30-DAY PREVALENCE OF DAILY USE OF MARIJUANA FOR EIGHTH, 10TH, AND 12TH GRADERS IN THE UNITED STATES, 1991–2002												
	1991	1992	1993	1994	1995	1996	1997	1998	1999	2000	2001	2002
8th grade	0.2	0.2	0.4	0.7	0.8	1.5	1.1	1.1	1.4	1.3	1.3	1.2
10th grade	0.8	0.8	1.0	2.2	2.8	3.5	3.7	3.6	3.8	3.8	4.5	3.9
12th grade	2.0	1.9	2.4	3.6	4.6	4.9	5.8	5.6	6.0	6.0	5.8	6.0

Source: Lloyd D. Johnston, Patrick O'Malley, and Jerald Bachman. *Monitoring the Future: National Results on Adolescent Drug Use. Overview of Key Findings, 2002.* NIH Publication No. 03-5374, Bethesda, Md.: National Institute on Drug Abuse, U.S. Department of Health and Human Service, National Institutes of Health, 2003.

were LSD and Ecstasy, and 3 percent of youths had used each drug.

As can be seen from the table below, African-American youths were the least likely to use hallucinogens (1.7 percent) and whites were the most likely (6.8 percent). In terms of percentages of lifetime use, whites were followed by Asians (5.2 percent) and Hispanics (4.1 percent). Part of the reason for this usage pattern is that researchers have found that African Americans and Hispanic youths were more likely than whites to perceive a great risk in using hallucinogens, such as LSD, even once or twice.

Factors Mitigating Against Drug Use

Researchers have found that some factors appear to have a positively protective effect against youths using drugs. These range from parental disapproval of drugs to students' own views of the risks of drugs to school programs.

Perception of parental approval When youths perceive that their parents disapprove of drug use, they are much more likely to avoid using drugs. For example, in the 2002 National Survey on Drug Use and Health, most youths (89.1 percent) said their parents would strongly disapprove of their trying marijuana once or twice. Among these adolescents, only 5.5 percent of them had used marijuana in the past month. In contrast, among those youths who

reported their perception that their parents would only somewhat disapprove or neither approve nor disapprove of their trying marijuana, 30.2 percent of this group had used marijuana in the past month.

Perception of a drug as a great risk Whether youths perceive a particular drug as risky or not also affects whether they use the drug. In the 2002 National Survey on Drug Use and Health, among youths who said that they perceived marijuana as a "great risk," only 1.9 percent said they had used the drug in the past month. Among adolescents who said marijuana presented a "moderate, slight, or no risk," the rate was 11.3 percent or nearly six times higher than when the youths perceived the drug as greatly risky. (See MARIJUANA to find out about the real risks behind this drug.)

Religious beliefs As part of the research for the National Survey on Drug Use and Health (NSDUH), researchers asked youths ages 12–17 about whether religious beliefs were important in their lives, if their religious beliefs influenced their decisions, and how often they attended religious services.

The researchers found that about 78 percent said their religious beliefs were very important in their lives, and a majority, 69 percent, said that their religious beliefs influenced how they made decisions. About 33 percent of the youths reported attending religious services 25 times or more in the past year.

Of the youths who said that their religious beliefs were very important to them, 9.2 percent reported taking an illicit drug in the past year, compared with about 21 percent of the individuals who did not consider their religious beliefs to be very important. As for the youths who said that their religious beliefs influenced their decisions, 8.2 percent of this group used an illicit drug in the past year, compared with 19 percent of the group not influenced by their religious beliefs.

When comparing the youths who attended 25 or more religious services with those who attended fewer or no religious services, the researchers found that about 7 percent of the more-religious youths reported taking an illicit drug within the past year, compared with about 14 percent of the less-religious group.

Although a religious commitment does not altogether remove drug use from the lives of youths, it

---

PERCENTAGES OF YOUTHS AGES 12 TO 17 REPORTING LIFETIME USE OF SPECIFIC HALLUCINOGENS, BY RACE/ETHNICITY, 2001

	White	Black	Asian	Hispanic
Any hallucinogen	6.8	1.7	5.2	4.1
PCP	1.2	0.2	0.2	0.6
LSD	3.9	0.5	2.3	2.1
Peyote	0.4	Under 0.1	0.2	0.3
Mescaline	0.4	0.1	0.6	0.3
Psilocybin (mushrooms)	2.7	0.4	0.7	1.4
Ecstasy (MDMA)	3.8	1.1	4.2	2.1

Source: National Household Survey on Drug Abuse (NHSDA). "Racial and Ethnic Differences in Youth Hallucinogen Use," *The NHSDA Report*. Rockville, Md.: Office of Applied Studies, Substance Abuse and Mental Health Services Administration, August 15, 2003.

clearly has a major effect on many youths, cutting the numbers who use drugs by half or greater.

Exposure to antidrug messages Most students are exposed to messages about alcohol and drugs outside their schools. According to the 2002 NSDUH, 83 percent of the students heard or saw alcohol or drug prevention messages outside of school. These messages had a slightly positive effect. Youths who said that they had heard or seen such messages had an 11.3 percent rate of illicit drug use, compared with the 13.2 percent rate of youths who said they had not heard or seen them.

Among youths who received education about drug or alcohol prevention in school, 78.8 percent said they had seen or heard such messages. Of those who said they had seen or heard the messages, the rate of past-month illicit drug use was 10.9 percent, compared with 14.6 percent for youths who did not see or hear them.

More than half (58 percent) of the youths had talked to at least one parent about the dangers of drug, alcohol, and tobacco abuse in the past year. Among those who had talked to a parent, the prevalence of illicit drug abuse was 11.3 percent. The prevalence was 12.1 percent among those who did not talk to a parent. (This is less than a 1 percent difference, but it may still mean some lives that were saved.)

Treatment Issues

Youths who abuse drugs may receive treatment in outpatient clinics or inpatient rehabilitation facilities. Finding facilities for some adolescent patients may be extremely difficult, particularly if they have other problems as well, such as psychiatric problems as well as problems with alcohol abuse or alcoholism. According to the 2002 NSDUH, only about 8 percent of adolescent patients with substance abuse problems receive treatment in treatment facilities, although the reasons for this are unknown.

See also COLLEGE STUDENTS; GHB; ILLEGAL DRUGS AND HEALTH PROBLEMS; TEENAGE AND YOUTH DRINKING; TEENAGE AND YOUTH GAMBLING; TEENAGE AND YOUTH SMOKING.

Biederman, Joseph, M.D., et al. "Patterns of Alcohol and Drug Use in Adolescents Can Be Predicted by Parental Substance Use Disorders," *Pediatrics* 106, no. 4 (October 2000): 792–797.

Kelly, Thomas M., Jack R. Cornelius, and Duncan B. Clark. "Psychiatric Disorders and Attempted Suicide Among Adolescents with Substance Use Disorders," *Drug and Alcohol Dependence* 73, no. 1 (2004): 87–97.

Johnston, Lloyd D., Patrick O'Malley, and Jerald Bachman. *Monitoring the Future: National Results on Adolescent Drug Use. Overview of Key Findings, 2002.* National Institute on Drug Abuse, U.S. Department of Health and Human Service, NIH Publication No. 03-5374, National Institutes of Health, 2003.

National Survey on Drug Use and Health. "Religious Beliefs and Substance Use Among Youths," *The NSDUH Report,* Rockville, Md.: Office of Applied Studies, Substance Abuse and Mental Health Services Administration (January 30, 2004), 1–3.

Substance Abuse and Mental Health Services Administration. *Results from the 2002 National Survey on Drug Use and Health: National Findings,* NHSDA Series H-22, Department of Health and Human Services Publication No. SMA 03-3836. Rockville, Md.: Office of Applied Studies, 2003.

teenage and youth gambling Adolescents ages 12–17 and their involvement in organized games of chance for money, such as lotteries, card games, horse races, and other opportunities for betting. It is nearly always illegal for adolescents to wager money. Some teenagers develop a problem with compulsive gambling. Compulsive gambling is also linked to other behavioral problems, such as excessive drinking, early sexual activity, and other high-risk behaviors.

In a study on teenage gambling among students in the eighth through the 12th grades among over 21,000 students in public and private schools in Vermont and published in a 1998 issue of *Pediatrics*, researchers found that 53 percent of the students had gambled in the past 12 months and 7 percent of them had problems with their gambling.

Some risk factors were related to compulsive gambling, including being male, daily MARIJUANA use, and frequent use of COCAINE and INHALANTS, never wearing seat belts in the car, and years of sexual activity. Those who gambled had more risk behaviors than those who had not gambled, and those who were compulsive gamblers had the greatest number of risk behaviors.

See also GAMBLING, PATHOLOGICAL; IMPULSE CONTROL DISORDER; TEENAGE AND YOUTH DRINKING; TEENAGE AND YOUTH DRUG ABUSE; TEENAGE AND YOUTH SMOKING.

Proimos, Jenny, et al. "Gambling and Other Risk Behaviors Among 8th–12th Grade Students," *Pediatrics* 102, no. 2 (August 1998). Available online. URL: http://pediatrics.aapublications.org/cji/content/fall/102/2/e 23. Accessed on March 15, 2004.

teenage and youth smoking Adolescents and children and their use of tobacco. Most adults who smoke report that they started when they were teenagers, according to the National Center for Health Statistics. Parents and pediatricians should actively discourage children and adolescents from smoking cigarettes, cigars, or pipes and from using SMOKELESS TOBACCO. They should also avoid tobacco themselves to act as role models for youths. A wide variety of school and government-based programs are aimed at stopping youths from smoking.

According to the American Academy of Pediatrics in their Committee on Substance Abuse, tobacco prevention efforts should start during a woman's pregnancy and continue through the child's pediatric visits. The pediatrician should also discuss smoking with teens. In their report, the Committee on Substance Abuse says, "The pediatrician can explore the teen's knowledge of short-term risks of smoking (such as cough and shortness of breath) and chewing tobacco (such as gingivitis and bad breath), clarify misperceptions, and reinforce and rehearse refusal skills. Teens who use tobacco should also be advised to quit."

The Committee on Substance Abuse says that smoking is associated with poor school performance, frequent absences from school, and dropping out of school. Adolescent smokers may also abuse alcohol and other drugs.

Children and adolescents who smoke may have a problem with low self-esteem and easy susceptibility to PEER PRESSURE. They may also have problems with DEPRESSION or ANXIETY DISORDERS. They may have a high rate of novelty seeking and rebelliousness.

Adolescents often begin smoking because they want to look older and they want to emulate or impress their peers.

Demographic Issues

In looking at a breakdown of age, gender and racial factors, researchers have found patterns among adolescents who smoke. Parents, physicians, educators and others may be able to use this information to help children and adolescents who are at risk for smoking and to work to prevent them from starting to smoke.

Age

Researchers found that most subjects started smoking when they were under the age of 17 years. (See table below.) Less than half of Americans who currently smoke started the habit when they were adults ages 18 and older. For this reason, many adults are concerned about teenage smoking as a health problem for individuals during their youth as well as a long-term problem in the future.

PERCENT DISTRIBUTION OF SMOKING INITIATION AMONG CURRENT SMOKERS AGED 18 YEARS AND OLDER BY AGE AND GENDER: UNITED STATES, 1997–1998

		Age First Smoked Fairly Regularly			
	Total	Less than 16 years	16–17 Years	18–20 Years	21 Years +
Both sexes					
18–24 years	100.0	37.6	34.1	24.0	4.0
25–44 years	100.0	30.4	26.0	26.9	16.7
45–64 years	100.0	27.5	20.6	29.2	22.7
65–74 years	100.0	26.3	22.1	24.7	26.9
75 years +	100.0	23.8	17.6	24.1	34.6
Men					
18–24 years	100.0	34.2	34.2	26.2	5.2
25–44 years	100.0	31.3	25.9	26.8	16.0
45–64 years	100.0	34.2	21.4	26.5	18.0
65–74 years	100.0	40.1	25.0	21.3	13.7
75 years +	100.0	37.0	21.2	22.5	19.3
Women					
18–24 years	100.0	41.8	34.4	21.2	2.6
25–44 years	100.0	29.5	26.1	27.0	17.4
45–64 years	100.0	19.7	19.7	32.5	28.2
65–74 years	100.0	15.6	19.8	27.3	37.2
75 years +	100.0	15.0	15.1	25.2	44.7

Source: Schoenborn, Charlotte A., Jackline L. Vickerie, and Patricia Barnes. *Cigarette Smoking Behavior of Adults: United States, 1997–98,* Advance data from Vital and Health Statistics Series, no. 331, Centers for Disease Control and Prevention, February 7, 2003.

In fact, in one study, researchers looked at the predictability of adolescent smoking to adult smoking. In a 2004 issue of the *American Journal of Public Health*, the researchers considered cigarette smoking (and SUBSTANCE ABUSE) among adults at age 35 compared to their behavior when they were seniors in high school. The researchers found that when the subjects had smoked in high school (but not on a daily basis), they were more than twelve times more likely to be smokers at age 35 than high school seniors who had never smoked.

In addition, among teenagers who had smoked on a daily basis when they were high school seniors, they were 42 times more likely to be smokers when they were age 35. Clearly, it is important to keep children and adolescents off tobacco, not only to protect their adolescent health but also their adult health.

Gender Males have a higher rate of smoking than women, although women of some races and ethnicities smoke more than men of other groups. For example, as can be seen from the table at right, 26.3 percent of American Indian/Alaska Native females ages 12–17 years reporting smoking in the past month. This is lower than the 29.5 percent rate for American Indian/Alaska Native males but is a higher rate than for males of every other race and ethnicity.

Race and ethnicity After American Indians and Alaska Natives, whites are the heaviest smokers. In fact, among teenagers who are American Indians or Alaska natives, teenage girls smoke more than teenage boys. An estimated 14.9 percent of white teenage males were smokers, compared with 17.2 percent of white teenage girls. In other races and ethnicities, however, males are heavier smokers than females. (See table at right.)

Factors Mitigating Against Smoking

Just as patterns occur among adolescents who are likely to smoke, researchers have also found that some factors appear to have a protective effect against youths using cigarettes. One such factor is the presence of religious beliefs. As part of the research for the National Survey on Drug Use and Health, researchers asked youths ages 12–17 about whether religious beliefs were important in their lives, if their religious beliefs influenced their

PERCENTAGE OF PERSONS AGES 12–17 YEARS REPORTING CIGARETTE USE DURING THE PRECEDING MONTH, BY RACE/ETHNICITY AND SEX, NATIONAL SURVEY ON DRUG USE AND HEALTH, UNITED STATES, 1999–2001

Race/Ethnicity	Male, %	Female, %	Total %
Non-Hispanic			
White	14.9	17.2	16.0
African American	8.2	5.9	7.0
American Indian/ Alaska Native	29.5	26.3	27.9
Hawaiian/Other Pacific Islander	7.0	Not available	11.0
Asian	8.8	7.3	8.1
Chinese	6.3	5.4	5.8
Filipino	5.8	8.9	7.4
Asian Indian	10.1	6.8	8.7
Korean	13.8	7.3	10.6
Vietnamese	Not available	8.0	6.8
Hispanic			
Mexican	11.4	10.2	10.8
Puerto Rican	11.2	10.4	10.8
Central or South American	9.9	9.3	9.6
Cuban	14.3	10.0	12.4
Total	13.3	14.2	13.8

Source: Centers for Disease Control and Prevention. "Prevalence of Cigarette Use Among 14 Racial/Ethnic Populations—United States, 1999–2001," *Morbidity and Mortality Weekly Report* 54, no. 3 (January 30, 2004): 51.

decisions, and how often they attended religious services.

The researchers found that about 78 percent said their religious beliefs were very important in their lives. A majority, 69 percent, said that their religious beliefs influenced how they made decisions. About 33 percent of the youths reported attending religious services 25 times or more in the past year.

Of the youths who reported that their religious beliefs were very important in their lives, about 10 percent reported smoking cigarettes in the past month, compared with 22 percent of the group for whom their religious beliefs were not important.

When considering the group that said their religious beliefs influenced their decisions, about 9 percent reported smoking cigarettes in the past month, compared with 22 percent of the group for whom religion did not play a role in their decision making.

When looking at the group of youths who attended 25 or more religious services in the past year, about 8 percent of this group reported smoking in the past month, compared with 16 percent of the group who attended fewer or no religious services.

Although the more-religious youths still had a small portion of individuals who smoked, it was dramatically lower than for the less-religious or nonreligious teens.

See also NICOTINE REPLACEMENT THERAPY; SMOKING AND HEALTH PROBLEMS; SMOKING CESSATION; TEENAGE AND YOUTH DRINKING; TEENAGE AND YOUTH DRUG ABUSE; TEENAGE AND YOUTH GAMBLING.

Committee on Substance Abuse, American Academy of Pediatrics. "Tobacco's Toll: Implications for the Pediatrician," *Pediatrics* 107, no. 4 (April 2001): 794–798.

Johnson, Jeffrey G., et al. "Association Between Cigarette Smoking and Anxiety Disorders During Adolescence and Early Adulthood," *Journal of the American Medical Association* 284, no. 18 (November 8, 2000): 2,348–2,351.

Merline, Alicia, et al. "Substance Use Among Adults 35 Years of Age: Prevalence, Adulthood Predictors, and Impact of Adolescent Substance," *American Journal of Public Health* 94, no. 1 (January 2004): 96–102.

National Survey on Drug Use and Health. "Religious Beliefs and Substance Use Among Youths," *The NSDUH Report,* Rockville, Md.: Office of Applied Studies, Substance Abuse and Mental Health Services Administration (January 30, 2004), 1–3.

television, addiction to Compulsion to watch television for many hours each day, even when the programs being watched are of little or no interest to the viewer. Some television addicts watch 60 or more hours per week. Although watching television does not create the same sort of physical changes that an addiction to drugs or alcohol would cause to the body, there are similar addictive elements. For example, compulsive viewers report that they watch television when they are sad or unhappy to change their mood, and they often watch far more hours than they intend. They may try to cut back on their hours of viewing but find doing so difficult or impossible. Others watch excessive television because they are bored. Constant television watching impedes a healthy social life and family life. Studies have shown that excessive television watching is also associated with OVEREATING/OBESITY.

According to researchers Robert Kubery and Mihaly Csikszentmihalyi in their 2002 article on television addiction for *Scientific American,* even average viewers watch television for about three hours a day. They performed a study in which they gave people beepers and contacted them randomly up to eight times a day to determine how television watching affected people. When the subjects heard the beep, they were to record what they were doing and how they felt, based on a scorecard. The researchers found that when people were contacted when they were watching television, they reported feelings of passivity and relaxation. The researchers added, "What is more surprising is that the sense of relaxation ends when the set is turned off, but the feelings of passivity and lowered alertness continue. Survey participants commonly reflect that television has somehow absorbed or sucked out their energy, leaving them depleted. They say they have more difficulty concentrating after viewing than before. In contrast, they rarely indicate such difficulty after reading. After playing sports or engaging in hobbies, people report improvements in mood. After watching TV, people's moods are about the same or worse than before."

It seems likely that the more dependent people are on television watching, the greater a problem they are developing and the more difficult it will be to break away. Therapy may help, as may medications such as antidepressants. There are also some suggestions uniquely targeted to those addicted to television watching that some experts offer, such as:

- Videotape what you want to watch and watch it later, instead of channel surfing.

- Limit the hours of television watching per day.

- Turn off the television set during the dinner hour and talk to other family members. Problems may come up, but they may also be ones that can be resolved.

- Get rid of the remote control. It encourages too much television watching and increases the risk for overweight and obesity.

See also IMPULSE CONTROL DISORDER; INTERNET ADDICTION DISORDER.

Goleman, Daniel. "How Viewers Grow Addicted to Television," Available online. URL: http://www.commercialalert.org/tvaddict.htm Downloaded on June 15, 2004.

Kubery, Robert and Mihaly Csikszentmihalyi. "Television Addiction is No Mere Metaphor," *Scientific American* 86, no. 2 (February 23, 2002): 74–77.

tobacco   A plant whose leaves are processed to make products to be used for smoking, such as cigarettes, cigars, and pipe tobacco. Tobacco is addictive. Its continued use in any form, including SMOKELESS TOBACCO, may lead to severe health problems such as CANCER, EMPHYSEMA, and chronic bronchitis. According to the Centers for Disease Control and Prevention, more than 440,000 people die per year from ailments directly related to cigarette smoking.

See also LUNG CANCER; NICOTINE REPLACEMENT THERAPY; ORAL CANCER; SMOKING CESSATION; SMOKING AND HEALTH PROBLEMS; ZYBAN.

tobacco settlement law   See MASTER SETTLEMENT AGREEMENT.

tolerance   A reduction in the effect that a given amount of alcohol or drug has on a person after chronic use of the substance over time. When a physical tolerance to a substance occurs, a greater amount of the substance is needed to achieve the same result as in the past. Individuals may build up a tolerance to substances such as alcohol and many illegal drugs. As a result, the alcoholic can consume much larger quantities of alcohol than others and remain conscious. He or she may not appear intoxicated at all, despite having consumed a large quantity of alcohol.

However, the presence of a tolerance to a substance alone does not necessarily mean that a person is addicted to the substance. Tolerance is only one element of addiction. For an addiction to be present, other elements must be present as well, such as a compulsive CRAVING for the substance, despite the negative consequences that may occur to the individual or others as a result of trying to obtain the substance. In addition, the addict has usually tried and failed to give up the use of the substance.

See also CROSS-TOLERANCE; SUBSTANCE ABUSE.

tramadol (Ultram)   A mild opioid drug that is not a scheduled drug in the United States as of this writing. However, some reports indicate that the drug should not be used in patients with a past history of opiate abuse. Tramadol is a prescribed painkiller that is taken orally. Doctors differ on whether they believe tramadol is an effective analgesic.

According to the position statement from the College on Problems of Drug Dependence in their 2003 article in *Drug and Alcohol Dependence*, there has been a study of high-risk populations who used tramadol, based on information from both informants and from systems provided through the Food and Drug Administration.

Said the authors, "The reported rate of abuse over a 3-year period was low, and 97% of tramadol abusers had a history of abusing opiates, alcohol, or other drugs." As a result, it seems clear that tramadol should not be prescribed to chronic pain patients with a history of opioid abuse or addiction.

Effects of Tramadol

Tramadol is a sedating drug. It may also cause headache, nausea and vomiting, dizziness, and drowsiness. Some patients may experience diarrhea, although constipation is more common. Increased perspiration may be seen. In a few cases, patients have reported musical hallucinations that have subsided when the drug was discontinued. Some patients have developed a dependence on addiction to tramadol.

See also OPIATES; PAIN; PAIN MANAGEMENT.

Zacny, James, et al. "College on Problems of Drug Dependence Taskforce on Prescription Opioid Non-Medical Use and Abuse: Position Statement," *Drug and Alcohol Dependence* 69, no. 3 (2003): 215–232.

treatment contract/medications   An agreement that a patient makes, with a physician or a treatment facility, regarding actions he or she agrees to comply with related to scheduled drugs that the physician may prescribe. Physicians who prescribe controlled drugs, especially OPIATES, may require such treatment contracts as a condition of treatment. In most such agreements, patients agree to obtain the scheduled drugs only from the physician with whom they have the treatment contract. (Other medications that the patient takes, such as medicine for diabetes or high blood pressure, may still be prescribed by their regular physician.)

The patient agrees not to give or sell the drugs to others. The treatment contract often calls for an agreement to random drug screening, if the physician requires it. The doctor may wish to go over each of these points orally at least one time to make sure the patient understands them. Some physicians or clinics require written contracts signed by both parties.

The purpose of these agreements is to try to educate patients as well as to screen them for the presence of addictive and/or illegal behaviors. It is also to shield physicians from accusations that they are lax in managing controlled drugs. How well patients comply with such agreements is unknown, however.

SAMPLE AGREEMENT: LONG-TERM CONTROLLED SUBSTANCES THERAPY FOR CHRONIC PAIN (A CONSENT FORM FROM THE AMERICAN ACADEMY OF PAIN MEDICINE)

The purpose of this agreement is to protect your access to controlled substances and to protect our ability to prescribe for you.

The long-term use of such substances as opioids (narcotic analgesics), benzodiazepine tranquilizers, and barbiturate sedatives is controversial because of uncertainty regarding the extent to which they provide long-term benefit. There is also the risk of an addictive disorder developing or of relapse occurring in a person with a prior addiction. The extent of this risk is not certain.

Because these drugs have potential for abuse or diversion, strict accountability is necessary when use is prolonged. For this reason the following policies are agreed to by you, the patient, as consideration for, and a condition of, the willingness of the physician whose signature appears below to consider the initial and/or continued prescription of controlled substances to treat your chronic pain.

1. All controlled substances must come from the physician whose signature appears below or, during his or her absence, by the covering physician, unless specific authorization is obtained for an exception. (Multiple sources can lead to untoward drug interactions or poor coordination of treatment.)
2. All controlled substances must be obtained at the same pharmacy, where possible. Should the need arise to change pharmacies, our office must be informed. The pharmacy that you have selected is _____. Phone: _____
3. You are expected to inform our office of any new medications or medical conditions, and of any adverse effects from any of the medications that you take.
4. The prescribing physician has permission to discuss all diagnostic and treatment details with dispensing pharmacists or other professionals who provide your health care for purposes of maintaining accountability.
5. You may not share, sell, or otherwise permit others to have access to these medications.
6. These drugs should not be stopped abruptly, as an abstinence syndrome will likely develop.
7. Unannounced urine or serum toxicology screens may be requested, and your cooperation is required. Presence of unauthorized substances may prompt referral for assessment for addictive disorder.
8. Prescriptions and bottles of these medications may be sought by other individuals with chemical dependency and should be closely safeguarded. It is expected that you will take the highest possible degree of care with your medication and prescription. They should not be left where others might see or otherwise have access to them.
9. Original containers of medications should be brought in to each office visit.
10. Since the drugs may be hazardous or lethal to a person who is not tolerant to their effects, especially a child, you must keep them out of reach of such people.
11. Medications may not be replaced if they are lost, get wet, are destroyed, left on an airplane, etc. If your medication has been stolen and you complete a police report regarding the theft, an exception may be made.

(continues)

12. Early refills generally will not be given.
13. Prescriptions may be issued early if the physician or the patient will be out of town when a refill is due. These prescriptions will contain instructions to the pharmacist that they not be filled prior to the appropriate date.
14. If the responsible legal authorities have questions concerning your treatment, as might occur, for example, if you were obtaining medications at several pharmacies, all confidentiality is waived and these authorities may be given full access to our records of controlled substances administration.
15. It is understood that failure to adhere to these policies may result in cessation of therapy with controlled substance prescribing by this physician or referral for further specialty assessment.
16. Renewals are contingent on keeping scheduled appointments. Please do not phone for prescriptions after hours or on weekends.
17. It should be understood that any medical treatment is initially a trial, and that continued prescription is contingent on evidence of benefit.
18. The risks and potential benefits of these therapies are explained elsewhere [and you acknowledge that you have received such explanation].
19. You affirm that you have full right and power to sign and be bound by this agreement, and that you have read, understood, and accept all of its terms.

_____

Physician Signature

_____

Date

_____

Patient Signature

_____

Date

Source: Copyright by the American Academy of Pain Medicine

See also ADDICTIVE BEHAVIORS; CONTROLLED SUBSTANCES ACT; DIVERSION PROGRAMS; NARCOTICS; PAIN; PAIN MANAGEMENT; PAIN MANAGEMENT CENTERS; SCHEDULED DRUGS.

treatment facilities   Inpatient or outpatient day treatment places where individuals who are addicted to drugs or alcohol can receive therapy in an attempt to change their addictive behavior patterns. Some inpatient facilities are short-term facilities, with programs lasting under 30 days, while other facilities offer long-term programs of 30 days or more. In 2000, about half of all SUBSTANCE ABUSE treatment facilities in the United States had contracts with managed care companies. These facilities were more likely to offer both detoxification and rehabilitation services than facilities that did not accept managed care.

Individuals who need to identify a substance abuse facility can use the Substance Abuse Treatment Facility Locator on the Internet, available at http://findtreatment.samhsa.gov.

Patients with a variety of addictions may receive treatment. However, the majority of patients who receive rehabilitative services are addicted to alcohol and/or to drugs. In 2000, four substances accounted for the wide majority (91 percent) of all admission to treatment facilities: ALCOHOL (45 percent), OPIATES, primarily HEROIN (17 percent), MARIJUANA/HASHISH (15 percent), and COCAINE (14 percent). (See table at top of page 248.)

Patients with ANOREXIA NERVOSA or BULIMIA NERVOSA may need hospitalization or assistance in a specialized treatment facility.

Most patients admitted for treatment are males, and the majority are white and under age 44, based on data provided from the Treatment Episode Data Set (TEDS) on demographic and substance abuse characteristics of about 1.6 million annual admissions to treatment for patients who have abused

ADMISSIONS TO SUBSTANCE ABUSE TREATMENT BY
PRIMARY SUBSTANCE OF ABUSE: 1995–2000, PERCENT DISTRIBUTION

	1995	1996	1997	1998	1999	2000
Total	100.0	100.0	100.0	100.0	100.0	100.0
Alcohol	50.5	50.2	48.4	47.2	46.7	45.3
Opiates	14.5	14.6	15.6	15.4	15.9	16.8
Cocaine	16.7	16.1	15.0	15.1	14.4	13.6
Marijuana/hashish	10.5	12.0	13.0	13.5	14.1	14.8
Stimulants	3.9	3.3	4.5	4.4	4.5	5.2
Other drugs	1.3	1.2	1.2	1.3	1.6	1.8
Tranquilizers	0.3	0.3	0.3	0.3	0.3	0.3
Sedatives/hypnotics	0.2	0.2	0.2	0.2	0.2	0.2
Hallucinogens	0.2	0.2	0.2	0.2	0.2	0.2
PCP	0.2	0.2	0.1	0.1	0.1	0.2
Inhalants	0.1	0.1	0.1	0.1	0.1	0.1
Other	0.2	0.2	0.3	0.4	0.6	0.8
None reported	2.7	2.5	2.5	3.0	2.7	2.5

Source: Substance Abuse and Mental Health Services Administration (SAMHSA). *Treatment Episode Data Set (TEDS) 1992–2000.* Rockville, Md.: Office of Applied Studies, SAMHSA, December 2002.

ADMISSIONS BY SEX, RACE/ETHNICITY AND AGE, 1995–2000, PERCENT DISTRIBUTION

	1995	1996	1997	1998	1999	2000
Sex						
Male	70.4	70.3	69.8	70.0	70.1	69.6
Female	29.6	29.7	30.2	30.0	29.9	30.4
Race/ethnicity						
White (non-Hispanic)	59.5	60.3	60.8	60.6	60.4	59.7
African American (non-Hispanic)	26.2	25.3	24.4	24.0	23.5	23.6
Hispanic	10.6	10.2	10.5	11.0	11.4	11.7
American Indian/Alaskan Native	2.3	2.5	2.5	2.5	2.4	2.4
Asian/Pacific Islander	0.6	0.6	0.7	0.7	0.8	0.9
Other	0.8	1.0	1.1	1.2	1.4	1.7
Age at Admission						
Under 18 years	7.8	8.4	8.9	8.8	8.5	8.4
18–24 years	14.0	13.6	14.3	14.9	15.6	16.3
25–34 years	36.1	34.0	32.2	30.4	28.5	27.1
35–44 years	29.7	30.8	31.2	31.7	32.1	32.0
45–54 years	9.3	10.1	10.4	11.2	12.0	12.9
55–64 years	2.4	2.5	2.4	2.5	2.6	2.6
65 years and older	0.7	0.7	0.7	0.6	0.7	0.7
Total	100.0	100.0	100.0	100.0	100.0	100.0

Source: Substance Abuse and Mental Health Services Administration (SAMHSA). *Treatment Episode Data Set (TEDS) 1992–2000.* Rockville, Md.: Office of Applied Studies, SAMHSA, December 2002.

alcohol and drugs. The TEDS data include facilities that are licensed or certified by the state substance abuse agency. Facilities that report TEDS data are also those agencies that receive state and federal funds for providing alcohol and drug treatment services. (See table at bottom of page 248.)

Youths Receiving Treatment for Substance Abuse

Each year, about 15,000 youths age 18 and under are referred to treatment referral sources. Of these youths, about 10 percent are referred by their schools. Most of the school-referred admissions involve patients for whom marijuana or alcohol is their primary substance of abuse. Students referred by their schools are more likely to be receiving treatment for the first time than if they were referred by other sources, such as the criminal justice system, health care providers, and other referral sources.

In 2002, the National Survey of Substance Abuse Treatment Services collected data on about 14,000 treatment facilities, including about 900 facilities that concentrated on treating individuals ages 18 and younger. This research revealed that the majority (73 percent) of the clients in these facilities were receiving treatment for both drug and alcohol abuse. This is in contrast to the lower percentage (55 percent) of adults age 18 and older who were receiving treatment for both alcohol and drug abuse.

The survey also showed that most of the adolescent treatment facilities offered individual therapy (97 percent), group therapy (94 percent), substance abuse assessment (90 percent), discharge planning (86 percent), and drug/alcohol urine screening (80 percent).

Outpatient Treatment

According to the Drug and Alcohol Services Information System (DASIS) in *The DASIS Report*, researchers analyzed the treatment outcomes for nearly 117,000 outpatients (not in a residential program) nationwide. Patients received treatment for a variety of addiction problems, including alcohol, opiates, cocaine, marijuana/hashish, stimulants, and other substances. The outpatient treatment completion rate was highest for patients whose problem was with alcohol (41 percent), followed by marijuana (32 percent), stimulants (30 percent), and opiates (27 percent). The patients least likely to complete treatment were patients who were users of cocaine (21 percent).

Among the patients who did not complete treatment, some were transferred to another facility, others left against professional advice, and some were terminated by the facility. (See table below.)

Inpatient Treatment

Some patients need 30 days or more to overcome their substance abuse problems, which is why both short-term and long-term facilities provide treatment. Of patients in long-term treatment, the majority are treated for alcohol abuse and dependence, followed by cocaine, opiates, and

DISCHARGES FROM OUTPATIENT TREATMENT BY REASON FOR DISCHARGE AND PRIMARY SUBSTANCE AT ADMISSION: 2000

Primary Substance at Admission	Total	Reasons for Discharge				
		Treatment Completed	Transferred to Another Treatment	Left Against Professional Advice	Terminated by Facility	Other
Alcohol	59,300	24,200	4,300	12,200	12,300	6,300
Opiates	8,400	2,300	600	2,500	2,300	700
Cocaine	13,700	2,800	1,000	3,600	4,800	1,500
Marijuana/hashish	26,400	8,400	2,100	6,500	6,700	2,700
Stimulants	6,000	1,800	900	1,600	900	800
Other/unknown	3,000	900	200	700	600	600
Total	116,800	40,400	9,100	27,100	27,600	12,600

Source: Drug and Alcohol Services Information System. "Discharges from Outpatient Treatment: 2000," *The DASIS Report* Office of Applied Studies, Substance Abuse and Mental Health Services Administration (November 21, 2003).

DISCHARGES FROM LONG-TERM RESIDENTIAL TREATMENT, BY REASON FOR DISCHARGE AND PRIMARY SUBSTANCE AT ADMISSION: 2000

Primary Substance at Admission	Total	Reasons for Discharge				
		Treatment Completed	Transferred to Another Treatment	Left Against Professional Advice	Terminated by Facility	Other
Alcohol	10,320	3,867	903	2,907	2,204	439
Opiates	3,949	1,131	143	1,511	989	175
Cocaine	6,063	1,766	425	1,772	1,851	249
Marijuana/hashish	3,342	1,058	352	789	1,016	127
Stimulants	2,079	631	49	462	371	122
Other/unknown	850	345	66	214	164	61
Total	26,603	8,798	2,382	7,655	6,595	1,173

Source: Drug and Alcohol Services Information System. "Discharges from Long-Term Residential Treatment: 2000," *The DASIS Report,* (February 20, 2004).

other substances. The largest numbers and percentages of individuals who successfully complete treatment are clients who were admitted for treatment of their alcohol problems. (See table at top of page.)

Psychiatric Problem in Addition to Substance Abuse Problem

Some patients admitted to treatment facilities were diagnosed with a psychiatric problem in addition to their substance abuse problem, primarily patients admitted for abuse of stimulants and tranquilizers.

SPECIAL POPULATIONS SERVED BY HOSPITAL INPATIENT FACILITIES

Special Population	Percent of Facilities
Persons with Co-occurring disorders	74
Adolescents	32
Seniors	31
Women only	28
Persons with HIV/AIDS	26
Men only	24
Gays/lesbians	19
Pregnant/postpartum women	19
Other	11

Source: Drug and Alcohol Services Information System. "Facilities Offering Hospital Inpatient Care," *The DASIS Report,* (June 20, 2003).

Hospital Treatment

Some patients with substance abuse problems require hospital care because they need medical attention while they undergo DETOXIFICATION from alcohol or drugs. About 1,000 hospitals treat patients with substance abuse problems. About half of them provide detoxification only, and about half offer both detoxification and rehabilitation. Some hospitals provide services for special populations of individuals with substance abuse problems. (See table below.)

See also ALCOHOLISM; DRUG ADDICTION; DUAL DIAGNOSIS.

Fiellin, David A., M.D., M. Carrington Reid, M.D., and Patrick O'Connor, M.D. "Outpatient Management of Patients with Alcohol Problems," *Annals of Internal Medicine* 133, no. 10 (November 21, 2000): 815–827.
Substance Abuse and Mental Health Services Administration. "Reasons for Not Receiving Substance Abuse Treatment," *The NSDUH Report* (November 7, 2003).
Substance Abuse and Mental Health Services Administration (SAMHSA). *Treatment Episode Data Set (TEDS) 1992–2000.* Rockville, Md.: Office of Applied Studies, SAMHSA, December 2002.

Twelve Steps An underlying, enduring, and principle policy of ALCOHOLICS ANONYMOUS, an important self-help organization that has helped millions of people with alcoholism worldwide to recover. Alcoholics Anonymous groups encourage but do not require individuals to work through each of the twelve steps as part of their recovery from ALCO-HOLISM. A key part of the success in refraining from drinking is believed to lie in reaching out to others with a similar problem. However, members who are not religious may substitute an alternate higher authority in their mind for the word *God*.

The Twelve Steps as outlined by Alcoholics Anonymous are as follows:

1. We admitted we were powerless over alcohol—that our lives had become unmanageable.

2. Came to believe that a Power greater than ourselves could restore us to sanity.

3. Made a decision to turn our will and our lives over to the care of God as we understood Him.

4. Made a searching and fearless inventory of ourselves.

5. Admitted to God, to ourselves, and to another human being the exact nature of our wrongs.

6. Were entirely ready to have God remove all these defects of character.

7. Humbly asked Him to remove our shortcomings.

8. Made a list of all persons we had harmed, and became willing to make amends to them all.

9. Made direct amends to such people wherever possible, except when to do so would injure them or others.

10. Continued to take personal inventory and when we were wrong promptly admitted it.

11. Sought through prayer and meditation to improve our conscious contact with God as we understood Him, praying only for knowledge of His will for us and the power to carry that out.

12. Having had a spiritual awakening as the result of these steps, we try to carry this message to alcoholics and to practice these principles in all our affairs.

The Twelve Steps are reprinted with permission of Alcoholics Anonymous World Services, Inc. (A.A.W.S.). Permission to reprint the Twelve Steps does not mean that A.A.W.S. has reviewed or approved the contents of this publication, or that A.A.W.S. necessarily agrees with the views expressed herein. A.A. is a program of recovery from alcoholism *only*—use of the Twelve Steps in connection with programs and activities which are patterned after A.A., but which address other problems, or in any other non-A.A. context, does not imply otherwise.

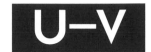

Ultram See TRAMADOL.

urine tests See DRUG TESTING; FALSE POSITIVES.

veterans, military Individuals who have served in the military services in the past, including in the Air Force, Army, Marine Corps, Navy, and Coast Guard, whether they were on active duty or were in the Reserves or the National Guard. Some military veterans develop addictions to alcohol and/or to drugs and they require treatment. The addiction may stem from the stress of serving in wartime conditions, or it may be caused by another problem, such as easy access to drugs or alcohol. In conditions such as combat, some veterans may develop a POSTTRAUMATIC STRESS DISORDER, which can lead to SUBSTANCE ABUSE. Sometimes determining the cause of the addiction may be difficult.

Veterans Receiving Treatment for Substance Abuse
The Drug and Alcohol Services Information System (DASIS) studied data about veterans admitted for substance abuse treatment over the period 1995–2000, reporting their findings in a 2003 issue of *The DASIS Report.* According to this report, there were more than 55,000 admissions of veterans for substance abuse treatment in 2000, including about 3,000 female veterans. (In past years, such as prior to the 1980s, most people in the service were males.) In 2000, 41 percent of the veterans who were admitted for treatment were 45 and older, compared with 32 percent in that age group in 1995.

The most common primary substance that was abused by male veterans was ALCOHOL (69 percent). Alcohol was also the most common substance abused by female veterans, although it was a lower percentage (56 percent). The next most common substance of abuse was COCAINE (14 percent for men and 21 percent for women). OPIATES were abused by about 9 percent of the female veterans and 8 percent of the male veterans. MARIJUANA was the drug of abuse for 7 percent of the women and 8 percent of the men in 2000.

Most of the veterans admitted for treatment were white, including 61 percent of the males in 2000 and 54 percent of the females. African Americans were the next largest group admitted for treatment, and they represented 25 percent of the male patients in 2000 and 32 percent of the female patients. Hispanics had a much lower rate of admission, or 6 percent of the males and 6 percent of the females in 2000. (Other races comprised the balance of admitted patients.)

See also ALCOHOLISM; ANTABUSE; TREATMENT FACILITIES.

Drug and Alcohol Services Information System. "Veterans in Substance Abuse Treatment: 1995–2000," *The DASIS Report* Substance Abuse and Mental Health Services Administration, November 7, 2003.

violence Physical and/or sexual actions against another person, including beating, rape, and other acts up to and including HOMICIDE (murder). Some addictive substances increase the rate of violence among users, such as ALCOHOL, some prescription medications, and illegal drugs such as ANABOLIC STEROIDS, COCAINE, CRACK COCAINE, and METHAMPHETAMINE. According to the NATIONAL INSTITUTE ON ALCOHOL ABUSE AND ALCOHOLISM (NIAAA), alcohol is often associated with violence. In fact, it is more associated with violence than other drugs are. It is a significant factor in 68 percent of manslaughters, 62 percent of assaults, 64 percent of murders and attempted murders, 48 percent of robberies, and 44 percent of burglaries.

Among family members, alcohol is associated with domestic violence. As many as 50–60 percent of male alcoholics undergoing treatment were violent with their female partners in the year before treatment occurred, according to the NIAAA. However, there are few studies of domestic violence among alcoholics. Alcohol is also associated with violence toward children and is estimated to be a factor in about 30 percent of all CHILD ABUSE cases, according to the NIAAA.

In one study of 256 women who were intentionally injured by others and went to emergency rooms as cases of domestic violence, reported in a 1999 issue of the *New England Journal of Medicine*, the researchers found that the women most at risk for injury were those with partners who abused or were addicted to alcohol and were either unemployed or employed off and on. Other risk factors for domestic violence were male partners who were former boyfriends or former or estranged husbands and men with less than a high school education.

A study in 1995, the National Study of Couples, funded by the NIAAA, surveyed more than 1,000 white, African-American, and Hispanic couples about incidents of domestic violence. It was reported in a 2001 issue of *Alcohol Research &*

Health. The study analyzed the demographics of domestic violence involving alcohol.

In this study, 23 percent of African-American couples, 17 percent of Hispanic couples, and 11.5 percent of whites couples reported an incident of "intimate partner" violence within the prior 12 months. It is also true that in some cases, the perpetrators of violence are females. The study also found that 30–40 percent of men and 27–34 percent of the women who caused the violence were drinking at the time of the act. The rates varied by race and ethnicity.

The researchers speculated that people might use alcohol as an excuse for violent behavior or that heavy drinking and violent behavior may be predicted by other factors, such as an impulsive personality.

See also IMPULSE CONTROL DISORDER; PROSTITUTION.

Abbey, Antonia, et al. "Alcohol and Sexual Assault," *Alcohol Research and Health* 25, no. 1 (2001): 43–51.

Caetano, Raul, M.D., John Schafer, and Carol B. Cunradi. "Alcohol-Related Intimate Partner Violence Among White, Black, and Hispanic Couples in the United States," *Alcohol Research & Health* 25, no. 1 (2001): 58–65.

Kyriacou, Demetrios N., M.D., et al. "Risk Factors for Injury to Women from Domestic Violence," *New England Journal of Medicine* 341, no. 25 (December 16, 1999): 1,892–1,898.

Wernicke's encephalopathy   A disease of the brain caused by a severe deficiency of thiamine (vitamin B1), usually caused by years of chronic ALCOHOLISM; rarely, however, other causes of thiamine deficiency may lead to this condition. Wernicke's encephalopathy was named after German neurologist Carl Wernicke. The disease leads to a malfunction of the central nervous system, balance disorder, and confusion. This condition is considered a medical emergency, and it can be fatal. The treatment is the administration of thiamine, either intravenously or intramuscularly. Some patients may improve within hours of receiving thiamine, while others may not significantly recover for months. Some patients never fully recover.

See also ALCOHOLIC HEALTH PROBLEMS.

Minocha, Anil and Christine Adamec. *The Encyclopedia of Digestive Diseases and Disorders.* New York: Facts On File, Inc., 2004.

withdrawal   The experience of the addicted person who is undergoing the process of ending the use of alcohol, tobacco, or drugs, which usually causes physical and emotional side effects. Although some individuals taper off the addicted substance, in many cases, they may cease to use the substance altogether and suddenly, for a variety of reasons. For example, they may be unable to obtain the drug or alcohol because they are incarcerated or cannot afford the substance, because their doctor refused to give them a prescription for the drug any longer, or for other unspecified reasons.

In some cases, withdrawal symptoms are very severe, as with the DELIRIUM TREMENS of the long-term alcoholic or the serious symptoms that can occur from the withdrawal from drugs such as HEROIN. For this reason, addicted patients should undergo DETOXIFICATION under the care of trained and experienced physicians.

Seizures or delirium tremens are more likely to be seen in patients who have repeatedly detoxified from alcohol in the past. If the patient is also feverish or has suffered a trauma, the physician should investigate whether the seizures have another origin.

Because withdrawal from alcohol or drugs can be dangerous and even fatal to the person, withdrawal symptoms should immediately be brought to the attention of a doctor.

Withdrawal may also occur when ending compulsive gambling, a shopping addiction, chronic overeating, or any one of the many types of addictive behaviors in which people engage. Although ending these behaviors will not cause a physical reaction as will a withdrawal from alcohol, tobacco, or drugs, the withdrawal from other behaviors may cause symptoms of DEPRESSION, ANXIETY, and other emotional difficulties, such as anger, distress, and even panic.

Withdrawal from Alcohol

An estimated 7.9 million people in the United States were alcoholics in 2002. Some of these individuals have tried to end their alcohol dependence through the help of their physicians, treatment centers, and self-help organizations such as ALCOHOLICS ANONYMOUS.

Medications are often given to patients withdrawing from alcohol to ease their craving for alcohol and prevent delirium tremens. NALTREXONE may be given, as may BENZODIAZEPINE medications. Anticonvulsant drugs such as carbamazepine may also be given to patients to prevent seizures and delirium tremens. However, patients with mild symptoms, or less than a score of an 8 on the Addiction Research Foundation Clinical Institute Withdrawal

Assessment for Alcohol (see figure at bottom of page) will not usually need medications because they will not develop withdrawal complications.

Say Dr. Thomas Kosten and Dr. Patrick O'Connor in their article on alcohol and drug withdrawal for a 2003 issue of the *New England Journal of Medicine,* "Without medication, alcohol-withdrawal symptoms might be expected to peak about 72 hours after the last use of alcohol, but medications can reduce symptoms within hours. In patients with delirium tremens, management with medication requires high doses of benzodiazepines (e.g., 5 to 10 mg of diazepam by intravenous injection, repeated in two to four hours if seizures occur). Unless delirium is present, medication is typically needed for no more than seven days after the last use of alcohol, although some patients will report withdrawal symptoms, including sleep problems, for several more weeks."

Many alcoholics will also need vitamin supplementation, particularly of thiamine and B vitamins, folate or folic acid, and often vitamin C as well.

Symptoms of withdrawal from alcohol According to Dr. Max Bayard and his colleagues in their article in *American Family Physician* in 2004, some minor withdrawal symptoms for an alcoholic that may occur within six to 12 hours after ending alcohol use include insomnia and tremulousness as well as mild anxiety, headache, palpitations, gastrointestinal upset, and palpitations.

Symptoms that may occur about 12–24 hours after alcohol cessation include fever, chills, severe tremor, and visual, auditory, or tactile HALLUCINATIONS. Withdrawal seizures may occur within 24–48 hours. Delirium tremens may occur within 48–72 hours after alcohol cessation. Patients at greater risk for severe withdrawal symptoms include those with the following profile:

- Those with abnormal liver function
- Elderly patients with long-term alcoholism
- Those who abused other drugs in addition to alcohol
- Those who have been detoxified at least several times before
- Patients with an intense craving for alcohol
- Patients with other serious health problems
- Patients with severe withdrawal symptoms when they presented for treatment
- Those with a past history of delirium tremens or seizures

Many physicians use the Addiction Research Foundation Clinical Institute Withdrawal Assessment for Alcohol to determine if patients are likely to undergo severe withdrawal effects. (See figure below.)

FIGURE: ADDICTION RESEARCH FOUNDATION CLINICAL INSTITUTE WITHDRAWAL ASSESSMENT FOR ALCOHOL

Patient _____   Date ___ ___ ____   Time _____
                                      y   m   d   (24-hour clock, midnight: 00:00)

Pulse or heart rate, taken for one minute: _____

NAUSEA AND VOMITING—Ask "Do you feel sick
   to your stomach? Have you vomited?" Observation.
0 no nausea and no vomiting
1 mild nausea with no vomiting
2
3
4 intermittent nausea with dry heaves
5
6
7 constant nausea, frequent dry heaves and vomiting

TACTILE DISTURBANCES—Ask "Have you any
   itching, pins and needles sensations, any burning,
   any numbness or do you feel bugs crawling on or
   under your skin" Observation.
0 none
1 very mild itching, pins and needles, burning or
   numbness
2 mild itching, pins and needles, burning or
   numbness
4 moderately severe hallucinations
5 severe hallucinations
6 extremely severe hallucinations
7 continuous hallucinations

(continues)

TREMOR—Arms extended and fingers spread apart. Observation.
0 no tremor
1 not visible, but can be felt fingertip to fingertip
2
3
4 moderate, with patient's arms extended
5
6
7 severe, even with arms not extended

PAROXYSMAL SWEATS—Observation.
0 no sweat visible
1 barely perceptible sweating, palms moist
2
3
4 beads of sweat obvious on forehead
5
6
7 drenching sweats

ANXIETY—Ask "Do you feel nervous?" Observation.
0 no anxiety, at ease
1 mildly anxious
2
3
4 moderately anxious or guarded, so anxiety is inferred
5
6
7 equivalent to acute panic states as seen in severe delirium or acute schizophrenic reactions

AGITATION—Observation
0 normal activity
1 somewhat more than normal activity
2
3
4 moderately fidgety and restless
5
6
7 paces back and forth during most of the interview, or constantly thrashes about

AUDITORY DISTURBANCE—Ask, "Are you more aware of sounds around you? Are they harsh? Do they frighten you? Are you hearing anything that is disturbing you? Are you hearing things you know are not there? Observation.
0 not present
1 very mild harshness or ability to frighten
2 mild harshness or ability to frighten
3 moderate harshness or ability to frighten
4 moderately severe hallucinations
5 severe hallucinations
6 extremely severe hallucinations
7 continuous hallucinations

VISUAL DISTURBANCES—Ask "Does the light appear to be too bright? Is its color different? Does it hurt your eyes? Are you seeing anything that is disturbing to you? Are you seeing things you know are not there? Observation.
0 not present
1 very mild sensitivity
2 mild sensitivity
3 moderate sensitivity
4 moderately severe hallucinations
5 severe hallucinations
6 extremely severe hallucinations
7 continuous hallucinations

HEADACHE, FULLNESS IN HEAD—Ask "Does your head feel different? Does it feel like there is a band around your head?" Do not rate for dizziness or lightheadedness. Otherwise, rate severity.
0 not present
1 very mild
2 mild
3 moderate
4 moderately severe
5 severe
6 very severe
7 extremely severe

ORIENTATION AND CLOUDING OF SENSORIUM— Ask "What day is this? Where are you? Who am I?"
0 oriented and can do serial additions
1 cannot do serial additions or is uncertain about date
2 disoriented for date by no more than 2 calendar days
3 disoriented for date by more than 2 calendar days
4 disoriented for place and/or person

Total CIWA-A Score _____
Rater's Initials_____
Maximum Possible Score: 67

A total score of 15 or more points indicates that the patient is at increased risk for severe withdrawal effects, such as confusion and seizures. (The scale is not copyrighted.)

Source: Richard Saitz, M.D. "Introduction to Alcohol Withdrawal," *Alcohol Health & Research World* 22, no. 1 (1998): 5–12.

Withdrawal from Opiates

Withdrawal from opiates can be very difficult for patients to undergo. Individuals need the help of their doctors and skilled professionals as well as the help and support of their families. Because the symptoms of opiate withdrawal can be severe and often alarming, some physicians or family members have been found to supply opiates inappropriately in response to the addicted individual's distress. This complicates further treatment and would be described as enabling behavior.

Patients withdrawing from opiates often have symptoms resembling a severe case of influenza, with runny nose, coughing, diarrhea, nausea and vomiting, and lack of appetite. If they become dehydrated, the situation can become life threatening. The higher the degree of addiction, the more severe the symptoms will be. Since most patients who are addicted are taking drugs illicitly, they generally obtain their drugs intermittently and thus the addiction level is not as high as when drugs are taken on a daily basis.

When receiving detoxification treatment, patients being medically withdrawn from opiates in a treatment facility may receive BUPRENORPHINE or METHADONE. They will also usually receive clonidine to aid in dealing with the severe anxiety symptoms that often accompany withdrawal from opioids.

See also ALCOHOLIC HEALTH PROBLEMS; ALCOHOLISM; BLACKOUTS, ALCOHOLIC; COCAINE; HEROIN; NARCOTICS; OPIATES; OxyContin; SCHEDULED DRUGS; TEENAGE AND YOUTH DRINKING; TREATMENT FACILITIES.

Bayard, Max, M.D., et al. "Alcohol Withdrawal Syndrome," *American Family Physician* 69, no. 6 (March 15, 2004): 1,443–1,450.

Jauhar, Pramod. "Current Drug Management of Alcohol Dependence Syndrome," Available online. URL: http://www.escriber.com/Assets/EscriberDownloads/Images/PinPalcholdep.PDF. Accessed on June 24, 2004.

Kosten, Thomas R., M.D. and Patrick G. O'Connor, M.D. "Management of Drug and Alcohol Withdrawal," *New England Journal of Medicine* 348, no. 18 (May 1, 2003): 1,786–1,795.

Krystal, John H., M.D., et al. "Naltrexone in the Treatment of Alcohol Dependence," *New England Journal of Medicine* 345, no. 24 (December 13, 2001): 1,745–1,739.

Saitz, Richard, M.D. "Introduction to Alcohol Withdrawal," *Alcohol Health & Research World* 22, no. 1 (1998): 5–12.

work   Work provides a sense of importance and even of identity to many people. Addictive behaviors may have a profound impact on both employees and their employers. Unemployed people are more likely to engage in BINGE DRINKING than employed individuals. Many employers have employee assistance programs in which workers who are identified as having a possible SUBSTANCE ABUSE problem are referred to counseling and treatment.

Based on data from the National Household Survey on Drug Abuse (NHSDA), reported in 2002 in *The NHSDA Report,* about 8 percent of workers in the United States are heavy drinkers and about 8 percent have also used illegal drugs within the past month. Younger workers (ages 18–25 years old) are the most likely of all age groups to have engaged in heavy drinking or illegal drug use. In addition, males are more likely to drink and use drugs than females. Individuals in some occupations, such as construction, are more likely to have high rates of both drinking and illegal drug use. (See table on page 259.)

Individuals who abuse or are addicted to drugs or alcohol are more likely to have had many employers and to miss work.

Abuse of Drugs and Alcohol Continues to Be a Problem

According to author and editor Joel Bennett in his introduction to *Preventing Workplace Substance Abuse: Beyond Drug Testing to Wellness,* the percentage of working adults who use illegal drugs or who are heavy drinkers has been a continuing problem despite the proliferation of DRUG TESTING programs in many workplaces. Bennett also points out that most testing programs test primarily or solely for illicit drugs and they ignore alcohol abuse, which may be a large problem at a corporation.

Some creative programs have been shown to be successful at reducing addictive behaviors. For example, Max Heirich and Cynthia J. Sieck described benefits stemming from the Wellness Outreach program. In this program, workers are screened for cardiovascular risks. Since individuals who are alcoholics or alcohol abusers are at an increased risk for cardiovascular problems, they are often automatically selected for such a program. When confidentiality is guaranteed, say Heirich and Sieck, workers are surprisingly candid about

PREVALENCE OF SUBSTANCE USE, ABUSE, OR DEPENDENCE AMONG FULL-TIME EMPLOYED WORKERS AGES 18 TO 49 YEARS: 2000

	Rates of Use (Percentage)				
	Estimated Population (Thousands)	Past Month, Heavy Alcohol Use	Past Month, Any Illegal Drug Use	Past Month, Dependence or Abuse of Alcohol	Past Month, Dependence or Abuse of Illegal Drugs
Total	87,672	8.1	7.8	7.4	1.9
Male	50,466	11.4	9.2	9.9	2.4
Female	37,206	3.6	5.9	4.0	1.2
Age groups					
18–25	15,190	13.5	14.9	13.5	5.3
26–34	24,464	8.7	7.9	8.2	1.8
35–49	48,017	6.0	5.5	5.1	1.0
Type occupation					
Executive, administrative, and managerial	14,822	6.5	6.5	6.9	1.1
Professional specialty	13,222	4.9	4.7	5.3	1.4
Technical and sales support	13,239	8.9	8.0	8.2	1.8
Administrative support	10,714	4.9	6.9	5.5	1.9
Services	10,047	7.7	9.7	8.0	2.3
Precision production, craft, and repair	10,786	12.6	11.2	9.2	2.5
Operators, fabricators, and laborers	12,428	11.2	8.6	9.3	3.0
Type industry					
Construction and mining	8,287	15.7	12.3	10.9	3.6
Manufacturing	14,610	9.4	6.7	6.7	1.7
Transportation, communications, and other public utilities	6,541	7.6	7.2	8.2	1.4
Wholesale and retail	15,881	9.2	10.8	10.5	2.9
Services—business and repairs	7,883	9.4	9.0	8.7	1.9
Finance, insurance, real estate, and other services (personal and recreation)	8,320	5.9	7.7	7.4	1.7
Services, professional	19,125	4.0	5.0	4.4	1.3
Government	4,252	6.3	3.7	3.3	0.6

Source: National Household Survey on Drug Abuse. "Substance Use, Dependence or Abuse Among Full-Time Workers," *The NHSDA Report,* September 6, 2002.

their problematic behaviors and they are also cooperative with counselors.

The Wellness Outreach program provides individual health assessments, individualized counseling, a reinforcement of healthy behaviors, and periodic follow-ups. Cardiovascular disease counseling and risk assessment proved to be an effective way to access adults who were at risk for problem drinking and also to alert them to their cardiovascular risks.

With this program, researchers found that a significant number of individuals changed their behaviors. For example in one study, 29 people (12.5 percent of the sample who were identified as at-risk drinkers) stopped drinking altogether, while 71 people (about 31 percent) decreased their drinking to levels that made them no longer at risk. Many patients experienced both lowering of their blood pressure and weight loss, and 19 percent lost 10 or more pounds.

The authors said, "Because of the clear relation of alcohol consumption levels to several CVD [cardiovascular] risks, cardiovascular wellness programs are a natural route for engaging employees in individualized alcohol education and prevention. As the EAP [employee assistance program] study demonstrates, proactive outreach and ongoing follow up can be an effective way to engage problem drinkers in healthy behavior change.

"General wellness screening provides an effective point of entrée to most of the work force, because many worksites find that 70% or more of their employees have one or more health risks. Assessment of alcohol consumption can be a non-stigmatizing part of the health assessments, and alcohol education can become part of feedback given at the end of the screening session."

See also EMPLOYEE ASSISTANCE PROGRAMS.

Bennett, Joel B. and Wayne E. K. Lehham, ed. *Preventing Workplace Substance Abuse: Beyond Drug Testing to Wellness.* Washington, D.C.: American Psychological Association, 2003.

Heirich, Max and Cynthia J. Sieck. "Helping At-Risk Drinkers Reduce Their Drinking: Cardiovascular Wellness Outreach at Work," in *Preventing Workplace Substance Abuse: Beyond Drug Testing to Wellness.* Washington, D.C.: American Psychological Association, 2003.

Office of Applied Studies. *Substance Use and Mental Health Characteristics by Employment Status.* Rockville, Md.: Substance Abuse and Mental Health Services Administration, June 1999.

Roman, Paul M. and Terry C. Blum. "The Workplace and Alcohol Problem Prevention," *Alcohol Research & Health* 26, no. 1 (2001): 49–57.

Z

zero-tolerance laws Refers to laws related to drug or alcohol use that rigidly require specific consequences to occur when they are broken despite the circumstances of the individual case. Zero tolerance laws include BLOOD ALCOHOL LEVEL laws, which exist in all states and the District of Columbia. These laws make it criminal for minor drivers (under age 21) to have alcohol in their bloodstream, even when the minor's blood alcohol level is well below the level for legal intoxication for an adult in that state. The primary purpose of these laws is to decrease the rate of fatalities and injuries caused by youthful drunken drivers.

State laws vary greatly from state to state. However, the blood alcohol levels above which the minor is deemed to have committed a criminal act range from any alcohol at all or 0.0 to alcohol above 0.02. These state laws were passed as a result of an amendment to the National Minimum Drinking Age of 1995, a federal law. All states were required to pass some form of zero-tolerance law related to minors' drinking and driving or they would lose federal funds.

The penalties for violating the zero-tolerance driving laws vary from state to state. They range from fines to community service to the loss of the individual's driver's license.

Zero-tolerance Work and School Policies

Some employers and some public and private schools have zero-tolerance policies. If employees or students violate these policies, the penalties are severe. For example, companies may fire employees who are found to be drinking or using drugs during working hours, and schools may suspend or expel those students who use alcohol or drugs on school grounds. These policies are actively promoted within the workplace or school so that individuals are very aware of them.

See also DRUG TESTING; WORK.

Zyban (bupropion) A prescribed drug that is used by individuals who wish to stop smoking. Bupropion is also marketed as Wellbutrin, a medication that is used as a drug to treat patients diagnosed with DEPRESSION. Clinical studies of Zyban have shown that it is effective in many individuals who wish to end their smoking habit. Some studies have shown that a combination of nicotine replacement therapy with bupropion is even more effective.

See also NICOTINE REPLACEMENT THERAPY; SMOKING CESSATION.

Hurt, Richard D., M.D., et al. "A Comparison of Sustained Release Bupropion and Placebo for Smoking Cessation," *New England Journal of Medicine* 337, no. 17 (October 23, 1997): 1,195–1,202.

Jorenby, Douglas E., et al. "A Controlled Trial of Sustained-Release Bupropion, A Nicotine Patch, Or Both for Smoking Cessation," *New England Journal of Medicine* 340, no. 9 (March 4, 1999): 685–691.

APPENDIXES

APPENDIX I
IMPORTANT ORGANIZATIONS

Al-Anon
1600 Corporate Landing Parkway
Virginia Beach, VA 23454
(757) 563-1600
http://www.al-anon.org

Alcoholics Anonymous World Services, Inc.
Grand Central Station
P.O. Box 459
New York, NY 10163
(212) 870-3400
http://www.alcoholics-anonymous.org

American Academy of Addiction Psychiatry
1010 Vermont Avenue NW
Suite 710
Washington, DC 20005
(202) 393-4484
http://www.aaap.org

American Academy of Pain Medicine
4700 West Lake Avenue
Glenview, IL 60025
(847) 375-4846
http://www.painmed.org

American Association for the Treatment of Opioid Dependence
217 Broadway
Suite 304
New York, NY 10007
(212) 566-5555
http://www.aatod.org

American Chronic Pain Association
P.O. Box 850
Rocklin, CA 95677
(916) 632-0922
http://www.theacpa.org

American Council for Drug Education
164 West 74th Street
New York, NY 10023
(800) 488–DRUG
http://www.acde.org

American Council on Alcoholism
1000 East Indian School Road
Phoenix, AZ 85014
(703) 248-9005
http://www.aca-usa.org

American Hospital Association (AHA)
One North Franklin
Chicago, IL 60606-3421
(312) 422-3000
http://www.aha.org

American Medical Association
515 North State Street
Chicago, IL 60610
(800) 621-8335
http://www.ama-assn.org

American Nurses Association
8515 Georgia Avenue
Suite 400
Silver Spring, MD 20910
(301) 628-5000
http://www.nursingworld.org

American Obesity Association
1250 24th Street NW
Suite 300
Washington, DC 20037
(202) 776-7711
http://www.obesity.org

American Pharmaceutical Association
2215 Constitution Avenue NW
Washington, DC 20037

(202) 628-4410
http://www.aphanet.org

American Psychiatric Association
1000 Wilson Boulevard
Suite 1825
Arlington, VA 22209-3901
(703) 907-7300
http://www.psych.org

American Psychological Association
750 First Street NE
Washington, DC 20002-4242
(202) 336-5500
http://www.apa.org

American Society of Addiction Medicine
4601 North Park Avenue
Upper Arcade #101
Chevy Chase, MD 20815
(301) 656-3920
http://www.asam.org

American Society of Human Genetics
9650 Rockville Pike
Bethesda, MD 20814
(301) 571-1825
http://www.faseb.org/genetics

Centers for Disease Control and Prevention (CDC)
1600 Clifton Road NE
Atlanta, GA 30333
(404) 371-5900
http://www.cdc.gov

Centers for Medicare and Medicaid Services
7500 Security Boulevard
Baltimore, MD 21244
(410) 786-3000
http://www.cms.hhs.gov

College on Problems of Drug Dependence
3420 North Broad Street
Philadelphia, PA 19140
(215) 707-1904
http://www.cpdd.vcu.edu/pages

Eating Disorder Referral and Information Center
2923 Sandy Pointe
Suite 6
Del Mar, CA 92014

(858) 792-7463
http://www.edreferral.com

Emergency Nurses Association
915 Lee Street
Des Plaines, IL 60016
(800) 900-9659
http://www.ena.org

Food and Drug Administration (FDA)
5600 Fishers Lane
Rockville, MD 20857
(888) 463-6332
http://www.fda.gov

Gam-Anon International Service Office, Inc.
P.O. Box 157
Whitestone, NY 11357
(718) 352-1671
http://www.gam-anon.org

Gamblers Anonymous
International Service Office
P.O. Box 17173
Los Angeles, CA 90017
(213) 386-8789
http://www.gamblersanonyomous.org

The Genetic Alliance
4301 Connecticut Avenue NW
Suite 404
Washington, DC 20008
(202) 966-5557
http://www.geneticalliance.org

Governors Highway Safety Association
750 First Street NE
Suite 720
Washington, DC 20002
(202) 789-0942
http://www.naghsr.org

Group for the Advancement of Psychiatry
P.O. Box 570218
Dallas, TX 75357
(972) 613-3044
http://www.groupadpsych.org

Hepatitis B Coalition/Immunization Action Coalition
1573 Selby Avenue
Suite 234
St. Paul, MN 55104

(651) 647-9009
http://www.immunize.org

Hepatitis B Foundation
700 East Butler Avenue
Doylestown, PA 18901
(215) 489-4900
http://www.hepb.org

Hepatitis Foundation International
504 Blick Drive
Silver Spring, MD 20904
(800) 891-0707
http://www.hepfi.org

The Higher Education Center for Alcohol and Other Drug Prevention
Education Development Center, Inc.
55 Chapel Street
Newton, MA 02458
(800) 676-1730
http://www.edc.org/hec/

Mothers Against Drunk Driving (MADD)
511 East John Carpenter Freeway
Suite 700
Irving, TX 75062
(800) GET-MADD (800-438-6233)
http://www.madd.org

Narcotics Anonymous World Services, Inc.
P.O. Box 9999
Van Nuys, CA 91409-9099
(818) 773-9999
http://www.na.org

National Association for Children of Alcoholics
11426 Rockville Pike
Suite 100
Rockville, MD 20852
(888) 555-4COAS
http://www.nacoa.net

National Association of Anorexia Nervosa and Associated Disorders
P.O. Box 7
Highland Park, IL 60035
(847) 831-3438
http://www.anad.org

National Association of Drug Court Professionals
4900 Seminary Road
Suite 320

Alexandria, VA 22311
(703) 575-9400
http://www.nadcp.org

National Association of State Controlled Substances Authorities
72 Brook Street
Quincy, MA 02170
(617) 472-0520
http://www.nascsa.org

National Center for Complementary and Alternative Medicine (NCCAM) Clearinghouse
National Institutes of Health (NIH)
P.O. Box 7923
Gaithersburg, MD 20907
(888) 644-6226
http://www.nccam.nih.gov

National Center on Addiction and Substance Abuse at Columbia University
633 Third Avenue
New York, NY 10017
(212) 841-5200
http://www.casacolumbia.org

National Center on Substance Abuse and Child Welfare
4940 Irvine Boulevard
Suite 202
Irvine, CA 92620
(714) 505-3525
http://www.ncsacw.samhsa.gov

National Clearinghouse for Alcohol and Drug Information
11426 Rockville Pike
Suite 200
Rockville, MD 20852
(800) 729-6686
http://www.health.org

National Clearinghouse on Child Abuse and Neglect Information
330 C Street SW
Washington, DC 20447
(703) 385-3206
http://nccanch.acf.hhs.gov

National Council on Alcoholism and Drug Dependence (NCADD)
20 Exchange Place
Suite 2902

New York, NY 10005
(800) NCA-CALL or (212) 269-7797
http://www.ncadd.org

National Drug Intelligence Center

319 Washington Street
Fifth Floor
Johnstown, PA 15901
(814) 532-4690
http://www.usdoj.gov/ndic

National Eating Disorders Organization

603 Stewart Street
Suite 803
Seattle, WA 98101
(800) 931-2237
http://www.edap.org

National Empowerment Center

599 Canal Street
Lawrence, MA 01840
(800) 769-3728
http://www.power2u.org

National Highway Traffic Safety Administration (NHTSA)

400 Seventh Street SW
Washington, DC 20590
(888) 327-4236
http://www.nhtsa.dot.gov

National Institute of Mental Health

NIMH Public Inquiries
6001 Executive Boulevard
Room 8184, MSC 9663
Bethesda, MD 20892
(301) 443-4513
www.nimh.nih.gov

National Institute on Alcohol Abuse and Alcoholism

5635 Fishers Lane
MSC 9304
Bethesda, MD 20892
http://www.niaaa.nih.gov

National Institute on Drug Abuse

National Institutes of Health
6001 Executive Boulevard
Room 5313
Bethesda, MD 20892
(301) 443-1124
http://www.nida.nih.gov

National Mental Health Association

2001 North Beauregard Street
12th Floor
Alexandria, VA 22311
(703) 684-7722
www.nmha.org

National Mental Health Consumers' Self-Help Clearinghouse

1211 Chestnut Street
Suite 1207
Philadelphia, PA 19107
(215) 751-1810 or (800) 553-4539
http://www.mhselfhelp.org

National Organization on Fetal Alcohol Syndrome (NOFAS)

900 17th Street NW
Suite 910
Washington, DC 20006
(202) 785-4585
http://www.nofas.org

National Self-Help Clearinghouse

365 Fifth Avenue
Suite 3300
New York, NY 10016
(212) 817-1822
http://www.selfhelpweb.org

National Sheriffs' Association

1450 Duke Street
Alexandria, VA 22314
(703) 836-7827
http://www.sheriffs.org

National Women's Health Network

514 10th Street NW
Suite 400
Washington, DC 20004
(202) 347-1140
http://www.womenshealthnetwork.org

Nicotine Anonymous

419 Main Street
PMB #370
Huntington Beach, CA 94159-1777
(415) 750-0328
http://www.nicotine-anonymous.org

Obsessive-Compulsive Foundation

676 State Street
New Haven, CT 06511

(203) 401-2070
http://www.ocfoundation.org

Office of Safe and Drug-Free Schools
U.S. Department of Education
400 Maryland Avenue SW
Washington, DC 20202
(202) 260-3954
http://www.ed.gov/about/offices/list/osdfs/index.html

Overeaters Anonymous
The World Service Office of Overeaters Anonymous
P.O. Box 44020
Rio Rancho, NM 87174-4020
(505) 891-2664
http://www.oa.org/ws

Social Security Administration (SSA)
Office of Public Inquiries
6401 Security Boulevard
Baltimore, MD 21235

(800) 772-1213
http://www.ssa.gov

Substance Abuse and Mental Health Services Administration (SAMSHA)
Department of Health and Human Services
5600 Fishers Lane
Rockville, MD 20857
(800) 729-6686
http://www.samhsa.gov

Weight-Control Information Network
1 Win Way
Bethesda, MD 20892
(800) WIN-8098

Weight Watchers International
175 Crossways Park West
Woodbury, NY 11797
(800) 651-6000
http://www.weightwatchers.com

APPENDIX II
STATE AND TERRITORIAL
SUBSTANCE ABUSE AGENCIES

This appendix includes lists of state and territorial offices that provide information on substance abuse, including treatment facilities within the state as well as general information.

ALABAMA

Substance Abuse Services Division
Department of Mental Health/Retardation
P.O. Box 301410
100 North Union Street
Montgomery, AL 36130
(334) 242-3961

ALASKA

Division of Alcoholism and Drug Abuse
Department of Health and Social Services
240 Main Street
Suite 700
Juneau, AK 99801
(907) 465-2071

AMERICAN SAMOA

Department of Human and Social Services
American Samoa Government
P.O. Box 997534
Pago Pago, AS 96799
(684) 633-2609

ARIZONA

Bureau of Substance Abuse Treatment & Prevention
Division of Behavioral Health Services
Department of Health Services
2122 East Highland Street
Suite 100
Phoenix, AZ 85016
(602) 381-8922

ARKANSAS

Department of Health, Alcohol and Drug Abuse Prevention
5800 West 10th Street
Freeway Medical Center
Suite 907
Little Rock, AR 72204
(501) 280-4515

CALIFORNIA

Department of Alcohol and Drug Programs
1700 K Street
Sacramento, CA 95814
(800) 879-2772

COLORADO

Alcohol and Drug Abuse Division
Department of Human Services
4055 South Lowell Boulevard
Denver, CO 80236
(303) 866-7480

CONNECTICUT

Department of Mental Health and Addiction Services
410 Capitol Avenue
4th Floor
P.O. Box 341431, MS #14COM
Hartford, CT 06134
(860) 418-6838

DELAWARE

Alcohol and Drug Services
Division of Substance Abuse and Mental Health
1901 North DuPont Highway
Administration Building, First Floor
New Castle, DE 19720
(302) 255-9399

DISTRICT OF COLUMBIA

**Addiction Prevention & Recovery
    Administration**
Department of Health
825 North Capitol Street NE
Suite 3132
Washington, DC 20002
(202) 442-9152

FEDERATED STATES OF MICRONESIA

Department of Health Services
The Federated States of Micronesia
P.O. Box Px70
Palikir Pohnpei, FM 96941
(691) 320-5520

FLORIDA

Substance Abuse Program Office
Florida Department of Children and Families
1317 Winewood Boulevard
Building 6, Room 334
Tallahassee, FL 32399

GEORGIA

**Division of Mental Health/Mental
    Retardation/Substance Abuse**
Two Peachtree Street NW
23rd Floor
Suite 23-204
Atlanta, GA 30303
(404) 657-2135

GUAM

Drug and Alcohol Treatment Services
Clinical Services Division
790 Governor Carlos Camacho Road
Tamunin, GU 96911
(671) 647-5440

HAWAII

Alcohol and Drug Abuse Division
Department of Health
Kakuhihewa Building
601 Kamokila Boulevard
Room 360
Kapolei, HI 96707
(808) 692-7506

IDAHO

Substance Abuse Program
Department of Health and Welfare
450 West State Street
5th Floor
P.O. Box 83720
Boise, ID 83720
(208) 334-5935

ILLINOIS

Office of Alcoholism and Substance Abuse
Department of Human Services
100 West Randolph
Suite 5-600
Chicago, IL 60601
(312) 814-3840

INDIANA

Division of Mental Health and Addiction
Family and Social Services Administration
402 West Washington Street
Room W353
Indianapolis, IN 46204
(317) 232-7800

IOWA

Iowa Department of Public Health
Lucas State Office Building, 4th Floor
321 East 12th Street
Des Moines, IA 50319
(515) 281-4417

KANSAS

**State Rehabilitative Services Health Care
    Policy**
DSOB 10th Floor North
915 Harrison Street
Topeka, KS 66612
(785) 291-3326

KENTUCKY

Division of Substance Abuse
Department for Mental Health/Mental Retardation
    Services
100 Fair Oaks Lane
4E-D
Frankfort, KY 40621
(502) 564-2880

LOUISIANA

Office for Addictive Disorders
Department of Health and Hospitals
1201 Capitol Access Road
4th Floor
P.O. Box 2790, Bin #18
Baton Rouge, LA 70821
(225) 342-6717

MAINE

Office of Substance Abuse
Department of Behavioral and Developmental Services
AMHI Complex, Marquardt Building
SHS #159, 3rd Floor
Augusta, ME 04333
(207) 287-2595

MARYLAND

Alcohol and Drug Abuse Administration
Department of Health and Mental Hygiene
55 Wade Avenue
Catonsville, MD 21228
(410) 402-8600

MASSACHUSETTS

Bureau of Substance Abuse Services
Department of Public Health
250 Washington Street
3rd Floor
Boston, MA 02108

MICHIGAN

Bureau of Mental Health and Substance Abuse Services
Department of Community Health
320 South Walnut
Lewis Cass Building, 6th Floor
Lansing, MI 48909
(517) 241-2596

MINNESOTA

Chemical Health Division
Department of Human Services
Human Services Building
444 Lafayette Road
St. Paul, MN 55155
(651) 582-1832

MISSISSIPPI

Division of Alcohol and Drug Abuse
Department of Mental Health
Robert E. Lee Office Building, 11th Floor
239 North Lamar Street
Jackson, MS 39201
(877) 210-8513

MISSOURI

Division of Alcohol and Drug Abuse
Missouri Department of Mental Health
1706 East Elm Street
P.O. Box 687
Jefferson City, MO 65102
(573) 751-4942

MONTANA

Addictive and Mental Disorders Division
Department of Public Health and Human Services
555 Fuller
P.O. Box 202905
Helena, MT 59620
(406) 444-3964

NEBRASKA

Office of Mental Health, Substance Abuse and Addiction Services
Department of Health and Human Services Systems
P.O. Box 98925
Lincoln, NE 68509
(402) 479-5583

NEVADA

Bureau of Alcohol and Drug Abuse
Department of Human Resources, Health Division
505 East King Street
Room 500
Carson City, NV 89701
(775) 684-4190

NEW HAMPSHIRE

Division of Alcohol and Drug Abuse Prevention and Recovery
Department of Health and Human Services
105 Pleasant Street
Concord, NH 03301
(800) 804-0909

NEW JERSEY

Division of Addiction Services
Department of Health and Senior Services
120 South Stockton Street
3rd Floor
P.O. Box 362
Trenton, NJ 08625
(609) 292-5760

NEW MEXICO

Behavioral Health Services Division
Department of Health
1190 Saint Francis Drive
Harold Runnels Building, Room 3300 North
Santa Fe, NM 87502
(505) 827-2601

NEW YORK

New York State Office of Alcoholism and Substance Abuse Services
1450 Western Avenue
Albany, NY 12203
(518) 473-3560

NORTH CAROLINA

Substance Abuse Services
Division of Mental Health/DD/Substance Abuse Services
325 North Salisbury Street
Suite 1156-P
3007 Mail Center
Raleigh, NC 27699
(919) 733-4670

NORTH DAKOTA

Division of Mental Health and Substance Abuse Services
Department of Human Services
600 South Second Street
Suite 1E
Bismarck, ND 58504
(701) 328-8920

OHIO

Ohio Department of Alcohol and Drug Addiction Services
280 North High Street
12th Floor

Two Nationwide Plaza
Columbus, OH 43215
(614) 466-3445

OKLAHOMA

Substance Abuse Program
Department of Mental Health and Substance Abuse Services
1200 Northeast 13th
Second Floor
P.O. Box 53277
Oklahoma City, OK 73152
(405) 522-3877

OREGON

Office of Mental Health and Addiction Services
Department of Human Services
500 Summer Street NE E86
Salem, OR 97301
(503) 945-5763

PALAU

Ministry of Health
Behavioral Health Division
P.O. Box 6027
Koror
Palau, PW 96940
(680) 488-1907

PENNSYLVANIA

Bureau of Drug and Alcohol Programs
Pennsylvania Department of Health
2 Kline Plaza
Suite B
Harrisburg, PA 17104
(717) 783-8200

PUERTO RICO

Mental Health and Anti-Addiction Services Administration
414 Barboza Avenue
P.O. Box 21414
San Juan, PR 00928
(787) 764-3795

RHODE ISLAND

Behavioral Health Care
Division of Behavioral Health

Department of Mental Health and Retardation
14 Harrington Road
Cranston, RI 02920
(401) 462-4680

SOUTH CAROLINA

South Carolina Department of Alcohol and Other Drug Abuse Services
101 Business Park Boulevard
Columbia, SC 29203
(803) 896-5555

SOUTH DAKOTA

Division of Alcohol and Drug Abuse
Department of Human Services
East Highway 34
Hillsview Plaza
c/o 500 East Capitol
Pierre, SD 57501
(605) 773-3123

TENNESSEE

Bureau of Alcohol and Drug Abuse Services
Tennessee Department of Health
Third Floor, Cordell Hull Building
425 Fifth Avenue North
Nashville, TN 37247
(615) 741-1921

TEXAS

Texas Commission on Alcohol and Drug Abuse
9001 North IH 35
Suite 105
P.O. Box 80529
Austin, TX 78708
(512) 349-6600

UTAH

Division of Substance Abuse and Mental Health
Utah Department of Human Services
120 North 200 West
Second Floor, Room 201
Salt Lake City, UT 84103
(801) 538-3939

VERMONT

Division of Alcohol and Drug Abuse Programs
Department of Health
108 Cherry Street

P.O. Box 70
Burlington, VT 05402
(802) 651-1550

VIRGINIA

Office of Substance Abuse Services
Department of Mental Health, Mental Retardation and Substance Abuse Services
P.O. Box 1797
1220 Bank Street
Richmond, VA 23218
(804) 786-3906

VIRGIN ISLANDS

Charles Harwood Hospital
Department of Mental Health
3500 Richmond Street
Christansted Saint Croix, VI 00820
(809) 773-1311

WASHINGTON

Division of Alcohol and Substance Abuse
Department of Social and Health Services
P.O. Box 45330
612 Woodland Square Loop SE
Building C
Olympia, WA 98504
(877) 301-4557

WEST VIRGINIA

Behavioral Health Assessment Unit
Department of Health and Human Resources
350 Capitol Street, Room 350
Charleston, WV 25301

WISCONSIN

Bureau of Substance Abuse Services
1 West Wilson Street
P.O. Box 7851
Madison, WI 53707
(608) 266-2717

WYOMING

Substance Abuse Division
2424 Pioneer Avenue
Suite 306
Cheyenne, WY 82002
(307) 777-3358

APPENDIX III
STATE CONTROLLED SUBSTANCES SCHEDULING AUTHORITIES

This appendix provides state contacts for authorities involved in scheduled drugs, such as narcotics.

ALABAMA

Department of Public Health
P.O. Box 30317
Montgomery, AL 36130
(334) 206-5300
http://www.adph.org/

ALASKA

Division of Occupational Licensing
P.O. Box 110806
Juneau, AK 99811
(907) 465-2589
http://www.dced.state.ak.us/occ/home.htm

ARIZONA

Board of Pharmacy
4425 West Olive Avenue
Suite 140
Glendale, AZ 85302
(623) 463-2727

ARKANSAS

Division of Pharmacy Services and Drug Control
Arkansas Department of Public Health
4815 West Markham Street
Slot 25
Little Rock, AR 72205
(501) 661-2325

CALIFORNIA

Board of Pharmacy
400 R Street
Suite 4070
Sacramento, CA 95814
(916) 445-5014

COLORADO

Board of Pharmacy
1560 Broadway
Suite 1310
Denver, CO 80202
(303) 894-7753

CONNECTICUT

Drug Control Division
Department of Consumer Protection
165 Capitol Avenue
Hartford, CT 06106
(860) 713-6050

DELAWARE

Board of Pharmacy
P.O. Box 637
Dover, DE 19901
(302) 739-4978

DISTRICT OF COLUMBIA

Bureau of Food, Drugs & Radiological Protection
Department of Health
51 N Street NE
Sixth Floor
Washington, DC 20002
(202) 535-2188

FLORIDA

Assistant Attorney General
Administrative Law Section
The Capitol, Room LL-04

Tallahassee, FL 32399
(850) 414-3300

GEORGIA

Georgia Drugs & Narcotics Agency
40 Pryor Street SW
Suite 2000
Atlanta, GA 30303
(404) 656-5100

HAWAII

Department of Public Safety
Bureau of Narcotic Enforcement
3375 Koapaka Street
Suite D100
Honolulu, HI 96819
(808) 837-8470

IDAHO

Board of Pharmacy
3380 Americana Terrace
Suite 320
Boise, ID 83706
(208) 334-2356

ILLINOIS

Illinois Prescription Monitoring Program
Department of Human Services
401 North Fourth Street
Room 133
Springfield, IL 62701
(217) 524-9074

INDIANA

Board of Pharmacy
Health Professions Bureau
402 West Washington Street
Room 041
Indianapolis, IN 46204
(317) 234-2067

IOWA

Controlled Drug Division
Board of Pharmacy Examiners
400 Southwest Eighth Street
Suite E
Des Moines, IA 50319
(515) 281-5944

KANSAS

Kansas State Board of Pharmacy
900 Jackson Avenue
Room 560
Topeka, KS 66612
(785) 296-4056

KENTUCKY

Department for Public Health
Drug Enforcement Branch
275 East Main Street HS2GW-B
Frankfort, KY 40621
(502) 564-7985

LOUISIANA

Louisiana Board of Pharmacy
Corporate Boulevard
Suite 8E
Baton Rouge, LA 70808
(225) 925-6496

MAINE

Board of Commissioners & Pharmacy
State House Station Number 35
Augusta, ME 04333
(207) 582-8723

MARYLAND

Maryland Board of Pharmacy
4201 Patterson Avenue
Baltimore, MD 21215
(410) 764-4794

MASSACHUSETTS

Drug Control Program
Department of Public Health, Division of Food and
  Drugs
305 South Street
Jamaica Plain, MA 02130
(617) 983-6700

MICHIGAN

Bureau of Health Services
Health Regulatory Division
P.O. Box 30454
6546 Mercantile Way
Suite 2
Lansing, MI 48909
(517) 335-1769

MINNESOTA

Board of Pharmacy
2829 University Avenue SE
Suite 530
Minneapolis, MN 55414
(612) 617-2201

MISSISSIPPI

**Pharmacy Department, Division of Public
  Health**
P.O. Box 1700
Jackson, MS 39205
(601) 713-3471

MISSOURI

Bureau of Narcotics & Dangerous Drugs
Department of Health and Senior Services
P.O. Box 570
Jefferson City, MO 65102
(573) 751-6321

MONTANA

Board of Pharmacy
P.O. Box 200513
Helena, MT 59620
(406) 841-2355

NEBRASKA

**Professional and Occupational Licensing
  Division**
Department of Health
P.O. Box 94986
Lincoln, NE 68509
(402) 471-2118

NEVADA

Board of Pharmacy
555 Double Eagle Court
Suite 1100
Reno, NV 89502
(775) 850-1440

NEW HAMPSHIRE

New Hampshire Board of Pharmacy
57 Regional Drive
Concord, NH 03301
(603) 271-2350

NEW JERSEY

Drug Control
Department of Law and Public Safety
P.O. Box 45045
Newark, NJ 07101
(973) 504-6561

NEW MEXICO

Division of Substance Abuse
Department of Health
P.O. Box 26110
1190 St. Francis Drive
Santa Fe, NM 87502-6110
(505) 827-2601

NEW YORK

Bureau of Controlled Substances
New York State Department of Health
433 River Street
Fifth Floor
Troy, NY 12180
(518) 402-0707

NORTH CAROLINA

Controlled Substances Regulatory Branch
Alcohol & Drug Abuse Services
3824 Barrett Drive
Suite 308
Raleigh, NC 27609
(919) 420-7932

NORTH DAKOTA

North Dakota Board of Pharmacy
P.O. Box 1354
Bismarck, ND 58502
(701) 328-9535

OHIO

Board of Pharmacy
77 South High Street
Room 1702
Columbus, OH 43215
(614) 466-4143

OKLAHOMA

Bureau of Narcotics and Dangerous Drugs
4545 North Lincoln Boulevard
Suite 11
Oklahoma City, OK 73105
(405) 521-2885

OREGON

Board of Pharmacy
State Office Building
800 Northeast Oregon
Suite 9
Portland, OR 97232
(503) 731-4032

PENNSYLVANIA

Bureau of Narcotic Investigations and Drug Control
106 Lowther Street
Lemoyne, PA 17043
(717) 783-2600

RHODE ISLAND

Compliance and Regulatory Section
Division of Drug Control
205 Cannon Office Building
3 Capitol Hill
Suite 205
Providence, RI 02908
(401) 222-2837

SOUTH CAROLINA

Bureau of Drug Control
Department of Health and Environmental Control
2600 Bull Street
Columbia, SC 29201

SOUTH DAKOTA

Department of Health
Licensure and Certification
615 East Fourth Street
Pierre, SD 57501
(605) 773-3356

TENNESSEE

Tennessee Board of Pharmacy
Davy Crockett Tower, Second Floor
500 James Robinson Parkway
Nashville, TN 37243
(615) 741-2718

TEXAS

Texas State Department of Health
1100 West 49th Street
Austin, TX 78756
(512) 719-0237

UTAH

Division of Professional Licensing
P.O. Box 146741
Salt Lake City, UT 84114
(801) 530-6721

VERMONT

Vermont Department of Health
P.O. Box 70
108 Cherry Street
Burlington, VT 05042
(802) 863-7281

VIRGINIA

Board of Pharmacy
6603 West Broad Street, Sixth Floor
Richmond, VA 23230
(804) 662-9911

WASHINGTON

Board of Pharmacy
P.O. Box 47863
Olympia, WA 98504
(360) 236-4825

WEST VIRGINIA

West Virginia Board of Pharmacy
232 Capitol Street
Charleston, WV 25301
(304) 558-0558

WISCONSIN

Department of Regulation and Licensing
Controlled Substances Board
P.O. Box 8935
Madison, WI 53708
(608) 266-8098

WYOMING

State Board of Pharmacy
1720 South Poplar Street
Suite 4
Casper, WY 82601
(307) 234-0294

APPENDIX IV
EXAMPLES OF SCHEDULED DRUGS

These are examples of drugs that are under the control of the Drug Enforcement Administration (DEA). Some of these drugs are illegal, and some are legal. (Illegal drugs are Schedule I drugs.) The Food and Drug Administration also has jurisdiction over legally prescribed medications. This table does not include all scheduled drugs and provides only a sample of the most common ones.

SCHEDULED DRUGS, SCHEDULES I THROUGH V			
Substance	DEA Number	Nonnarcotic (N = Nonnarcotic)	Other Names for Drug
Schedule I Drugs			
3,4-Methyenedioxymethamphetamine	7405	N	MDMA, Ecstasy, XTC
3-Methylfentanyl	9813		China white, fentanyl
4-Methoxyamphetamine	7395	N	PMA
Acetylmethadol	9601		Methadyl acetate
Alpha-ethyltryptamine	9604	N	ET, trip
Diethyltryptamine	7434	N	DET
Gamma-hydroxybutryic acid	2010	N	GHB
Heroin	9200		Diacetylmorphine
Lysergic acid diethylamide	9631	N	LSD, lysergide
Marijuana	7360	N	Cannabis, marijuana
Mescaline	7381	N	Peyote
Psilocybin	7438	N	Psilocin, magic mushrooms
Schedule II Drugs			
Amphetamine	1100	N	Dexedrine, Biphetamine
Fentanyl	9801		Innovar, Sublimaze
Hydromorphone	9150		Dilaudid, dihydromorphine
Meperidine	9230		Demerol, Mepergan
Methadone	9250		Dolophine, Methadose
Methylphenidate	1105	N	Ritalin
Morphine	9300		MS-Contin, Roxanol
Opium tincture	9630		Laudanum
Oxycodone	9143		OxyContin, Percocet, Tylox, Roxicodone, Roxicet
Oxymorphone	9652		Numorphan
Phencyclidine	7471	N	PCP, Sernvylan
Secobarbital	2315	N	Seconal, Tuinal

Substance	DEA Number	Nonnarcotic (N = Nonnarcotic)	Other Names for Drug
Schedule III Drugs			
Anabolic steroids	4000	N	Body-building drugs
Buprenorphine	9064		Buprenex, Temgesic
Butalbital	2100	N	Fiornal, Butalbital with aspirin
Codeine combination product	9804		Empirin, Fiorinal, Tylenol, APAP, all with codeine
Ketamine	7285	N	Ketaset, Ketalar, special
Mesterolone	4000	N	Proviron
Opium combination product 25	9809		Paregoric, other combinations
Schedule IV Drugs			
Alprazolam	2882	N	Xanax
Chlordiazepoxide	2744	N	Librium, Libritabs
Clonazepam	2737	N	Klonopin, clonopin
Dextropropoxyphene dosage forms	9278		Darvone, propoxyphene
Diazepam	2765	N	Valium, Valrelease
Flunitrazepam	2763	N	Rohypnol, Narcozep
Lorazepam	2885	N	Ativan
Meprobamate	2820	N	Miltown, Equanil, Deprol, Meprospan
Midazolam	2884	N	Versed
Nitrazepam	2834	N	Mogadan
Pemoline	1530	N	Cylert
Phenobarbital	2285	N	Luminal, Donnatal
Phentermine	1640	N	Ionamin, Fastin, Adipex
Sibutramine	1675	N	Meridia
Temazepam	2925	N	Restoril
Triazolam	2887	N	Halcion
Zaleplon	2781	N	Sonata
Zolpidem	2783	N	Ambien, Stilnoct, Ivadal
Schedule V Drugs			
Diphenoxylate preparations			Lomotil, Logen
Opium preparations			Parapectolin, Kapectolin

Source: Drug Enforcement Administration. "Drug Scheduling," Available online. URL: http://www. usdoj.gov/dea/pubs/ scheduling.html Downloaded on May 31, 2004.

APPENDIX V
STATE MENTAL HEALTH AGENCIES

ALABAMA

Department of Mental Health and Mental Retardation
RSA Union Building
100 North Union Street
Montgomery, AL 36130-3417
(334) 242-3454
(800) 367-0955
http://www.mh.state.al.us

ALASKA

Division of Mental Health and Developmental Disabilities
Department of Health and Social Services
P.O. Box 110620
Juneau, AK 99811-0620
(907) 465-3370
(800) 465-4828 or (907) 465-2225 (TDD)
http://www.hss.state.ak.us/dbh/

ARIZONA

Department of Health Services
Division of Behavioral Health Services
150 North 18th Avenue
#200
Phoenix, AZ 85007
(602) 364-4558
http://www.hs.state.az.us/bhs/index.htm

ARKANSAS

Division of Mental Health Services
Department of Human Services
4313 West Markham Street
Little Rock, AR 72205-4096
(501) 686-9164 or (501) 686-9176 (TDD)
http://www.state.ar.us/dhs/dmhs/

CALIFORNIA

Department of Mental Health
Health and Welfare Agency
1600 Ninth Street
Room 151
Sacramento, CA 95814
(916) 654-3565 or (800) 896-4042 or
    (800) 896-2512 (TDD)
http://www.dmh.cahwnet.gov

COLORADO

Colorado Mental Health Services
3824 West Princeton Circle
Denver, CO 80236
(303) 866-7400
http://www.cdhs.state.co.us/ohr/mhs/

CONNECTICUT

Department of Mental Health and Addictions Services
410 Capitol Avenue
Hartford, CT 06106
(860) 418-6700 or (800) 446-7348 or
    (888) 621-3551 (TDD)
http://www.dmhas.state.ct.us

DELAWARE

Division of Substance Abuse and Mental Health
Department of Health and Social Services
1901 N. DuPont Highway
Main Building
New Castle, DE 19720
(302) 255-9427
http://www.state.de.us/dhss/dsamh/dmhhome.htm

DISTRICT OF COLUMBIA

Department of Mental Health Services
77 P Street NE
4th Floor
Washington, DC 20002
(202) 673-7440
http://dmh.dc.gov/dmh/site/default.asp

FLORIDA

Department of Children and Families
1317 Winewood Boulevard
Building 1, Room 202
Tallahassee, FL 32399-0700
(850) 487-1111
http://www.state.fl.us/cf_web/

GEORGIA

**Division of Mental Health, Mental Retardation
and Substance Abuse**
Department of Human Resources
2 Peachtree Street, NW
Suite 22-224
Atlanta, GA 30303
(404) 657-2168
http://www2.state.ga.us/departments/dhr/mhmrsa/
index.html

HAWAII

Behavioral Health Services Administration
Department of Health
P.O. Box 3378
Honolulu, HI 96801
(808) 586-4419
http://www.state.hi.us/doh/about/behavior.html

IDAHO

Department of Health and Welfare
450 West State Street
Boise, ID 83720-0036
(208) 334-5500
http://www2.state.id.us/dhw/index.htm

ILLINOIS

Office of Mental Health
Department of Human Services
319 East Madison Street
Centrum Building, Third Floor
Springfield, IL 62701
(217) 785-6023
http://www.dhs.state.il.us

INDIANA

Division of Mental Health
Department of Family and Social Services
  Administration
402 West Washington Street
Room W-353
Indianapolis, IN 46204-2739
(317) 232-7844

IOWA

**Division of Mental Health and Developmental
  Disabilities**
Hoover State Office Building
1305 East Walnut Street
Des Moines, IA 50319-0114
(515) 281-3573

KANSAS

**Department of Social and Rehabilitation
  Services**
Docking State Office Building
915 SW Harrison Street
Topeka, KS 66612
(785) 296-3959
http://www.srskansas.org

KENTUCKY

**Department for Mental Health and Mental
  Retardation Services**
Cabinet for Human Resources
100 Fair Oaks Lane
Frankfort, KY 40621-0001
(502) 564-4527
http://mhmr.chs.ky.gov/Default.asp

LOUISIANA

Office of Mental Health
P.O. Box 4049
Bin #12
Baton Rouge, LA 70821-4049
(225) 342-2540
http://www.dhh.state.la.us/OMH/index.htm

MAINE

Adult Mental Health Services
Department of Behavioral and Developmental Services
40 State House Station
Augusta, ME 04333
(207) 287-4200 or (888) 568-1112
http://www.state.me.us/dmhmrsa

MARYLAND

Department of Health and Mental Hygiene
201 West Preston Street
Baltimore, MD 21201
(410) 767-6860 or (877) 463-3464 or
    (800) 735-2258 (TDD)
http://www.dhmh.state.md.us

MASSACHUSETTS

Department of Mental Health
25 Staniford Street
Boston, MA 02114
(617) 626-8000 or (617) 727-9842 (TDD)
http://www.state.ma.us/dmh/_MainLine/
    MissionStatement.HTM

MICHIGAN

Department of Community Health
Lewis-Cass Building
320 South Walnut Street
Sixth Floor
Lansing, MI 48913
(517) 373-3500 or (517) 373-3573 (TDD)
http://www.michigan.gov/mdch

MINNESOTA

Department of Human Services
Mental Health Program Division
Human Services Building
444 Lafayette Road
Saint Paul, MN 55155-3828
(651) 297-3510
http://www.dhs.state.mn.us/Contcare/
    mentalhealth/default.htm

MISSISSIPPI

Department of Mental Health
Robert E. Lee Building
Suite 1101
239 North Lamar Street
Jackson, MS 39201
(601) 359-1288 or (601) 359-6230 (TDD)
http://www.dmh.state.ms.us

MISSOURI

Department of Mental Health
P.O. Box 687
Jefferson City, MO 65102
(800) 364-9687 or (573) 526-1201 (TDD)
http://www.dmh.missouri.gov

MONTANA

Addictive and Mental Disorders Division
Department of Public Health and Human Services
555 Fuller
Helena, MT 59620
(406) 444-4928
http://www.dphhs.state.mt.us

NEBRASKA

**Office of Mental Health, Substance Abuse and
    Addictions Services**
P.O. Box 98925
Lincoln, NE 68509
(402) 479-5166
http://www.hhs.state.ne.us/beh/mhsa.htm

NEVADA

**Mental Health & Developmental Services
    Division**
Department of Human Resources
Kinkead Building, Room 602
505 East King Street
Carson City, NV 89701
(775) 684-5943
http://www.mhds.state.nv.us

NEW HAMPSHIRE

Division of Behavioral Health
Department of Health and Human Services
State Office Park South
105 Pleasant Street
Concord, NH 03301
(603) 271-8140 or (800) 735-2964 (TDD) or
    (800) 852-3345
http://www.dhhs.state.nh.us

NEW JERSEY

Division of Mental Health Services
50 East State Street
Capitol Center, Post Office 727
Trenton, NJ 08625-0727
(609) 777-0702
http://www.state.nj.us/humanservices/dmhs

NEW MEXICO

Behavioral Health Services Division
Harold Runnels Building
1190 Saint Francis Drive
Room North 3300
Santa Fe, NM 87505-6110

(505) 827-2601 or (800) 362-2013
(consumer hotline)
http://www.nmcares.org

NEW YORK

Office of Mental Health
44 Holland Avenue
Albany, NY 12229
(518) 474-4403 or (800) 597-8481 (toll-free)
http://www.omh.state.ny.us

NORTH CAROLINA

**Division of Mental Health, Developmental
Disabilities, and Substance Abuse Services**
Department of Health & Human Resources
3001 Mail Service Center
Raleigh, NC 27699-3001
(919) 733-7011
http://www.dhhs.state.nc.us/mhddsas

NORTH DAKOTA

**Division of Mental Health & Substance Abuse
Services**
600 South Second Street
Suite 1D
Bismarck, ND 58504-5729
(701) 328-8940 or (800) 755-2719

OHIO

Department of Mental Health
30 East Broad Street
Eighth Floor
Columbus, OH 43215
(614) 466-2337
http://www.mh.state.oh.us

OKLAHOMA

**Department of Mental Health and Substance
Abuse Services**
P.O. Box 53277, Capitol Station
Oklahoma City, OK 73152
(405) 522-3908 or (800) 522-9054 or (800) 522-
7233 (Domestic Violence Safeline)
http://www.odmhsas.org

OREGON

Oregon Department of Human Services
Mental Health and Addiction Services
500 Summer Street NE
E86

Salem, OK 97301
(503) 945-5763 or (503) 947-5330 (TDD)
http://www.dhs.state.or.us/mentalhealth/

PENNSYLVANIA

**Office of Mental Health and Substance Abuse
Services**
P.O. Box 2675
Harrisburg, PA 17105-2675
(717) 787-6443 or (877) 356-5355
http://www.dpw.state.pa.us/omhsas/dpwmh.asp

RHODE ISLAND

**Department of Mental Health, Mental
Retardation and Hospitals**
14 Harrington Road
Cranston, RI 02920
(401) 462-3201
http://www.mhrh.state.ri.us

SOUTH CAROLINA

Department of Mental Health
P.O. Box 485
2414 Bull Street
Columbia, SC 29202
(803) 898-8581
http://www.state.sc.us/dmh

SOUTH DAKOTA

Division of Mental Health
Department of Human Services
Hillsview Plaza, East Highway 34
c/o 500 East Capitol
Pierre, SD 57501-5070
(605) 773-5991 or (800) 265-9684
http://www.state.sd.us/dhs/dmh

TENNESSEE

**Department of Mental Health and
Developmental Disabilities**
Third Floor, Cordell Hull Building
425 Fifth Avenue North
Nashville, TN 37243
(615) 532-6500
http://www.state.tn.us/mental/

TEXAS

**Texas Department of Mental Health and
Mental Retardation**
Central Office
909 West Forty Fifth Street

Austin, TX 78751
(512) 454-3761 or (800) 252-8154
http://www.mhmr.state.tx.us

UTAH

Division of Mental Health
Department of Human Services
120 North 200 West, Fourth Floor
Suite 415
Salt Lake City, UT 84103
(801) 538-4270
http://www.hsmh.state.ut.us

VERMONT

Department of Developmental and Mental Health Services
Weeks Building
103 South Main Street
Waterbury, VT 05671-1601
(802) 241-2610
http://www.state.vt.us/dmh

VIRGINIA

Department of Mental Health, Mental Retardation and Substance Abuse Services
P.O. Box 1797
Richmond, VA 23218
(804) 786-3921 or (804) 371-8977 (TDD)
http://www.dmhmrsas.state.va.us/

WASHINGTON

Mental Health Division
Department of Social and Health Services
P.O. Box 45320

Olympia, WA 98504-5320
(360) 902-0790 or (800) 446-0259
http://www.wa.gov/dshs/

WEST VIRGINIA

Bureau for Behavioral Health and Health Facilities
Department of Health and Human Resources
350 Capitol Street
Room 350
Charleston, WV 25301-3702
(304) 558-0627
http://www.wvdhhr.org/

WISCONSIN

Bureau of Community Mental Health
Department of Health and Family Services
P.O. Box 7851
1 West Wilson Street
Room 433
Madison, WI 53702-7851
(608) 267-7792
http://www.dhfs.state.wi.us/mentalhealth

WYOMING

Mental Health Division
Department of Health
6101 Yellowstone Road
Room 259-B
Cheyenne, WY 82002
(307) 777-7094
http://mhd.state.wy.us/

APPENDIX VI

USE OF SELECTED SUBSTANCES IN THE PAST MONTH BY PERSONS 12 YEARS OF AGE AND OLDER, BY AGE, SEX, RACE, AND HISPANIC ORIGIN: UNITED STATES, SELECTED YEARS, 1999–2001 (PERCENT OF POPULATION)

	Any Illicit Drug			Marijuana			Heavy Alcohol Use		
	1999	2000	2001	1999	2000	2001	1999	2000	2001
Age									
12–13 years	3.9	3.0	3.8	1.5	1.1	1.5	0.2	0.2	0.2
14–15 years	9.8	9.8	10.9	6.9	6.9	7.6	1.6	1.8	1.7
16–17 years	15.4	16.4	17.6	13.2	13.7	14.9	5.4	6.0	5.7
18–25 years	16.4	15.9	18.8	14.2	13.6	16.0	13.3	12.8	13.6
26–34 years	6.8	7.6	8.8	5.4	5.9	6.8	7.5	7.6	7.8
35 years+	3.4	3.3	3.5	2.2	2.3	2.4	4.2	4.1	4.2
Sex									
Male	8.1	7.7	8.7	6.5	6.2	7.0	9.2	8.7	9.2
Female	4.6	5.0	5.5	3.1	3.5	3.8	2.4	2.7	2.6
Race and ethnicity									
White Only	6.2	6.4	7.2	4.7	4.9	5.6	6.2	6.2	6.4
Black or African American only	7.5	6.4	7.4	5.9	5.2	5.6	3.6	4.0	4.1
American Indian and Alaska Native only	10.4	12.6	9.9	6.9	10.1	8.0	5.8	7.2	7.1
Native Hawaiian and Other Pacific Islander only	Not available	6.2	7.5	Not available	2.5	7.1	Not available	Not available	4.0
Asian only	3.2	2.7	2.8	2.3	2.3	1.4	2.5	1.4	1.5
2 or more races	10.3	14.8	12.6	8.5	12.5	9.6	7.7	5.2	6.7
Hispanic or Latino, any race	6.1	5.3	6.4	4.2	3.6	4.2	5.4	4.4	4.4

Source: Fried, V. M., et al. *Chartbook on Trends in the Health of Americans. Health, United States, 2003.* Hyattsville, Md.: National Center for Health Statistics, 2003.

APPENDIX VII
PERCENT DISTRIBUTION OF CURRENT CIGARETTE SMOKING STATUS FOR ADULTS AGED 18 YEARS AND OVER, BY SELECTED CHARACTERISTICS: UNITED STATES, AVERAGE ANNUAL 1997–1998

Selected Characteristic	Total	Nonsmoker	Nondaily Smoker	Daily Smoker
Age				
18–24 years	100.0	71.7	6.1	22.2
25–44 years	100.0	72.0	5.4	22.7
45–64 years	100.0	75.3	3/5	21.2
65–74 years	100.0	85.0	2.3	12.7
75 years and older	100.0	93.2	1.0	5.8
Race and ethnicity				
Hispanic	100.0	81.1	5.8	13.2
White non-Hispanic	100.0	74.6	3.9	21.5
African-American non-Hispanic	100.0	74.5	5.7	19.7
Asian/Pacific Islander, non-Hispanic	100.0	85.9	3.1	11.0
Education				
Less than high school graduate	100.0	65.6	5.1	29.2
GED diploma	100.0	55.7	4.1	40.2
High school graduate	100.0	71.8	4.3	24.0
Some college, no degree	100.0	75.7	4.8	19.5
Associate of arts degree	100.0	77.3	4.4	18.3
Bachelor of arts or science degree	100.0	87.3	3.6	9.1
Master's, doctorate, or medical degree	100.0	91.6	3.5	4.9
Poverty status				
Below poverty level	100.0	66.4	5.4	28.2
Poverty–1.99 times poverty level	100.0	68.9	4.6	26.5
2.00–3.99 times poverty level	100.0	74.2	4.2	21.6
4.00 times poverty level or more	100.0	81.5	3.9	14.5
Marital Status				
Never married	100.0	73.9	5.7	20.4
Married	100.0	79.2	3.5	17.3
Cohabiting	100.0	60.1	5.8	34.1
Divorced or separated	100.0	63.7	5.4	30.9
Widowed	100.0	68.8	4.7	26.6

Selected Characteristic	Total	Nonsmoker	Nondaily Smoker	Daily Smoker
Region				
Northeast	100.0	76.1	4.4	19.4
Midwest	100.0	74.0	4.5	21.5
South	100.0	74.6	4.1	21.3
West	100.0	80.0	4.2	15.8

Source: Schoenborn, Charlotte A., Jackline L. Vickerie, and Patricia Barnes. *Cigarette Smoking Behavior of Adults: United States, 1997–98,* Advance data from Vital and Health Statistics Series, no. 331, Centers for Disease Control and Prevention, February 7, 2003.

APPENDIX VIII
CIGARETTE SMOKING AMONG MEN, WOMEN, HIGH SCHOOL STUDENTS, AND MOTHERS DURING PREGNANCY: PERCENTAGES, UNITED STATES, 1990–2001

Year	Men	Women	High School Students	Mothers During Pregnancy
1990	28.0	22.9	—	18.4
1991	27.6	23.5	27.5	17.8
1992	28.1	24.6	—	16.9
1993	27.3	22.6	30.5	15.8
1994	27.6	23.1	—	14.6
1995	26.5	22.7	34.8	13.9
1996	—	—	—	13.6
1997	27.1	22.2	36.4	13.2
1998	25.9	22.1	—	12.9
1999	25.2	21.6	34.8	12.6
2000	25.2	21.1	—	12.2
2001	24.7	20.8	28.5	12.0

— Data not available

APPENDIX IX

USE OF SELECTED SUBSTANCES BY HIGH SCHOOL SENIORS, EIGHTH AND 10TH GRADERS, ACCORDING TO SEX AND RACE, UNITED STATES, SELECTED YEARS 1991–2002

Substance, Sex, Race, and Grade in School	1991	1995	1998	1999	2000	2001	2002
Cocaine							
All seniors	1.4	1.8	2.4	2.6	2.1	2.1	2.3
Male	1.7	2.2	3.0	3.3	2.7	2.5	2.7
Female	0.9	1.3	1.7	1.8	1.6	1.6	1.8
White	1.3	1.7	2.7	2.8	2.2	2.3	2.8
African American	0.8	0.4	0.4	0.5	1.0	0.6	0.2
All 10th graders	0.7	1.7	2.1	1.9	1.8	1.3	1.6
Male	0.7	1.8	2.3	2.2	2.1	1.5	1.6
Female	0.6	1.5	1.8	1.6	1.4	1.2	1.4
White	0.6	1.7	2.0	1.9	1.7	1.2	1.7
African American	0.2	0.4	0.8	0.3	0.4	0.3	0.4
All eighth graders	0.5	1.2	1.4	1.3	1.2	1.2	1.1
Male	0.7	1.1	1.5	1.4	1.3	1.1	1.1
Female	0.4	1.2	1.2	1.2	1.1	1.2	1.1
White	0.4	1.0	1.0	1.1	1.1	1.1	1.0
African American	0.4	0.4	0.6	0.3	0.5	0.4	0.5
Inhalants							
All seniors	2.4	3.2	2.3	2.0	2.2	1.7	1.5
Male	3.3	3.9	2.9	2.5	2.9	2.3	2.2
Female	1.6	2.5	1.7	1.5	1.7	1.1	0.6
White	2.4	3.7	2.6	2.1	2.1	1.8	1.3
African American	1.5	1.1	1.0	0.4	2.1	1.3	1.2
All 10th graders	2.7	3.5	2.9	2.6	2.6	2.5	2.4
Male	2.9	3.8	3.2	2.9	3.0	2.5	2.3
Female	2.6	3.2	2.6	2.2	2.2	2.4	2.4
White	2.9	3.9	3.3	2.9	2.8	2.5	2.6
African American	2.0	1.2	1.1	0.8	1.5	0.9	1.5
All eighth graders	4.4	6.1	4.8	5.0	4.5	4.0	3.8

(continues)

(continued)

Substance, Sex, Race, and Grade in School	1991	1995	1998	1999	2000	2001	2002
Male	4.1	5.6	4.8	4.6	4.1	3.6	3.5
Female	4.7	6.6	4.7	5.3	4.8	4.3	3.9
White	4.5	7.0	5.3	5.6	4.5	4.1	3.9
African American	2.3	2.3	2.2	2.3	2.3	2.6	2.7
MDMA* (Ecstasy)							
All seniors	—	—	1.5	2.5	3.6	2.8	2.4
Male	—	—	2.3	2.6	4.1	3.7	2.6
Female	—	—	0.8	2.5	3.1	2.0	2.1
White	—	—	1.3	2.1	2.5	2.6	2.3
African American	—	—	0.2	0.0	1.9	0.9	0.5
All 10th graders	—	—	1.3	1.8	2.6	2.6	1.8
Male	—	—	1.4	1.7	2.5	3.5	1.6
Female	—	—	1.1	1.9	2.5	1.6	1.8
White	—	—	1.3	2.1	2.5	2.6	2.3
African American	—	—	0.7	0.3	1.8	1.0	0.5
All eighth graders	—	—	0.9	0.8	1.4	1.8	1.4
Male	—	—	1.0	0.9	1.6	1.9	1.5
Female	—	—	0.7	0.7	1.2	1.8	1.3
White	—	—	0.9	0.9	1.4	2.0	1.0
African American	—	—	0.4	0.4	0.8	1.1	0.6

* MDMA methylenedioxymethamphetamine
Source: Fried, V. M., et al. *Chartbook on Trends in the Health of Americans. Health, United States, 2003.* Hyattsville, Md.: Washington, D.C. National Center for Health Statistics, 2003.

APPENDIX X

PERCENTAGE OF HIGH SCHOOL STUDENTS WHO USED COCAINE AND WHO INJECTED ILLEGAL DRUGS, BY SEX, SELECTED U.S. STATES, YOUTH RISK BEHAVIOR SURVEY, 2003

State Surveys	Lifetime Cocaine Use		Current Cocaine Use		Lifetime Illegal Injected Drug Use	
	Female	Male	Female	Male	Female	Male
Alabama	7.0	7.1	2.7	3.6	0.5	2.8
Alaska	5.2	7.7	1.7	3.2	1.0	2.2
Arizona	13.5	11.9	6.6	5.1	1.7	2.4
Delaware	6.4	8.3	2.4	5.0	0.9	2.4
Florida	6.8	9.3	2.9	5.1	1.7	4.1
Georgia	6.3	7.8	2.5	3.7	1.6	1.9
Idaho	5.4	6.7	1.3	2.6	1.3	1.7
Indiana	7.1	8.7	2.6	3.6	0.8	2.4
Kentucky	9.3	9.8	3.0	4.5	2.7	3.4
Maine	5.2	11.0	1.9	4.7	1.7	3.3
Massachusetts	6.9	9.8	n/a	n/a	1.5	2.9
Michigan	7.8	9.3	3.2	4.5	2.3	2.4
Mississippi	4.7	6.7	1.6	3.0	1.2	3.2
Missouri	6.7	6.4	2.4	2.7	1.5	1.0
Montana	8.8	8.6	3.0	4.3	2.0	2.8
Nebraska	7.0	6.7	2.4	3.3	1.2	2.7
Nevada	12.3	9.6	5.1	3.7	3.3	3.4
New Hampshire	10.0	10.3	3.4	4.6	1.3	2.2
New York	5.7	6.6	2.0	2.8	0.8	2.1
North Carolina	7.6	9.0	2.8	2.6	1.5	3.3
North Dakota	7.6	11.4	n/a	n/a	n/a	n/a
Ohio	8.0	8.4	3.6	3.2	1.5	2.9
Oklahoma	8.4	9.8	2.8	3.9	1.6	3.1
Rhode Island	5.0	7.4	3.2	5.2	1.5	3.9
South Dakota	7.2	7.6	2.9	4.2	1.2	3.4
Tennessee	8.0	10.2	3.6	5.0	1.6	3.6
Texas	10.2	13.7	4.3	6.5	1.2	2.5
Utah	5.0	9.1	2.2	6.0	1.6	4.9

(continues)

(continued)

State Surveys	Lifetime Cocaine Use		Current Cocaine Use		Lifetime Illegal Injected Drug Use	
	Female	Male	Female	Male	Female	Male
Vermont	n/a	n/a	3.5	6.5	1.7	3.1
West Virginia	12.1	9.8	5.4	4.7	1.4	3.1
Wisconsin	8.9	10.8	3.5	4.5	n/a	n/a
Wyoming	10.5	10.8	3.8	4.6	3.1	2.9

n/a: not available

Source: Centers for Disease Control and Prevention. "Youth Risk Behavior Surveillance—United States, 2003," *Morbidity and Mortality Weekly Report* 53, no. SS-2 (May 21, 2004): 60.

APPENDIX XI
PERCENTAGE OF HIGH SCHOOL STUDENTS WHO USED MARIJUANA, BY SEX, SELECTED U.S. STATES, YOUTH RISK BEHAVIOR SURVEY, 2003

State	Lifetime Marijuana Use		Current Marijuana Use	
	Female	Male	Female	Male
Alabama	35.0	37.1	16.9	18.4
Alaska	42.7	51.6	21.2	25.9
Arizona	42.1	48.6	22.7	24.7
Delaware	47.2	50.3	25.0	29.5
Florida	37.8	43.5	19.1	23.7
Georgia	33.1	43.1	15.4	23.7
Idaho	28.1	32.8	11.9	17.3
Indiana	37.7	48.8	18.9	25.3
Kentucky	41.1	45.4	19.5	22.5
Maine	n/a	n/a	20.9	31.4
Massachusetts	44.2	49.3	24.9	30.6
Michigan	41.2	46.7	22.5	25.5
Mississippi	30.7	46.9	14.5	27.0
Missouri	39.8	42.9	20.4	23.1
Montana	41.5	46.3	19.9	25.8
Nebraska	32.9	36.2	16.0	20.5
Nevada	48.9	44.4	22.2	22.3
New Hampshire	45.0	54.0	28.2	32.9
New York	32.5	41.6	17.4	23.8
North Carolina	38.4	46.9	20.7	27.9
North Dakota	n/a	n/a	20.7	27.9
Ohio	36.5	37.4	21.2	21.6
Oklahoma	36.8	48.3	19.0	25.2
Rhode Island	43.8	44.4	26.4	28.6
South Dakota	34.7	38.6	20.8	22.2
Tennessee	38.4	48.3	19.8	27.3
Texas	35.5	45.9	16.5	24.0
Utah	19.1	24.0	8.6	14.0
Vermont	n/a	n/a	26.3	30.0

(continues)

(continued)

State	Lifetime Marijuana Use		Current Marijuana Use	
	Female	Male	Female	Male
West Virginia	43.2	44.1	22.7	23.6
Wisconsin	35.5	40.5	19.2	24.3
Wyoming	36.1	42.4	17.4	23.4

n/a: not available

Source: Centers for Disease Control and Prevention. "Youth Risk Behavior Surveillance—United States, 2003," *Morbidity and Mortality Weekly Report* 53, no. SS-2 (May 21, 2004): 58.

APPENDIX XII
PERCENTAGE OF HIGH SCHOOL STUDENTS WHO DRANK ALCOHOL, BY SEX, SELECTED U.S. STATES, YOUTH RISK BEHAVIOR SURVEY, 2003

State	Lifetime Alcohol Use		Current Alcohol Use		Episodic Heavy Drinking*	
	Female	Male	Female	Male	Female	Male
Alabama	72.4	69.1	40.5	39.9	21.9	26.4
Alaska	75.3	74.6	37.4	39.6	23.4	29.1
Arizona	80.1	76.6	51.0	50.7	31.8	35.5
Delaware	80.8	76.0	46.9	43.7	23.9	29.3
Florida	74.1	73.0	43.8	41.9	20.5	25.9
Georgia	70.9	73.5	36.0	39.5	16.4	23.2
Idaho	61.4	61.8	34.0	35.4	21.7	25.0
Indiana	78.2	77.4	45.4	44.5	27.8	29.9
Kentucky	79.7	73.6	44.2	46.3	32.3	33.4
Maine	n/a	n/a	41.3	42.8	22.6	31.5
Massachusetts	78.0	74.6	46.0	45.4	25.2	28.6
Michigan	77.5	74.2	45.6	42.3	26.8	27.9
Mississippi	75.1	76.3	40.0	44.0	22.1	27.3
Missouri	80.4	75.2	48.5	49.7	30.5	30.5
Montana	79.5	82.5	48.9	49.6	34.9	39.1
Nebraska	79.3	77.6	49.3	43.8	31.6	32.6
Nevada	78.0	73.3	46.3	40.5	28.9	26.7
New Hampshire	76.3	74.5	46.9	47.1	27.9	33.5
New York	75.2	73.3	45.0	43.1	23.0	27.5
North Carolina	n/a	n/a	37.3	41.5	16.7	25.1
North Dakota	n/a	n/a	55.8	52.6	38.7	40.1
Ohio	75.3	75.9	40.7	43.7	22.5	30.4
Oklahoma	76.8	80.4	44.1	51.1	28.5	39.2
Rhode Island	77.2	73.8	46.6	42.2	25.2	28.0
South Dakota	75.8	76.1	49.9	50.4	36.4	40.0
Tennessee	73.0	75.1	39.5	42.7	21.6	29.3
Texas	78.9	74.9	43.3	42.5	23/7	27.4
Utah	42.3	44.1	19.5	22.8	13.6	14.8
Vermont	n/a	n/a	42.0	43.9	24.5	28.2

(continues)

(continued)

State	Lifetime Alcohol Use		Current Alcohol Use		Episodic Heavy Drinking*	
	Female	Male	Female	Male	Female	Male
West Virginia	78.8	73.7	45.6	43.3	32.7	34.2
Wisconsin	n/a	n/a	47.1	47.3	25.8	30.3
Wyoming	76.4	76.1	49.0	49.2	33.8	35.7

* Current episodic heavy drinking is drinking five or more drinks in a row on one or more days in the past 30 days preceding the survey.
n/a: not available
Source: Centers for Disease Control and Prevention. "Youth Risk Behavior Surveillance—United States, 2003," *Morbidity and Mortality Weekly Report* 53, no. SS-2 (May 21, 2004): 58.

APPENDIX XIII

PERCENTAGE OF HIGH SCHOOL STUDENTS WHO USED SMOKELESS TOBACCO, SMOKED CIGARS, AND USED ANY TOBACCO, BY SEX, SELECTED U.S. STATES, YOUTH RISK BEHAVIOR SURVEY, 2003

State	Current Smokeless Tobacco Use		Current Cigar Use		Current Tobacco Use*	
	Female	Male	Female	Male	Female	Male
Alabama	0.7	19.7	10.0	15.7	28.3	34.7
Alaska	6.2	15.6	3.5	11.7	23.1	26.6
Arizona	1.3	8.4	8.7	20.0	23.0	28.3
Delaware	0.9	5.8	8.5	15.6	26.8	26.1
Florida	1.3	8.1	8.2	18.5	19.7	25.7
Georgia	1.3	13.9	9.3	18.5	20.6	31.7
Idaho	2.0	9.0	4.0	12.9	15.0	20.3
Indiana	1.2	13.1	8.0	21.0	27.0	34.0
Kentucky	3.4	23.5	12.6	24.2	37.6	44.5
Maine	0.9	7.4	5.0	16.5	20.4	26.6
Massachusetts	1.7	6/4	6.3	17.3	24.0	26.7
Michigan	2.9	10.0	8.3	18.5	26.3	28.5
Mississippi	1.0	15.5	11.4	25.7	26.0	41.2
Missouri	0.9	10.3	9.2	17.4	28.0	31.4
Montana	5.3	20.4	9.4	18.4	27.1	34.4
Nebraska	2.8	17.0	11.7	24.2	28.0	33.5
Nevada	1.1	6.1	n/a	n/a	n/a	n/a
New Hampshire	1.1	7.3	5.2	21.0	21.4	29.8
New York	1.6	6.7	3.9	13.0	21.4	24.1
North Carolina	n/a	n/a	n/a	n/a	n/a	n/a
North Dakota	4.1	15.9	8.5	17.0	31.9	26.0
Ohio	3.0	12.8	9.6	16.9	26.2	20.1
Oklahoma	1.7	23.0	9.6	24.7	25.9	42.1
Rhode Island	2.0	7.0	6.4	14.2	23.4	23.2
South Dakota	6.7	23.5	6.8	20.5	31.4	40.4
Tennessee	2.7	21.4	10.1	22.8	30.4	40.5
Texas	1.6	11.6	10.0	18.9	24.8	12.4
Utah	1.2	4.9	3.5	10.9	8.0	12.4
Vermont	1.3	8.7	6.0	17.4	25.1	28.6

(continues)

(continued)

State	Current Smokeless Tobacco Use		Current Cigar Use		Current Tobacco Use*	
	Female	Male	Female	Male	Female	Male
West Virginia	3.3	23.3	8.1	18.3	33.3	36.7
Wisconsin	2.4	13.1	n/a	n/a	n/a	n/a
Wyoming	5.0	21.1	6.3	22.5	36.9	36.9

* Current tobacco use is smoked cigarettes or cigars or used chewing tobacco, snuff, or dip on one or more of the 30 days preceding the survey.
n/a: not available
Source: Centers for Disease Control and Prevention. "Youth Risk Behavior Surveillance—United States, 2003," *Morbidity and Mortality Weekly Report* 53, no. SS-2 (May 21, 2004): 54.

APPENDIX XIV
PERCENTAGES OF LIFETIME USERS OF SPECIFIC HALLUCINOGENS, 2001

Hallucinogen	Total	Ages 12–17	Ages 18–25	Ages 26+
PCP*	12.5	5.7	22.1	11.9
LSD†	9.0	3.1	15.3	2.9
Peyote	2.3	0.4	1.8	2.6
Mescaline	3.5	0.3	2.5	4.1
Psilocybin	6.6	2.1	12.2	6.3
Ecstasy (MDMA‡)	3.6	3.2	13.1	2.0

* phencyclidine
†lysergic acid diethylamide
‡methylenedioxymethamphetamine
Source: National Household Survey on Drug Abuse. Rockville, Md.: Office of Applied Studies, Substance Abuse and Mental Health Services Administration, 2001.

APPENDIX XV
RECEIVED SUBSTANCE USE TREATMENT IN THE PAST YEAR AMONG PERSONS AGES 12 OR OLDER, BY DEMOGRAPHIC CHARACTERISTICS: PERCENTAGES, 2002

Demographic Characteristic	Substance for Which Treatment Was Received in Past Year			
	Any Illicit Drug	Alcohol	Both Any Illicit Drug and Alcohol	Any Illicit Drug or Alcohol
Total	0.9	1.0	0.6	1.5
Age				
12–17	1.0	0.9	0.7	1.5
18–25	1.3	1.5	0.8	2.2
26 or older	0.7	1.0	0.5	1.4
Gender				
Male	1.1	1.5	0.8	2.1
Female	0.6	0.5	0.3	0.9
Race and ethnicity				
White	0.8	1.1	0.5	1.4
African American	1.6	1.3	1.1	2.2
American Indian or Alaska Native	2.6	2.8	2.0	4.8
Native Hawaiian or other Pacific Islander	0.4	0.3	0.3	0.5
Asian	0.2	0.2	0.1	0.2
Two or more races	1.5	0.9	0.7	2.1
Hispanic or Latino	0.9	0.8	0.5	1.3

Source: Substance Abuse and Mental Health Services Administration (SAMHSA). *Results from the 2002 National Survey on Drug Use and Health: National Findings.* NSDA Series H-22, DHHS Publication No. SMA 03-3836. Rockville, Md.: Office of Applied Studies, SAMHSA, September 2003.

APPENDIX XVI
NEEDED AND RECEIVED TREATMENT FOR AN ILLICIT DRUG PROBLEM IN THE PAST YEAR AMONG PERSONS AGES 12 AND OLDER, BY DEMOGRAPHIC CHARACTERISTICS: PERCENTAGES

Demographic Characteristic	Needed Treatment for an Illicit Drug Problem in the Past Year			
	Total	Received Treatment at a Specialty Facility	Did not Receive Treatment at a Specialty Facility	Received Treatment at a Specialty Facility Among Persons Who Needed Treatment
Total	3.3	0.6	2.7	18.2
Age				
12–17	5.7	0.6	5.1	10.1
18–25	8.6	0.9	7.7	10.7
26 or older	2.0	0.5	1.5	26.9
Gender				
Male	4.3	0.7	3.6	17.0
Female	2.4	0.5	1.9	20.4
Race or ethnicity				
White	3.0	0.5	2.5	17.9
African American	4.7	1.1	3.6	22.8
Hispanic or Latino	4.0	0.6	3.4	14.9

Source: Substance Abuse and Mental Health Services Administration (SAMHSA). *Results from the 2002 National Survey on Drug Use and Health: National Findings.* NSDA Series H-22, DHHS Publication No. SMA 03-3836. Rockville, Md.: Office of Applied Studies, SAMHSA, September 2003.

APPENDIX XVII
NEEDED AND RECEIVED TREATMENT FOR AN ALCOHOL PROBLEM IN THE PAST YEAR AMONG PERSONS AGES 12 AND OLDER, BY DEMOGRAPHIC CHARACTERISTICS: PERCENTAGES

Demographic Characteristic	Needed Treatment for an Alcohol Problem in the Past Year			Received Treatment at a Specialty Facility
	Total	Received Treatment at a Specialty Facility	Did not Receive Treatment at a Specialty Facility	
Total	7.9	0.7	7.3	8.3
Age				
12–17	6.0	0.5	5.6	8.1
18–25	18.0	0.9	17.1	4.8
26 or older	6.4	0.6	5.8	10.0
Gender				
Male	11.2	1.0	10.2	8.7
Female	4.9	0.4	4.5	7.5
Race or ethnicity				
White	8.0	0.7	7.4	8.4
African American	7.4	0.9	6.6	11.8
Two or more races	10.3	0.7	9.6	6.7
Hispanic or Latino	8.6	0.5	8.1	5.5

Source: Substance Abuse and Mental Health Services Administration (SAMHSA). *Results from the 2002 National Survey on Drug Use and Health: National Findings.* NSDA Series H-22, DHHS Publication No. SMA 03-3836. Rockville, Md.: Office of Applied Studies, SAMHSA, September 2003.

APPENDIX XVIII
SUBSTANCE ABUSE CLIENTS IN SPECIALTY TREATMENT UNITS ACCORDING TO SUBSTANCE ABUSED, GEOGRAPHIC DIVISION, AND STATE, UNITED STATES, 1998–2002, CLIENTS PER 100,000 POPULATION

Geographic Division and State	All Clients			Clients with Both Alcoholism and Drug Abuse			Alcoholism Only Clients			Drug Abuse Only Clients		
	1998	2000	2002	1998	2000	2002	1998	2000	2002	1998	2000	2002
United States	461.9	434.9	488.0	228.6	211.5	235.4	109.8	98.0	103.1	123.5	125.4	149.4
New England	703.7	617.6	648.9	365.5	289.9	291.6	160.8	118.5	126.3	177.4	210.1	231.0
Maine	809.2	462.0	613.0	406.2	241.7	309.3	290.2	152.8	165.9	112.7	67.5	137.9
New Hampshire	338.4	324.1	303.1	174.6	180.7	141.3	132.5	95.8	118.2	31.3	47.6	43.6
Vermont	507.0	536.3	456.2	278.2	275.0	261.3	166.4	198.6	124.0	62.4	62.7	70.9
Massachusetts	824.4	671.4	682.9	461.2	331.1	328.2	171.8	126.4	129.4	191.4	213.8	225.4
Rhode Island	768.0	704.2	689.2	355.4	257.6	212.2	155.0	107.8	143.1	257.5	338.8	334.0
Connecticut	585.5	674.5	754.0	258.4	280.0	303.2	101.0	86.2	104.9	226.1	308.3	345.9
Middle Atlantic	554.3	556.7	650.0	259.7	272.9	319.9	86.7	79.1	82.8	207.9	204.7	247.3
New York	773.0	779.0	925.5	330.2	376.7	456.7	114.2	102.6	115.8	328.6	299.7	353.1
New Jersey	367.1	349.2	461.5	178.6	150.3	189.0	56.3	48.2	47.8	132.2	150.7	224.7
East North Central	473.8	421.0	475.8	224.5	194.1	219.9	141.1	121.4	127.5	108.3	105.5	128.4
Ohio	452.5	409.9	408.2	253.9	226.6	233.0	119.7	105.2	96.0	79.0	78.2	79.2
Indiana	339.7	313.9	548.9	148.8	159.3	277.0	116.4	90.4	148.8	74.5	64.2	123.1
Illinois	466.5	419.8	453.4	230.2	179.0	184.4	113.3	104.3	104.9	122.9	136.4	164.1
Michigan	614.6	541.6	547.4	249.3	217.5	224.8	198.8	171.5	154.9	166.5	152.7	167.7
Wisconsin	431.8	351.6	456.9	189.0	157.4	195.9	172.3	139.2	171.6	70.5	55.0	89.3
West North Central	355.0	322.2	344.9	199.9	179.9	199.3	97.3	79.3	79.4	57.8	63.0	66.3
Minnesota	264.0	205.9	229.6	140.4	100.2	128.7	67.1	54.7	54.3	56.5	51.0	46.6
Iowa	300.9	229.0	334.6	150.5	117.1	189.7	107.9	76.1	88.4	42.4	35.8	56.5
Missouri	387.0	378.9	404.4	249.2	216.9	237.3	73.7	73.1	75.6	64.1	88.9	91.5
North Dakota	549.3	251.6	330.9	258.7	120.4	176.3	224.0	114.4	116.0	66.6	16.8	38.6
South Dakota	445.9	290.6	407.8	201.9	148.4	216.1	211.2	115.9	149.3	32.8	26.4	42.4

(continues)

(continued)

Geographic Division and State	All Clients			Clients with Both Alcoholism and Drug Abuse			Alcoholism Only Clients			Drug Abuse Only Clients		
	1998	2000	2002	1998	2000	2002	1998	2000	2002	1998	2000	2002
Nebraska	396.2	323.1	374.2	220.2	162.5	238.5	122.4	96.6	76.5	53.6	64.0	59.3
Kansas	411.6	544.7	408.9	231.0	351.7	235.0	109.1	111.1	95.3	71.6	81.9	78.6
South Atlantic	382.0	406.1	427.0	191.7	199.9	196.4	94.2	99.1	88.6	96.0	107.1	142.0
Delaware	603.5	589.8	623.2	306.3	371.3	473.3	127.5	122.5	60.5	169.6	96.0	89.4
Maryland	557.6	696.6	808.1	256.0	293.3	327.5	117.2	133.0	153.2	184.3	270.3	327.4
District of Columbia	1,447.8	1,395.4	1,309.5	879.7	616.3	569.2	199.6	195.8	135.3	368.5	583.2	605.0
Virginia	364.5	388.1	391.3	184.9	205.9	185.6	102.3	103.1	98.4	77.3	79.2	107.2
West Virginia	295.8	317.4	304.6	103.5	123.2	157.8	142.0	143.2	89.0	50.3	51.0	57.9
North Carolina	402.0	471.8	407.1	214.6	237.6	203.1	115.5	140.6	96.6	71.9	93.6	107.4
South Carolina	306.6	414.1	339.0	116.3	191.5	162.6	112.6	138.0	102.5	77.6	84.6	73.9
Georgia	252.0	199.3	276.9	115.5	100.5	135.6	65.4	47.5	67.6	71.1	51.3	73.6
Florida	365.1	352.3	398.4	199.1	185.0	171.3	70.2	71.8	65.2	95.8	95.4	162.0
East South Central	327.8	307.8	301.5	151.8	136.7	141.1	89.1	79.9	70.0	86.9	91.1	90.4
Kentucky	442.4	534.6	541.6	199.1	236.8	247.5	161.4	178.1	162.1	81.9	119.6	132.1
Tennessee	280.0	195.5	201.2	110.9	77.8	94.0	71.4	42.4	33.2	97.7	75.3	74.1
Alabama	244.8	233.0	254.1	117.1	81.7	110.4	47.4	37.7	43.2	80.3	113.6	100.5
Mississippi	391.3	328.7	237.6	221.7	199.0	134.3	86.7	80.0	58.1	83.0	49.7	45.2
West South Central	329.3	268.8	244.3	186.1	150.0	129.9	63.8	42.2	37.6	79.5	76.6	76.8
Arkansas	326.1	141.2	175.5	190.6	73.7	95.6	66.6	22.2	28.7	68.9	45.4	51.3
Louisiana	472.6	311.2	327.6	268.8	157.8	160.6	88.0	42.3	55.2	115.8	111.1	111.8
Oklahoma	315.2	260.9	309.6	125.4	143.2	179.6	96.7	70.6	65.7	93.2	47.0	64.3
Texas	299.7	278.0	224.2	177.3	159.9	119.5	52.1	39.9	30.3	70.3	78.2	74.4
Mountain	584.8	596.8	630.2	278.1	261.2	291.0	175.1	194.5	178.2	131.7	141.2	161.0
Montana	321.9	244.1	318.0	172.8	108.2	190.7	107.8	96.8	83.6	41.3	39.1	43.7
Idaho	278.4	257.2	359.7	178.6	169.5	223.0	58.4	55.9	82.5	41.3	31.9	54.3
Wyoming	406.2	523.9	450.6	193.0	317.7	253.7	160.2	154.5	138.8	53.0	51.7	58.1
Colorado	722.4	843.4	909.4	326.7	333.5	406.5	267.3	351.1	350.4	128.4	158.7	152.5
New Mexico	714.0	669.7	678.7	296.6	281.7	308.6	275.3	215.3	183.7	142.1	172.7	186.4
Arizona	532.6	661.0	668.3	236.5	277.4	276.1	137.9	201.8	148.2	158.2	181.9	244.0
Utah	704.7	409.6	490.4	351.7	206.4	286.9	145.4	79.4	88.2	207.5	123.8	115.4
Nevada	548.4	464.5	428.3	322.2	229.3	170.8	116.7	90.1	95.5	109.5	145.1	162.0
Pacific	525.1	466.4	628.1	256.1	229.8	309.6	120.1	98.2	145.0	148.2	138.4	173.5
Washington	674.8	676.4	745.9	398.4	391.7	429.4	182.7	169.1	189.2	93.7	115.6	127.3
Oregon	653.4	759.7	815.9	347.8	431.4	461.9	138.5	149.4	160.6	167.0	178.9	193.4
California	491.4	401.7	597.3	223.7	180.7	275.3	106.2	79.0	136.6	161.5	142.0	185.4
Alaska	583.0	536.1	564.1	287.8	250.2	317.7	252.2	228.7	198.9	43.0	57.2	47.5
Hawaii	299.6	254.3	346.6	169.1	128.1	169.1	64.6	38.3	72.1	66.0	87.9	105.4

Notes: Estimates for 1998 and 2000 were revised from previous editions of *Chartbook on Trends in the Health of Americans.* Rates for the 1990s are based on postcensus estimates of the resident population 12 years of age and over as of July 1. Client data are as of October 1.
Treatment rates at the state level can vary from year to year for a variety of reasons, including failure of large facilities to respond to the survey in some years and normal variation in the number of people in treatment on a given day.
Source: Fried, V. M., et al. *Chartbook on Trends in the Health of Americans. Health, United States, 2003.* Hyattsville, Md.: National Center for Health Statistics, 2003, p. 266.

BIBLIOGRAPHY

Abbey, Antonia, et al. "Alcohol and Sexual Assault," *Alcohol Research & Health* 25, no. 1 (2001): 43–51.

Aboujaoude, E., N. Gamel, and L. M Koran. "A 1-year Naturalistic Follow-up of Patients with Compulsive Shopping Disorder," *Journal of Clinical Psychiatry* 64, no. 8 (August 2003): 946–950.

Acker, Caroline Jean. *Creating the American Junkie: Addiction Research in the Classic Era of Narcotic Control.* Baltimore, Md.: Johns Hopkins University Press, 2002.

Ahmad, Khabir. "Asia Grapples with Spreading Amphetamine Abuse," *The Lancet* 361, no. 9372 (May 31, 2003): 1,878–1,879.

Annas, George J., M.D. "Reefer Madness—The Federal Response to California's Medical Marijuana Law," *New England Journal of Medicine* 337, no. 6 (August 7, 1997): 435–439.

Annas, George J., M.D. "Testing Poor Pregnant Women for Cocaine—Physicians as Police Investigators," *New England Journal of Medicine* 344, no. 22 (May 31, 2001): 1,729–1,732.

Anthony, James C. and Fernando Echeagaray-Wagner. "Epidemiologic Analysis of Alcohol and Tobacco Use: Patterns of Co-Occurring Consumption and Dependence in the United States," *Alcohol Research & Health* 24, no. 4 (2000): 201–208.

Arnold, Paul D., and Margaret A. Richter. "Is Obsessive-Compulsive Disorder an Autoimmune Disease?" *Canadian Medical Association Journal* 165, no. 10 (2001): 1,353–1,358.

Avants, S. Kelly, et al. "A Randomized Controlled Trial of Auricular Acupuncture for Cocaine Dependence," *Archives of Internal Medicine* 160, no. 21 (August 14–28, 2000): 2,305–2,312.

Baden, Lindsey R., M.D., et al. "Quinolones and False-Positive Urine Screening for Opiates by Immunoassay Technology," *Journal of the American Medical Association* 286, no. 24 (December 26, 2001): 3,115–3,119.

Bagnardi, Vincenzo, et al. "Alcohol Consumption and the Risk of Cancer: A Meta-Analysis," *Alcohol Research & Health* 25, no. 4 (2001): 263–270.

Ballantyne, Jane C., M.D., and Jianren Mao, M.D. "Opioid Therapy for Chronic Pain," *New England Journal of Medicine* 349, no. 20 (November 13, 2003): 1,943–1,953.

Bamber, Diane, Ian M. Cockerill, and Douglas Carroll. "The Pathological Status of Exercise Dependence," *British Journal of Sports Medicine* 34, no. 2 (2000): 125–132.

Barkley, Russell A., et al. "Does the Treatment of Attention Deficit/Hyperactivity Disorder with Stimulants Contribute to Drug Use/Abuse? A 12-Year Prospective Study," *Pediatrics* 111, no. 1 (January 2003): 97–109.

Bassuk, Ellen L., M.D., et al. "Prevalence of Mental Health and Substance Use Disorders Among Homeless and Low-Income Housed Mothers," *American Journal of Psychiatry* 155, no. 11 (November 1998): 1,561–1,564.

Bayard, Max, et al. "Alcohol Withdrawal Syndrome," *American Family Physician* 69, no. 6 (March 15, 2004): 1,443–1,450.

Becker, Anne E., M.D. "Eating Disorders," *New England Journal of Medicine* 340, no. 14 (April 8, 1999): 1,092–1,098.

Bejerot, S., and M. Humble. "Low Prevalence of Smoking Among Patients with Obsessive-Compulsive Disorder," *Comprehensive Psychiatry* 40, no. 4 (July/August 1999): 268–272.

Bennett, Joel B., and Wayne E. Lehham. *Preventing Workplace Substance Abuse: Beyond Drug Testing to Wellness.* Washington, D.C.: American Psychological Association, 2003.

Biederman, J., et al. "Protective Effects of ADHD Pharmacotherapy on Subsequent Substance

Abuse: A Longitudinal Study," *Pediatrics* 104, no. 2 (August 1999): e20.

Biederman, Joseph, M.D., et al. "Patterns of Alcohol and Drug Use in Adolescents Can Be Predicted by Parental Substance Use Disorders," *Pediatrics* 106, no. 4 (October 2000): 792–797.

Bierut, Laura Jean, M.D., et al. "Co-Occurring Risk Factors for Alcohol Dependence and Habitual Smoking: Results from the Collaborative Study on the Genetics of Alcoholism," *Alcohol Research & Health* 24, no. 4 (2000): 233–241.

Bierut, Laura Jean, M.D., et al. "Defining Alcohol-Related Phenotypes in Humans: The Collaborative Study on the Genetics of Alcoholism," *Alcohol Research & Health* 26, no. 3 (2002): 208–213.

Black, Donald W., M.D., and Trent Moyer. "Clinical Features and Psychiatric Comorbidity of Subjects with Pathological Gambling Behavior," *Psychiatric Services* 49, no. 11 (November 1998): 1,434–1,439.

Black, Donald W., M.D., et al. "Family History and Psychiatric Comorbidity in Persons with Compulsive Buying: Preliminary Findings," *American Journal of Psychiatry* 155, no. 7 (July 1998): 960–963.

Bloomfield, Kim, et al. "International Comparisons of Alcohol Consumption," *Alcohol Research & Health* 27, no. 1 (2003): 95–109.

Blow, Frederic C., and Kristen Lawton Barry. "Use and Misuse of Alcohol Among Older Women," *Alcohol Research & Health* 26, no. 4 (2002): 308–315.

Bobo, Janet K., and Corinne Husten, M.D. "Sociocultural Influences on Smoking and Drinking," *Alcohol Research & Health* 24, no. 4 (2000): 225–232

Bovasso, Gregory B. "Cannabis Abuse as a Risk Factor for Depressive Symptoms," *American Journal of Psychiatry* 158, no. 12 (December 2001): 2,033–2,037.

Brewer, Robert D., et al. "The Risk of Dying in Alcohol-Related Automobile Crashes Among Habitual Drunk Drivers," *New England Journal of Medicine* 331, no. 8 (August 25, 1994): 513–517.

Brookoff, Daniel, et al. "Testing Reckless Drivers for Cocaine and Marijuana," *New England Journal of Medicine* 331, no. 8 (August 25, 1994): 518–522.

Caetano, Raul, M.D., John Schafer, and Carol B. Cunradi. "Alcohol-Related Intimate Partner Violence Among White, Black, and Hispanic Couples in the United States," *Alcohol Research & Health* 25, no. 1 (2001): 58–65.

Cami, Jodi, M.D., and Magi Farre, M.D. "Drug Addiction," *New England Journal of Medicine* 349, no. 10 (September 4, 2003): 975–986.

Campbell, Lucien B. and Henry J. Bemporad. "An Introduction to Federal Guideline Sentencing," Available online. URL: http://www.ussc.gov/TRAINING/intro8.pdf. Accessed on June 18, 2004.

Carnes, Patrick. *Don't Call It Love: Recovery from Sexual Addiction.* New York, N.Y.: Bantam Books, 1991.

Centers for Disease Control and Prevention. "State-Specific Prevalence of Selected Chronic Disease-Related Characteristics—Behavioral Risk Factor Surveillance System, 2001," *Morbidity and Mortality Weekly Report* 52, no. SS-8 (August 22, 2003): 1–80.

Centers for Disease Control and Prevention. "Viral Hepatitis Surveillance: Disease Burden from Hepatitis A, B, and C in the United States," Available online. URL: http://www.cdc.gov/ncidod/diseases/hepatitis/resource/dz_burden02.htm. Accessed on October 1, 2004.

Chen, Wei Jung A., et al. "Alcohol and the Developing Brain: Neuroanatomical Studies," *Alcohol Research & Health* 27, no. 2 (2003): 174–180.

Clark, Duncan B., M.D., Michael Banyukov, and Jack Cornelius, M.D. "Childhood Antisocial Behavior and Adolescent Alcohol Use Disorders," *Alcohol Research & Health* 26, no. 2 (2002): 109–115.

Clark, Kathryn Anderson, et al. "Treatment Compliance among Prenatal Care Patients with Substance Abuse Problems," *American Journal of Drug and Alcohol Abuse.* Available online. URL: http://www.findarticles.com/cf_dls/m0978/1_27/75119727/print.jhtml. Accessed February 27, 2004.

Clark, Robin E., Judith Freeman Clark, with Christine Adamec. *The Encyclopedia of Child Abuse, 2nd ed.* New York: Facts On File, Inc., 2000.

Cnattingius, Sven, M.D., et al. "Caffeine Intake and the Risk of First-Trimester Spontaneous Abortion," *New England Journal of Medicine* 343, no. 25 (December 21, 2000): 1,839–1,945.

Collins, R. Lorraine and Lily D. McNair. "Minority Women and Alcohol Use," *Alcohol Research & Health* 26, no. 4 (2002): 251–256.

Committee on Adolescence, American Academy of Pediatrics. "Care of the Adolescent Sexual Assault Victim," *Pediatrics* 107, no. 6 (June 2001): 1,476–1,479.

Committee on Nutrition, American Academy of Pediatrics. "Prevention of Pediatric Overweight and Obesity," *Pediatrics* 112, no. 2 (August 2003): 424–430.

Committee on Substance Abuse, American Academy of Pediatrics. "Tobacco's Toll: Implications for the Pediatrician," *Pediatrics* 107, no. 4 (April 2001): 794–798.

Committee to Identify Strategies to Raise the Profile of Substance Abuse and Alcoholism Research, Division of Neuroscience and Behavioral Health, Division of Health Promotion and Disease Prevention, Institute of Medicine. *Dispelling the Myths About Addiction: Strategies to Increase Understanding and Strengthen Research.* Washington, D.C.: National Academy Press, 1997.

Condren, Rita M., John O'Connor, and Roy Browne. "Prevalence and Patterns of Substance Misuse in Schizophrenia: A Catchment Area Case-Control Study," *Psychiatric Bulletin* 25, no. 1 (2001): 17–20.

Coombs, Robert Holman. *Drug-Impaired Professionals.* Cambridge, Mass.: Harvard University Press, 1997.

Cooper, M. Lynne. "Alcohol Use and Risky Sexual Behavior Among College Students and Youth: Evaluating the Evidence," *Journal of Studies on Alcohol* Supplement 14 (2002): 101–117.

Cornuz, Jacques, M.D. "Efficacy of Resident Training in Smoking Cessation: A Randomized, Controlled Trial of a Program Based on Application of Behavioral Theory and Practice with Standardized Patients," *Annals of Internal Medicine* 136, no. 6 (March 19, 2002): 429–437.

Crum, R. M., and J. C. Anthony. "Cocaine Use and Other Suspected Risk Factors for Obsessive-Compulsive Disorder: A Prospective Study with Data from the Epidemiologic Catchment Area Surveys," *Drug Alcohol Dependence* 31, no. 3 (1993): 281–295.

Curry, Susan J., et al. "Use and Cost Effectiveness of Smoking-Cessation Services Under Four Insurance Plans in a Health Maintenance Organization," *New England Journal of Medicine* 339, no. 10 (September 3, 1998): 673–679.

Dalla, Rochelle L. "Exposing the 'Pretty Woman' Myth: A Qualitative Examination of the Lives of Female Streetwalking Prostitutes," Available online. URL: http://articles.findarticles.com/p/articles/mi_m2372/is_4_37/ai_72272308/print. Accessed June 14, 2004.

Deas, Deborah, M.D., and Suzanne Thomas. "Comorbid Psychiatric Factors Contributing to Adolescent Alcohol and Other Drug Use," *Alcohol Research & Health* 26, no. 2 (2002): 116–121.

Dees, W. Les, Vinod K. Srivasta, and Jill K. Hiney. "Alcohol and Female Puberty: The Role of Intraovarian Systems," *Alcohol Research & Health* 25, no. 4 (2001): 271–275.

Dervaux, Alain, M.D., et al. "Is Substance Abuse in Schizophrenia Related to Impulsivity, Sensation Seeking, or Anhedonia?" *American Journal of Psychiatry* 158, no. 3 (2001): 492–494.

Diagnostic and Statistical Manual of Mental Disorders, Fourth Edition. Text Revision, DSM-IV-TR. Washington, D.C.: American Psychiatric Association, 2000.

DiClemente, Carlo C. *Addiction and Change: How Addictions Develop and Addicted People Recover.* New York: The Guilford Press, 2003.

Donovan, Dennis M., and Alan G. Marlatt. *Assessment of Addictive Behaviors.* New York: The Guilford Press, 1988.

Drake, Robert E., M.D., and Kim T. Mueser. "Co-Occurring Alcohol Use Disorder and Schizophrenia," *Alcohol Research & Health* 26, no. 2 (2002): 99–102.

Drobes, David J. "Concurrent Alcohol and Tobacco Dependence: Mechanisms and Treatment," *Alcohol Research & Health* 26, no. 2 (2002): 136–142.

Drug and Alcohol Services Information System. "Women in Treatment for Smoked Cocaine: 2000," Available online. URL: http://www.oas.samhsa.gov/2k3/FemCrack/FemCrack.htm. Accessed October 7, 2004.

Drug Enforcement Administration, Office of Diversion Control. *Steroid Abuse in Today's Society: A*

Guide for Understanding Steroids and Related Substances. Washington, D.C.: U.S. Department of Justice, March 2004.

Dube, Shanta R., et al. "Childhood Abuse, Household Dysfunction, and the Risk of Attempted Suicide Through the Life Span: Findings from the Adverse Childhood Experiences Study," *Journal of the American Medical Association* 286, no. 24 (December 26, 2001): 3,089–3,096.

Dube, Shanta R., et al. "Childhood Abuse, Neglect, and Household Dysfunction and the Risk of Illicit Drug Use: The Adverse Childhood Experiences Study," *Pediatrics* 111, no. 3 (March 2003): 564–572.

Einstat, Stephanie A., M.D. "Domestic Violence," *New England Journal of Medicine* 341, no. 12 (September 16, 1999): 886–892.

Elia, Josephine, M.D., Paul J. Ambrosini, M.D., and Judith L. Rapoport, M.D. "Treatment of Attention-Deficit-Hyperactivity Disorder," *New England Journal of Medicine* 340, no. 10 (March 11, 1999): 780–788.

Ellickson, Phyllis, Joan S. Tucker, and David J. Klein. "Ten-Year Prospective Study of Public Health Problems Associated with Early Drinking," *Pediatrics* 111, no. 5 (May 2003): 949–955.

Ellinwood, Everett H., M.D., George King, and Tong H. Lee, M.D. "Chronic Amphetamine Use and Abuse," Available online. URL: http://www.acnp.org/g4/GN401000166/CH162.htm. Accessed on June 2, 2004.

Emanuele, Mary Ann, M.D., Frederick Wezeman, and Nicholas V. Emanuele, M.D. "Alcohol and the Male Reproductive System," *Alcohol Research & Health* 25, no. 4 (2001): 282–287.

Emanuele, Mary Ann, M.D., Frederick Wezeman, and Nicholas V. Emanuele, M.D. "Alcohol's Effects on Female Reproductive Function," *Alcohol Research & Health* 26, no. 4 (2002): 274–281.

Engwall, Douglas, Robert Hunter, and Marvin Steinberg. "Gambling and Other Risk Behaviors on University Campuses," *Journal of American College of Health* 52, no. 6 (May/June 2004): 245–255.

Epstein, Joan, et al. "Serious Mental Illness and Its Co-occurrence with Substance Use Disorders, 2002," Available online. URL: http://oas.samhsa.gov/CoD/CoD.htm. Accessed on October 7, 2004.

Farrell, M., et al. "Psychosis and Drug Dependence: Results from a National Survey of Prisoners," *British Journal of Psychiatry* 181 (2002): 393–398.

Federation of Families for Children's Mental Health and Keys for Networking. *Blamed and Ashamed: The Treatment Experiences of Youth with Co-occurring Substance Abuse and Mental Health Disorders.* Alexandria, Va.: Federal of Families for Children's Mental Health, 2001.

Fiellin, David A., M.D. and Patrick G. O'Connor, M.D. "Office-Based Treatment of Opiod-Dependent Patients," *New England Journal of Medicine* 347, no. 11 (September 12, 2002): 817–823.

Fiellin, David A., M.D., M. Carrington Reid, M.D., and Patrick O'Connor, M.D. "Outpatient Management of Patients with Alcohol Problems," *Annals of Internal Medicine* 133, no. 10 (November 21, 2000): 815–827.

Fischer, Mariellen and Russell A. Barkley. "Childhood Stimulant Treatment and Risk for Later Substance Abuse," *Journal of Clinical Psychiatry* 64, Supplement 11 (2003): 19–23.

Fisher, Bonnie S., Francis T. Cullen, and Michael G. Turner. "The Sexual Victimization of College Women." Available online. URL: http://www.ncjrs.org/pdffiles/nji/182369.pdf. Accessed on October 7, 2004.

Foley, Kathleen M., M.D. "Opioids and Chronic Neuropathic Pain," *New England Journal of Medicine* 348, no. 13 (March 27, 2003): 1,279–1,281.

Fried, V. M., et al. *Chartbook on Trends in the Health of Americans. Health, United States, 2003.* Hyattsville, Md.: National Center for Health Statistics, 2003.

Fudala, Paul J., et al. "Office-Based Treatment of Opiate Addiction with a Sublingual-Tablet Formulation of Buprenorphine and Naloxone," *New England Journal of Medicine* 349, no. 10 (September 4, 2003): 949–958.

Fuller, Tamara L. and Susan J. Wells. "Predicting Maltreatment Recurrence Among CPS Cases with Alcohol and Other Drug Involvement," *Children and Youth Services Review* 25, no. 7 (2003): 553–569.

Galvan, Frank H. and Raul Caetano, M.D. "Alcohol Use and Related Problems Among Ethnic Minorities in the United States," *Alcohol Research & Health* 27, no. 1 (2003): 87–94.

Garbutt, James C., M.D., et al. "Pharmacological Treatment of Alcohol Dependence," *Journal of the American Medical Association* 281, no. 14 (April 14, 1999): 1,318–1,325.

Garfinkel, Doron, M.D., et al. "Facilitation of Benzodiazepeine Discontinuation by Melatonin: A New Clinical Approach," *Archives of Internal Medicine* 159, no. 20 (November 8, 1999): 2,456–2,460.

Garman, J. G., et al. "Occurrence of Exercise Dependence in a College-Aged Population," *Journal of American College Health* 52, no. 5 (March/April 2004): 221–228.

Gebhart, Fred. "Doctor Shopping: New Strategies Are Being Developed in Various States to Catch Offenders," Available online. URL: http://www.findarticles.com/cf_dls/m3045/22_146/96925876/print.jhtml. Accessed on December 23, 2003.

General Accounting Office. "Prescription Drugs: OxyContin Abuse and Diversion and Efforts to Address the Problem," Available online. URL: http://www.gao.gov.new.items.do4110.pdf. Accessed October 7, 2004.

Gfoerer, Joseph C., Li-Tzy Wu, and Michael Penne. "Initiation of Marijuana Use: Trends, Patterns, and Implications," Available online. URL: http://www.oas.samhsa.gov/mjinitiation/toc.htm. Accessed October 7, 2004.

Gmel, Gerhard and Jurgen Rehm. "Harmful Alcohol Use," *Alcohol Research & Health* 27, no. 1 (2003): 52–62.

Goodwin, Renee D., et al. "The Relationship Between Anxiety and Substance Use Disorders Among Individuals with Severe Affective Disorders," *Comprehensive Psychiatry* 43, no. 4 (July/August 2002): 245–252.

Grant, Bridget F., et al. "The 12-Month Prevalence and Trends in DSM-IV Alcohol Abuse and Dependence: United States, 1991–1992 and 2001–2002," *Drug and Alcohol Dependence* 74, no. 3 (2004): 223–234.

Grant, Jon E., M.D., Matt G. Kushner, and Suck Won Kim, M.D. "Pathological Gambling and Alcohol Use Disorder," *Alcohol Research & Health* 26, no. 2 (2002): 143–150.

Greenfield, David N. "The Net Effect: Internet Addiction and Compulsive Internet Use," Available online. URL: http://www.virtual-addiction.com/a_neteffect.com. Accessed on June 12, 2004.

Greenfield, David N. *Virtual Addiction: Help for Netheads, Cyberfreaks, and Those Who Love Them.* Oakland, Calif.: New Harbinger Publications, Inc., 1999.

Grilo, Carlos M., Rajita Sinha, and Stephanie O'Malley. "Eating Disorders and Alcohol Use Disorders," *Alcohol Research & Health* 26, no. 2 (2002): 151–160.

Grisso, Jeanne Ann, M.D., et al. "Violent Injuries Among Women in an Urban Area," *New England Journal of Medicine* 341, no. 25 (December 16, 1999): 1,899–1,905.

Gross, Cary P., M.D., et al. "State Expenditures for Tobacco-Control Programs and the Tobacco Settlement," *New England Journal of Medicine* 347, no. 14 (October 8, 2002): 1,080–1,086.

Hall, Gladys W., et al. "Pathological Gambling Among Cocaine-Dependent Outpatients," *American Journal of Psychiatry* 157, no. 7 (July 2000): 1,127–1,133.

Hanna, Gregory L., et al. "Genome-Wide Linkage Analysis of Families with Obsessive-Compulsive Disorder Ascertained Through Pediatric Probands," *American Journal of Medical Genetics* 114 (2002): 541–552.

Hans, S. L. "Demographic and Psychosocial Characteristics of Substance-Abusing Pregnant Women," *Clinical Perinatology* 26, no. 1 (March 1999): 55–74.

Harbison, Kent G. "New Law Avoids Unnecessary Punishment of Impaired Physicians," Available online. URL: http://www.fredlaw.com/articles/health/heal_9409_kghmm.html. Accessed on December 20, 2003.

Hasin, Deborah. "Classification of Alcohol Use Disorders," *Alcohol Research & Health* 27, no. 1 (2003): 5–17.

Hasin, Deborah S. and Bridget F. Grant. "Major Depression in 6050 Former Drinkers," *Archives of General Psychiatry* 59, no. 9 (September 2002): 794–800.

Hasin, Deborah, et al. "Effects of Major Depression on Remission and Relapse of Substance Dependence," Archives of General Psychiatry 59, no. 4 (April 2002): 375–380.

Hausenblas, Heather, and Danielle Symons Downs. "Exercise Dependence: A Systematic Review," *Psychology of Sport and Exercise* 3 (2002): 89–123.

Hausenblas, Heather, and Danielle Symons Downs. "Relationship Among Sex, Imagery, and Exercise

Dependence Symptoms," *Psychology of Addictive Behaviors* 16, no. 2 (2002): 169–172.

Hedley, Allison A., et al. "Prevalence of Overweight and Obesity and U.S. Children Adolescents, and Adults, 1999–2002," *Journal of the American Medical Association* 291, no. 23 (2004): 2,847–2,850.

Hendler, Nelson, M.D. "Pain Clinics," in *Pain Management Secrets: Questions and Answers Reveal the Secrets to Successful Pain Management, 2nd ed.* Philadelphia, Pa.: Hanley & Belfus, Inc., 2003.

Heiberg Brix, Thomas, M.D., et al. "Cigarette Smoking and Risk of Clinically Overt Thyroid Disease," *Archives of Internal Medicine* 160, no. 5 (March 13, 2000): 661–666.

Heron, Dawn, M.D. and Nathan A. Shapira, M.D. "Time to Log Off: New Diagnostic Criteria for Problematic Internet Use," Available online. URL: http://www.currentpsychiatry.com/2003_04/0403_internet.asp. Accessed on October 22, 2003.

Hingson, R., et al. "Age of First Intoxication, Heavy Drinking, Driving After Drinking and Risk of Unintentional Injury Among U.S. College Students," *Journal of Studies on Alcohol* 64, no. 1 (2003): 23–31.

Hodgkins, Candace C., et al. "Adolescent Drug Addiction Treatment and Weight Gain," *Journal of Addictive Diseases* 23, no. 3 (2004): 55–65.

Hollander, Eric, M.D., et al. "Short-Term Single-Blind Fluvoxamine Treatment of Pathological Gambling," *American Journal of Psychiatry* 155, no. 12 (December 1998): 1,781–1,783.

Honigman, R. J., K. A. Phillips, and D. J. Castle. "A Review of Psychosocial Outcomes for Patients Seeking Cosmetic Surgery," *Plastic Reconstructive Surgery* 113, no. 4 (April 1, 2004): 1,229–1,237.

Hu, Frank B., M.D., et al. "Television Watching and Other Sedentary Behaviors in Relation to Risk of Obesity and Type 2 Diabetes Mellitus in Women," *Journal of the American Medical Association* 289, no. 14 (April 9, 2003): 1,785–1,791.

Hurt, Richard D., M.D., et al. "A Comparison of Sustained Release Bupropion and Placebo for Smoking Cessation," *New England Journal of Medicine* 337, no. 17 (October 23, 1997): 1,195–1,202.

Ibanez, Angela, M.D., et al. "Psychiatric Comorbidity in Pathological Gamblers Seeking Treatment," *American Journal of Psychiatry* 158, no. 10 (October 2001): 1,733–1,735.

Jauhar, Pramod. "Current Drug Management of Alcohol Dependence Syndrome," Available online. URL: http://www.escriber.com/Assets/EscriberDownloads/Images/PinPalcholdep.PDF. Accessed on June 24, 2004.

Jenike, Michael, M.D. "Obsessive-Compulsive Disorder," *New England Journal of Medicine* 350, no. 3 (January 15, 2004): 259–265.

Johnson, Jeannette L., and Michelle Leff, M.D. "Children of Substance Abusers: Overview of Research Findings," *Pediatrics* 103 Supplement (1999): 1,085–1,099.

Johnson, Jeffrey G., et al. "Association between Cigarette Smoking and Anxiety Disorders During Adolescence and Early Adulthood," *Journal of the American Medical Association* 284, no. 18 (November 8, 2000): 2,348–2,351.

Johnson, Rolley E., et al. "A Comparison of Levomethadyl Acetate, Buprenorphine, and Methadone for Opioid Dependence," *New England Journal of Medicine* 343, no. 18 (November 2, 2000): 1,290–1,297.

Johnston, Lloyd D., Patrick O'Malley, and Jerald Bachman. *Monitoring the Future: National Results on Adolescent Drug Use. Overview of Key Findings, 2002.* NIH Publication No. 03-5374, Bethesda, Md.: National Institute on Drug Abuse, U.S. Department of Health and Human Service, National Institutes of Health, 2003.

Johnston, Lloyd D., Patrick O'Malley, and Jerald Bachman. *Monitoring the Future: National Results on Adolescent Drug Use. Overview of Key Findings, 2002.* NIH Publication No. 03-5374, Bethesda, Md.: National Institute on Drug Abuse, U.S. Department of Health and Human Service, National Institutes of Health, 2003.

Jordan, Joe, Ann Hamer, and Kathy L. Katchum. "Carisoprodol (Soma) and Sedative Quantities to be Restricted on November 15, 2002," Available online. URL: http://pharmacy.oregonstate.edu/drug_policy/news/4_8/4_8.html. Accessed on August 13, 2004.

Jorenby, Douglas E., et al. "A Controlled Trial of Sustained-Release Bupropion, a Nicotine Patch, or Both for Smoking Cessation," *New England Journal of Medicine* 340, no. 9 (March 4, 1999): 685–691.

Kandel, Joseph, M.D., and Christine Adamec. *The Encyclopedia of Senior Health and Well-Being.* New York, N.Y.: Facts On File, Inc., 2003.

Kelly, Thomas M., Jack R., Cornelius, and Duncan B. Clark. "Psychiatric Disorders and Attempted Suicide among Adolescents with Substance Abuse Disorders," *Drug and Alcohol Dependence* 73, no. 1 (2004): 87–97.

Kendler, Kenneth S., M.D. and Carol A. Prescott. "Caffeine Intake, Tolerance, and Withdrawal in Women: A Population-Based Twin Study," *American Journal of Psychiatry* 156, no. 2 (February 1999): 223–228.

Kessler, Ronald C., M.D., et al. "The Epidemiology of Major Depressive Disorder: Results from the National Comorbidity Survey Replication (NCS-R)," *Journal of the American Medical Association* 289, no. 23 (June 18, 2003): 3,095–3,105.

King, Charles, III, and Michael Siegel, M.D. "The Master Settlement Agreement with the Tobacco Industry and Cigarette Advertising in Magazines," *New England Journal of Medicine* 35, no. 7 (August 16, 2001): 504–511.

Klump, K. L., et al. "Genetic and Environmental Influences on Anorexia Nervosa Syndromes in a Population-Based Twin Sample," *Psychological Medicine* 31, no. 4 (2001): 737–740.

Komro, Kelli A. and Traci L. Toomey. "Strategies to Prevent Underage Drinking," *Alcohol Research & Health* 26, no. 1 (2002): 5–14.

Kosten, Thomas R., M.D. and Patrick G. O'Connor, M.D. "Management of Drug and Alcohol Withdrawal," *New England Journal of Medicine* 348, no. 18 (May 1, 2003): 1,786–1,795.

Kovacs, Elizabeth J. and Kelly A. N. Messingham. "Influence of Alcohol and Gender on Immune Response," *Alcohol Research & Health* 26, no. 4 (2002): 257–263.

Krantz, Mori J., M.D. and Philip S. Mehler, M.D. "Treating Opioid Dependence: Growing Implications for Primary Care," *Archives of Internal Medicine* 164, no. 3 (February 9, 2004): 277–288.

Kropenske, Vickie and Judy Howard. *Protecting Children in Substance-Abusing Families.* Washington, D.C.: U.S. Department of Health and Human Services, Administration for Children and Families, National Center on Child Abuse and Neglect, 1994.

Krystal, John H., M.D., et al. "Naltrexone in the Treatment of Alcohol Dependence," *New England Journal of Medicine* 345, no. 24 (December 13, 2001): 1,739–1,745.

Kumpfer, Karol L. "Outcome Measures of Interventions in the Study of Children of Substance-Abusing Parents," *Pediatrics* 103, Supplement (1999): 1,128–1,144.

Kyriacou, Demetrios N., M.D., et al. "Risk Factors for Injury to Women from Domestic Violence," *New England Journal of Medicine* 341, no. 25 (December 16, 1999): 1,892–1,898.

Ladd, George T. and Nancy M. Petry. "Disordered Gambling Among University-Based Medical and Dental Patients: A Focus on Internet Gambling," *Psychology of Addictive Behaviors* 16, no. 1 (2002): 76–79.

Lande, R. Gregory. "Caffeine-Related Psychiatric Disorders," Available online. URL: http://www. emedicine.com/med/topic3115.htm. Accessed April 11, 2004.

Lasser, Karen, M.D., et al. "Smoking and Mental Illness: A Population-Based Prevalence Study," *Journal of the American Medical Association* 284, no. 20 (November 22–29, 2000): 2,606–2,610.

Leitzmann, Michael F., M.D., et al. "A Prospective Study of Coffee Consumption and the Risk of Symptomatic Gallstone Disease in Men," *Journal of the American Medical Association* 281, no. 22 (June 9, 1999): 2,106–2,112.

Lerman, Caryn, et al. "Individualizing Nicotine Replacement Therapy for the Treatment of Tobacco Dependence," *Annals of Internal Medicine* 14, no. 6 (March 16, 2004): 426–433.

Lieber, Charles S., M.D. "Alcohol and Hepatitis C," *Alcohol Research & Health* 25, no. 4 (2001): 245–254.

Lieber, Charles Saul, M.D. "Medical Disorders of Alcoholism," *New England Journal of Medicine* 333, no. 16 (October 19, 1995): 1,058–1,065.

Little, Hilary J. "Behavioral Mechanisms Underlying the Link Between Smoking and Drinking," *Alcohol Research & Health* 24, no. 4 (2000): 215–224.

Littrell, Robert A., Therese Sage, and William Miller. "Meprobamate Dependence Secondary to Carisoprodol Use—Soma," Available online. URL: http://www.findarticles.com/p/articles/

mi_m0978/is-n1_v19/ai_13497394. Accessed August 13, 2004.

Longo, Lance P., M.D. and Brian Johnson, M.D. "Addiction: Part I. Benzodiazepines—Side Effects, Abuse Risks and Alternatives," Available online. URL: http://www.aafp.org/afp/20000401/2121. html. Accessed on February 11, 2004.

Lynskey, Michael T., et al. "Escalation of Drug Use in Early-Onset Cannabis Users vs. Co-Twin Controls," *Journal of the American Medical Association* 289, no. 4 (January 22–29, 2003): 427–433.

MacCoun, Robert J. and Peter Reuter. *Drug War Heresies: Learning from Other Vices, Times & Places.* Cambridge: Cambridge University Press, 2001.

Malone, Stephen M., William G. Iacono, and Matt McGue. "Drinks of the Father: Father's Maximum Number of Drinks Consumed Predicts Externalizing Disorders, Substance Abuse, and Substance Abuse Disorders in Preadolescent and Adolescent Offspring," *Alcoholism: Clinical and Experimental Research* 26, no. 12 (2002): 1,823–1,832.

Mann, J. John, M.D. "A Current Perspective of Suicide and Attempted Suicide," *Annals of Internal Medicine* 136, no. 4 (February 19, 2002): 302–311.

Martin, Christopher S. and Ken C. Winters. "Diagnosis and Assessment of Alcohol Use Disorders Among Adolescents," *Alcohol Health & Research World* 22, no. 2 (1998): 95–106.

Martin, Peter R., M.D., Charles K. Singleton, and Susanne Hiller-Sturmhofel. "The Role of Thiamine Deficiency in Alcoholic Brain Disease," *Alcohol Research & Health* 27, no. 3 (2003): 134–142.

Martin, Susan E., Kendall Bryant, and Nora Fitzgerald. "Self-Reported Alcohol Use and Abuse by Arrestees in the 1998 Arrestee Drug Abuse Monitoring Program," *Alcohol Research & Health* 25, no. 1 (2001): 72–79.

Marzuk, Peter M., M.D., et al. "Fatal Injuries After Cocaine Use as a Leading Cause of Death Among Young Adults in New York City," *New England Journal of Medicine* 332, no. 26 (June 29, 1995): 1,753–1,757.

McClanahan, Susan F., et al. "Pathways into Prostitution Among Female Jail Detainees and Their Implications for Mental Health Services," *Psychiatric Services* 50, no. 12 (December 1999): 1,606–1,613.

McGue, Matt, et al. "Origins and Consequences of Age at First Drink. I. Associations with Substance-Use Disorders, Disinhibitory Behavior and Psychopathology, and P3 Amplitude," *Alcoholism: Clinical and Experimental Research* 25, no. 8 (2001): 1,156–1,165.

McGue, Matt, et al. "Origins and Consequences of Age at First Drink. II. Familial Risk and Heritability," *Alcoholism: Clinical and Experimental Research* 25, no. 7 (July 2001): 1,166–1,173.

Mehler, Philip S., M.D. "Bulimia Nervosa," *New England Journal of Medicine* 349, no. 9 (August 28, 2003): 675–881.

Mendelson, Jack H., M.D. and Nancy K. Mello. "Management of Cocaine Abuse and Dependence," *New England Journal of Medicine* 335, no. 15 (April 11, 1996): 965–972.

Menon, K. V., M.D., Gregory J. Gores, M.D., and Vijay H. Shah, M.D. "Pathogenesis, Diagnosis, and Treatment of Alcoholic Liver Disease," *Mayo Clinic Proceedings* 76, no. 10 (2001): 1,021–1,029.

Merline, Alicia, et al. "Substance Use Among Adults 35 Years of Age: Prevalence, Adulthood Predictors, and Impact of Adolescent Substance," *American Journal of Public Health* 94, no. 1 (January 2004): 96–102.

Millstein, Susan G. and Arik V. Marcell, M.D. "Screening and Counseling for Adolescent Alcohol Use Among Primary Care Physicians in the United States," *Pediatrics* 111, no. 1 (January 2003): 114–122.

Minocha, Anil, M.D. and Adamec Christine. *The Encyclopedia of Digestive Diseases and Disorders.* New York: Facts On File Inc., 2004.

Mitchell, Peter. "Internet Addiction: Genuine Diagnosis or Not?" *Lancet* 355, no. 9204 (February 19, 2000): 632.

Mitka, Mike. "Experts Debate Widening Use of Opioid Drugs for Chronic Nonmalignant Pain," *Journal of the American Medical Association* 289, no. 18 (May 14, 2003): 2,347–2,348.

Moeller, F. Gerard, M.D. "Psychiatric Aspects of Impulsivity," *American Journal of Psychiatry* 158, no. 11 (November 2001): 1,783–1,793.

Moeller, F. Gerard, M.D. and Dougherty, Donald M. "Antisocial Personality Disorder, Alcohol, and Aggression," *Alcohol Research & Health* 25, no. 1 (2001): 5–11.

Mohler-Kuo, Meichun, et al. "Correlates of Rape While Intoxicated in a National Sample of College Women," *Journal of Studies on Alcohol* 65, no. 1 (2004): 37–45.

Mokdad, Ali H., et al. "Prevalence of Obesity, Diabetes, and Obesity-Related Health Risk Factors, 2001," *Journal of the American Medical Association* 289, no. 1 (January 1, 2003): 76–79.

Mondimore, Francis Mark, M.D. *Bipolar Disorder: A Guide for Patients and Families.* Baltimore, Md.: Johns Hopkins University Press, 1999.

Morrison, James, M.D. and Peter Wickersham. "Physicians Disciplined by a State Medical Board," *Journal of the American Medical Association* 279, no. 23 (June 17, 1998): 1,889–1,893.

Mukamal, Kenneth J., M.D. and Eric B. Rimm. "Alcohol's Effects on the Risk for Coronary Heart Disease," *Alcohol Research & Health* 25, no. 4 (2001): 255–261.

Musto, David F. *The American Disease: Origins of Narcotic Control,* 3rd ed. New York, N.Y.: Oxford University Press, 1999.

Nakken, Craig. *The Addictive Personality: Understanding the Addictive Process and Compulsive Behavior.* Center City, Minn.: Hazelden Information & Educational Services, 1996.

National Cancer Institute. "Clearing the Air: Quit Smoking Today," Available online. URL: http://www.smokefree.gov/pubs/cleaning_the_air.pdf. Accessed October 8, 2004.

National Center for Health Statistics. "Summary Health Statistics for U.S. Adults: National Health Interview Survey, 1999." Available online. URL: http://www.cdc.gov/nchs/data/series/sr_10/sr10_212.pdf. Accessed October 8, 2004.

National Center on Addiction and Substance Abuse at Columbia University. "Food for Thought: Substance Abuse and Eating Disorders." Available online. URL: http://www.casacolumbia.org/pdshopprov/files/food_for_thought.pdf. Accessed October 8, 2004.

National Center on Addiction and Substance Abuse at Columbia University. "National Survey of American Attitudes on Substance Abuse VIII: Teens and Parents," Available online. URL:http://www.casacolumbia.org/absolutenm/templates/PressReleases.asp?articleid=348&zoneid =46. Accessed October 8, 2004.

National Center on Addiction and Substance Abuse at Columbia University. "Report on Teen Cigarette Smoking and Marijuana Use," Available online. URL: http://www.casacolumbia.org/absolutenm/templates/articles.asp?articleid=334&zoneid=31. Accessed October 8, 2004.

National Center on Birth Defects and Developmental Disabilities, Centers for Disease Control and Prevention, Department of Health and Human Services. "Fetal Alcohol Syndrome: Guidelines for Referral and Diagnosis," Available online. URL: http://www.cdc.gov/ncbddd/fas/documents/FAS_guidelines_accessible.pdf. Accessed October 8, 2004.

National Drug Intelligence Center. "Drugs, Youth, and the Internet," Available online. URL: http://www.usdoj.gov/ndic/pubs2/2161/. Accessed October 8, 2004.

National Drug Intelligence Center. "Methadone Abuse Increasing," Available online. URL: http://www.usdoj.gov/ndic/pubs2/6292/. Accessed October 8, 2004.

National Drug Intelligence Center. "National Drug Threat Assessment 2003." Available online. URL: http://www.usdoj.gov/ndic/pubs3/3300. Accessed October 8, 2004.

National Emphysema Treatment Trial Research Group. "A Randomized Trial Comparing Lung-Volume-Reduction Surgery with Medical Therapy for Severe Emphysema," *New England Journal of Medicine* 348, no. 21 (May 22, 2003): 2,059–2,073.

National Institute of Mental Health. "Eating Disorders: Facts About Eating Disorders and the Search for Solutions," Available online. URL: http://www.nimh.nih.gov/publicat/eatingdisorders.cfm. Accessed March 15, 2004.

National Institute on Alcohol Abuse and Alcoholism. "Alcohol: A Women's Health Issue," Available online. URL: http://www.niaaa.nih.gov/publications/brochurewomen/women.htm. Accessed October 8, 2004.

National Institute on Alcohol Abuse and Alcoholism. "The Genetics of Alcoholism," Available online. URL: http://www.niaaa.nih.gov/publications/aa60.htm. Accessed October 8, 2004.

National Institute on Alcohol Abuse and Alcoholism. "Underage Drinking: A Major Public

Health Challenge," Available online. URL: http://www.niaaa.nih.gov/publications/aa59.htm. Accessed October 8, 2004.

National Institute on Drug Abuse. "Principles of Drug Addiction Treatment: A Research-Based Guide," Available online. URL: http://www.nida.nih.gov/PODAT/PODATindex.html. Accessed October 8, 2004.

National Institute on Drug Abuse. "Marijuana Abuse," Available online. URL: http://www.nida.nih.gov/ResearchReports/marijuana/. Accessed October 8, 2004.

National Institute on Drug Abuse. "Prescriptions Drugs: Abuse and Addiction," Available online. URL: http://www.nida.nih.gov/ResearchReports/Prescription/Prescription.html. Accessed October 8, 2004.

National Institute on Drug Abuse. "Preventing Drug Use with Children and Adolescents: A Research-Based Guide for Parents, Educators, and Community Leader," 2nd ed. Available online. URL: http://www.drugabuse.gov/pdf/prevention/RedBook.pdf. Accessed October 8, 2004.

National Survey on Drug Use and Health. "Drugged Driving: 2002 Update," Available online. URL: http://www.oas.samhsa.gov/2k3/DrugDriving/DrugDriving.cfm. Accessed on October 8, 2004.

Naylor, Adam H. "Drug Use Patterns Among High School Athletes and Nonathletes," *Adolescence* 36, no. 144 (Winter 2001): 627–639.

Nephew, Thomas M., et al. "Apparent Per Capita Alcohol Consumption: National, State, and Regional Trends, 1977–2000," Available online. URL: http://www.niaaa.nih.gov/publications/Cons97.pdf. Accessed October 8, 2004.

Ness, Roberta B., M.D., et al. "Cocaine and Tobacco Use and the Risk of Spontaneous Abortion," *New England Journal of Medicine* 340, no. 5 (February 4, 1999): 333–339.

O'Brien, Robert, et al. *The Encyclopedia of Understanding Alcohol and Other Drugs.* New York: Facts On File, Inc., 1999.

O'Connor, Patrick G., M.D. and Richard S. Schottenfeld, M.D. "Patients with Alcohol Problems," *New England Journal of Medicine* 338, no. 9 (February 26, 1998): 592–602.

O'Connor, Patrick G., M.D. and Thomas R. Kosten, M.D. "Rapid and Ultrarapid Opioid Detoxification Techniques," *Journal of the American Medical Association* 279, no. 3 (January 21, 1998): 229–234.

Office of Applied Studies, Drug and Alcohol Services Information System. "Characteristics of Homeless Admissions to Substance Abuse Treatment: 2000," Available online. URL: http://www.oas.samhsa.gov/2k3/homelessTX/homelessTX.cfm. Accessed October 8, 2004.

Office of Applied Studies, Drug and Alcohol Services Information System. "Older Adults in Substance Abuse Treatment: 2001," Available online. URL: http://www.oas.samhsa.gov/2k4/OlderAdultsTX/olderAdultsTX.cfm. Accessed October 8, 2004.

Office of National Drug Policy Information Clearinghouse. "MDMA (Ecstasy)," Available online. URL: http://www.nida.nih.gov/Infofax/ecstasy.html. Accessed October 8, 2004.

O'Malley, Patrick M. and Lloyd D. Johnston. "Epidemiology of Alcohol and Other Drug Use Among College Students," *Journal of Studies on Alcohol* Supplement 14 (2002): 23–39.

O'Malley, Stephanie S., et al. "Initial and Maintenance Naltrexone Treatment for Alcohol Dependence Using Primary Care vs. Specialty Care," *Archives of Internal Medicine* 163, no. 14 (July 28, 2003): 1,695–1,704.

Pallanti, S., et al. "Lithium and Valproate Treatment of Pathological Gambling: A Randomized Single-Blind Study," *Journal of Clinical Psychiatry* 63, no. 7 (2002): 559–564.

Petit, William, M.D. and Christine Adamec. *The Encyclopedia of Endocrine Diseases and Disorders.* New York: Facts On File, Inc., 2005.

Petrakis, Ismene L., M.D., et al. "Comorbidity of Alcoholism and Psychiatric Disorders: An Overview," *Alcohol Research & Health* 26, no. 2 (2002): 81–89.

Petry, Nancy M. and Christopher Armentano. "Prevalence, Assessment, and Treatment of Pathological Gambling: A Review," *Psychiatric Services* 50, no. 8 (August 1999): 1,021–1,027.

Phillips, David P., Nicholas Christenfeld, and Natalie M. Ryan. "An Increase in the Number of Deaths in the United States in the First Week of the Month: An Association with Substance Abuse and Other Causes of Death," *New England Journal of Medicine* 341, no. 2 (July 8, 1999): 93–98.

Phillips, Katharine A. and David J. Castle. "Body Dysmorphic Disorder in Men," *British Medical Journal* 323, no. 7320 (November 3, 2001): 1,015–1,016.

Potenza, Marc N., M.D., Thomas R. Kosten, M.D., and Bruce J. Rounsaville, M.D. "Pathological Gambling," *Journal of the American Medical Association* 286, no. 2 (July 11, 2001): 141–144.

Prescott, Carol A. "Sex Differences in the Genetic Risk for Alcoholism," *Alcohol Research & Health* 26, no. 4 (2002): 264–273.

Proimos, Jenny, et al. "Gambling and Other Risk Behaviors Among 8th- to 12th Grade Students," Available online. URL: http://www.pediatrics.aapublications.org/cji/content/fall/102/2/e23. Accessed March 15, 2004.

Register, Thomas C., J. Mark Cline, and Carol A. Shively. "Health Issues in Postmenopausal Women Who Drink," *Alcohol Research & Health* 26, no. 4 (2002): 299–307.

Rehm, Jurgen, et al. "Alcohol-Related Morbidity and Mortality," *Alcohol Research & Health* 27, no. 1 (2003): 39–51.

Rehn, Nina, Robin Room, and Griffith Edwards. *Alcohol in the European Region—Consumption, Harm and Policies.* Copenhagen, Denmark: World Health Organization Regional Office for Europe, 2001.

Rigotti, Nancy A., M.D., Jae Eun Lee, and Henry Wechsler. "U.S. College Students' Use of Tobacco Products: Results of a National Survey," *Journal of the American Medical Association* 284, no. 6 (August 9, 2000): 699–705.

Roberts, Linda J., and Barbara S. McCrady. "Alcohol Problems in Intimate Relationships: Identification and Intervention: A Guide for Family Therapists," Available online. URL: http://www.niaaa.nih.gov/publications/niaaa_guide/. Accessed on October 8, 2004.

Roman, Paul M. and Terry C. Blum. "The Workplace and Alcohol Problem Prevention," *Alcohol Research & Health* 26, no. 1 (2002): 49–57.

Ross, G. Webster, M.D. "Association of Coffee and Caffeine Intake with the Risk of Parkinson Disease," *Journal of the American Medical Association* 283, no. 20 (May 24–31, 2000): 2,674–2,679.

Rowbotham, Michael C., M.D., et al. "Oral Opioid Therapy for Chronic Peripheral and Central Neuropathic Pain," *New England Journal of Medicine* 348, no. 13 (March 27, 2003): 1,223–1,232.

Roy, Alec M., M.D. "Characteristics of Cocaine-Dependent Patients Who Attempt Suicide," *American Journal of Psychiatry* 158, no. 8 (August 2001): 1,215–1,219.

Sampson, H. Wayne. "Alcohol and Other Factors Affecting Osteoporosis Risk in Women," *Alcohol Research & Health* 26, no. 4 (2002): 292–298.

Sanchez, Devonne R. and Blake Harrison. "The Methamphetamine Menace," *Legisbrief,* 12, no. 1 (January 2004): 1–2.

Sattar, S. Pirzada, M.D. "Benzodiazepines for Substance Abusers: Yes or No?" Available online. URL: http://www.currentpsychiatry.com/2003-05/0505-benzodiazepines.asp. Accessed on February 11, 2004.

Schnoll, Sidney H., M.D. and Michael F. Weaver, M.D. "Pharmacology: Gender-Specific Considerations in the Use of Psychoactive Medications," Available online. URL: http://www.nida.nih.gov/WHGD/DARHW-Download2.html. Accessed on October 8, 2004.

Schoenborn, Charlotte A., Jackline L. Vickerie, and Patricia Barnes. "Cigarette Smoking Behavior of Adults: United States, 1997–98," Available online. URL: http:www.ihs.gov/medicalprograms/mch/w/whsubst.asp. Accessed on October 8, 2004.

Schoenborn, Charlotte A., and Patricia F. Adams. "Alcohol Use Among Adults: United States, 1997–98," Available online. URL: http://www.ihs.gov/medicalprograms/mch/w/whsubst.asp. Accessed on October 8, 2004.

Schydlower, Manuel, M.D. *Substance Abuse: A Guide for Health Professionals,* 2nd ed. Elk Grove Village, Ill.: American Academy of Pediatrics, 2001.

Sees, Karen L., et al. "Methadone Maintenance vs. 180-Day Psychosocially Enriched Detoxification for Treatment of Opioid Dependence: A Randomized Controlled Trial," *Journal of the American Medical Association* 283, no. 10 (March 8, 2000): 1,303–1,310.

Sevarino, Kevin A. *Treatment of Substance Use Disorders.* New York: Brunner-Routledge, 2002.

Shader, Richard I. and David J. Greenblatt. "Use of Benzodiazepines in Anxiety Disorders," *New*

England Journal of Medicine 328, no. 19 (May 13, 1993): 1,398–1,405.

Shivani, Ramesh, M.D., R. Jeffrey Goldsmith, M.D., and Robert M. Anthenelli, M.D. "Alcoholism and Psychiatric Disorders: Diagnostic Challenges," *Alcohol Research & Health* 26, no. 2 (2002): 90–98.

Shrier, Lydia A., M.D., et al. "Substance Use Problems and Associated Psychiatric Symptoms Among Adolescents in Primary Care," *Pediatrics* 111, no. 6 (June 2003): 28–30.

Singer, Lynn, T., et al. "Cognitive and Motor Outcomes of Cocaine-Exposed Infants," *Journal of the American Medical Association* 287, no. 15 (April 17, 2002): 1,952–1,960.

Sjoberg, Rickard L. and Frank Lindblad, M.D. "Limited Disclosure of Sexual Abuse in Children Whose Experiences Were Documented by Videotape," *American Journal of Psychiatry* 159, no. 2 (2002): 312–314.

Smith, Bradley H., Brooke Molina, and William E. Pelham, Jr. "The Clinically Meaningful Link Between Alcohol Use and Attention Deficit Hyperactivity Disorder," *Alcohol Research & Health* 26, no. 2 (2002): 122–129.

Smoller, Jordan W., M.D. "Prevalence and Correlates of Panic Attacks in Postmenopausal Women," *Archives of Internal Medicine* 163, no. 17 (September 22, 2003): 2,041–2,050.

Sokhkhah, Ramon, M.D. and Timothy E. Wilens, M.D. "Pharmacotherapy of Adolescent Alcohol and Other Drug Use Disorders," *Alcohol Health & Research World* 22, no. 2 (1998): 122–126.

Sokol, Robert J., M.D., Virginia Delaney-Black, M.D., and Beth Nordstrom. "Fetal Alcohol Spectrum Disorder," *Journal of the American Medical Association* 290, no. 22 (December 10, 2003): 2,996–2,999.

Sonne, Susan C., and Kathleen T. Brady, M.D. "Bipolar Disorder and Alcoholism," Available online.URL:http://www.niaaa.nih.gov/publications/arh26-2/103-108.htm. Accessed on May 19, 2004.

Sorensen, James L., et al. *Drug Abuse Treatment Through Collaboration: Practice and Research Partnerships That Work.* Washington, D.C.: American Psychological Association, 2003.

Spillane, Joseph F. *Cocaine: From Medical Marvel to Modern Menace in the United States, 1884–1920.*

Baltimore, Md.: Johns Hopkins University Press, 2000.

Stein, Dan J., M.D., et al. "Hypersexual Disorder and Preoccupation with Internet Pornography," *American Journal of Psychiatry* 158, no. 10 (2001): 1,590–1,594.

Streissguth, Ann P., et al. "Risk Factors for Adverse Life Outcomes in Fetal Alcohol Syndrome and Fetal Alcohol Effects," *Journal of Developmental and Behavioral Pediatrics* 25, no. 4 (2004): 228–238.

Substance Abuse and Mental Health Services Administration. "Alcohol Use by Persons Under the Legal Drinking Age of 21," Available online. URL: http://www.oas.samhsa.gov/2k3/UnderageDrinking/UnderageDrinking.cfm. Accessed October 8, 2004.

Substance Abuse and Mental Health Services Administration, "Reasons for Not Receiving Substance Abuse Treatment," Available online. URL: http://www.oas.samhsa.gov/2k3/SAnoTX/SAnoTX.cfm. Accessed October 11, 2004.

Substance Abuse and Mental Health Services Administration. "Results from the 2003 National Survey on Drug Use and Health: National Findings," Available online. URL: http://www.oas.samhsa.gov/nhsda/2k3nsduh/2k3results.htm. Accessed October 11, 2004.

Substance Abuse and Mental Health Services Administration. "Substance Use and Mental Health Characteristics by Employment Status," Available online. URL: http://www.oas.samhsa.gov/NHSDA/A10.pdf. Accessed October 11, 2004.

Substance Abuse and Mental Health Services Administration, "Veterans in Substance Abuse Treatment: 1995–2000," Available online. URL: http://www.oas.samhsa.gov/2k3/VetsTX/VetsTX.cfm. Accessed October 11, 2004.

Substance Abuse and Mental Health Services Administration, Office of Applied Studies. "Emergency Department Trends from the Drug Abuse Warning Network, Final Estimates 1995–2002," Available online. URL: http://www.dawninfo.samhsa.gov/pubs_94_02/edpubs/2002final/. Accessed October 8, 2004.

Substance Abuse and Mental Health Services Administration, Office of Applied Studies. "Treatment Episode Data Set (TEDS) Highlights—2002: National Admissions to Substance Abuse Treatment Services," Available online. URL: http://www.dasis.samhsa.gov/teds02/2002_teds_highlights.pdf. Accessed October 11, 2004.

Sullivan, Michael and John Wodarski. "Rating College Students' Substance Abuse: A Systematic Literature Review," *Brief Treatment and Crisis Intervention* 4, no. 1 (Spring 2004): 71–91.

Swift, Robert M., M.D. "Drug Therapy for Alcohol Dependence," *New England Journal of Medicine* 340, no. 9 (May 13, 1999): 1,482–1,490.

Swofford, Cheryl D. "Double Jeopardy: Schizophrenia and Substance Use," *American Journal of Drug and Alcohol Abuse*, Available online. URL: http://www.findarticles.com/p/articles/mi_m0978/is_3_26/ai_65803039/print. Accessed on September 1, 2004.

Terry, Ken. "Impaired Physicians Speak No Evil? (Reporting an Impaired Colleague)," Available online. URL: http://www.findarticles.com/cf_dls/m3229/19_79/93212856/print.jhtml. Accessed on December 20, 2003.

Thombs, Dennis L. *Introduction to Addictive Behaviors*, 2nd ed. New York: The Guilford Press, 1999.

Thun, Michael J., M.D., et al. "Alcohol Consumption and Mortality Among Middle-Aged and Elderly U.S. Adults," *New England Journal of Medicine* 337, no. 24 (December 11, 1997): 1,705–1,714.

"Treatment Helps Addicted Physicians," *Journal of the American Medical Association* 286, no. 24 (December 26, 2001): 3,071.

Trimpey, Jack. *Rational Recovery: The New Cure for Substance Addiction*. New York: Pocket Books, 1996.

Tucker, Jalie, Dennis M. Donova, and G. Alan Marlatt. *Changing Addictive Behavior: Bridging Clinical and Public Health Strategies*. New York: The Guilford Press, 1999.

Tyas, Suzanne L. "Alcohol Use and the Risk of Developing Alzheimer's Disease," *Alcohol Research & Health* 25, no. 4 (2001): 299–306.

United Nations Office on Drugs and Crime. "Mexico 2003: Country Profile," Available online. URL: http://www.unodc.org/mexico/en/country-profile.html. Accessed October 11, 2004.

U.S. Department of Health and Human Services. "The Health Consequences of Smoking: A Report of the Surgeon General," Available online. URL: http://www.surgeongeneral.gov/library/smokingconsequences/. Accessed October 11, 2004.

U.S. Food and Drug Administration. "Statement of William K. Hubbard, Associate Commission for Policy and Planning Before the Committee on Government Reform, U.S. House of Representatives Hearing on Internet Drug Sales, March 18, 2004," Available online. URL: http://www.fda.gov/ola/2004/internetdrugs0318.html. Accessed September 8, 2004.

U.S. General Accounting Office Testimony Before the Permanent Subcommittee on Investigations. "Internet Pharmacies: Hydrocodone, an Addictive Narcotic Pain Medication Is Available Without a Prescription Through the Internet: Statement of Robert J. Cramer, Managing Director, Office of Special Investigations, June 17, 2004," Available online. URL: http://www.gao.gov/cgi-bin/getrpt?GAO-04-892t. Accessed October 11, 2004.

Vastag, Brian. "Addiction Poorly Understood by Clinicians," *Journal of the American Medical Association* 290, no. 10 (September 10, 2003): 1,299–1,303.

Veale, David. "Outcome of Cosmetic Surgery and 'DIY' Surgery in Patients with Body Dysmorphic Disorder," *Psychiatric Bulletin* 24, (2000): 218–221.

Verghese, Abraham, M.D. "Physicians and Addiction," *New England Journal of Medicine* 346, no. 20 (May 16, 2002): 1,510–1,511.

Vermeiren, Robert, M.D., et al. "Violence Exposure and Substance Use in Adolescents: Findings from Three Countries," *Pediatrics* 111, no. 3 (March 2003): 535–540.

Warner, Elizabeth A. "Cocaine Abuser," *Annals of Internal Medicine* 119, no. 3 (August 1993): 226–235.

Warren, Kenneth R. and Laurie L. Foudin. "Alcohol-Related Birth Defects—The Past, Present, and Future," *Alcohol Research & Health* 25, no. 3 (2001): 153–158.

Weathermon, Ron and Crabb, David W., M.D. "Alcohol and Medication Interactions," *Alcohol Research & Health* 23, no. 1 (1999): 40–54.

Wechsler, Henry and Toben F. Nelson. "Binge Drinking and the American College Student: What's Five Drinks?" *Psychology of Addictive Behaviors* 15, no. 4 (2001): 287–291.

Wechsler, Henry. "Binge Drinking on America's College Campuses: Findings from the Harvard School of Public Health College Alcohol Study." Available online. URL: http://www.hsph.harvard.edu/cas/Documents/monograph_2000/cas_mono_2000.pdf. Accessed on June 26, 2004.

Weir, Hannah K., et al. "Annual Report to the Nation on the Status of Cancer, 1975–2000, Featuring the Uses of Surveillance Data for Cancer Prevention and Control," *Journal of the National Cancer Institute* 95, no. 17 (September 3, 2003): 1,276–1,299.

Weitzman, Elissa R. "Poor Mental Health, Depression, and Associations with Alcohol Consumption, Harm, and Abuse in a National Sample of Young Adults in College," *Journal of Nervous & Mental Disease* 192, no. 4 (April 2004): 269–277.

Wellford, Charles. "When It's No Longer A Game: Pathological Gambling in the United States," *National Institute of Justice Journal,* issue no. 247 (April 2001): 15–18.

White, Aaron M. "What Happened? Alcohol, Memory Blackouts, and the Brain," *Alcohol Research & Health* 27, no. 2 (2003): 186–196.

White, Aaron M., David W. Jamieson-Drake, and H. Scott Swartwelder. "Prevalence and Correlates of Alcohol-Induced Blackouts Among College Students: Results of an E-Mail Survey," *Journal of American College Health* 51, no. 3 (2002): 117–131.

Whooley, Mary A., M.D. and Gregory E. Simon, M.D. "Managing Depression in Medical Outpatients," *New England Journal of Medicine* 343, no. 26 (December 28, 2000): 1,942–1,950.

Wilens, Timothy E., M.D. "Impact of ADHD and Its Treatment on Substance Abuse in Adults," *Journal of Clinical Psychiatry* 65, Supplement 3 (2004): 38–45.

Windle, Michael. "Alcohol Use Among Adolescents and Young Adults," *Alcohol Research & Health,* 27, no. 1 (2003): 7,985.

World Health Organization. Available online. URL: http://whqlibdoc.who.int/hq/2001/WHO_MSD_MSB_01.5.pdf. Accessed October 7, 2004.

Wright, D. "State Estimates of Substance Use from the 2002 National Survey on Drug Use and Health," Available online. URL: http://www.oas.samhsa.gov/nhsda.htm. Accessed on October 11, 2004.

Yehuda, Rachel. "Post-Traumatic Stress Disorder," *New England Journal of Medicine* 346, no. 2 (January 10, 2002): 108–114.

Yoon, Young-Hee, et al. "Accidental Alcohol Poisoning Mortality in the United States, 1996–1998," *Alcohol Research & Health* 27, no. 1 (2003): 110–118.

Young, Kimberly S. "Internet Addiction: The Emergence of a New Clinical Disorder," Available online. URL: http://www.netaddiction.com/articles/newdisorder.htm. Accessed on June 13, 2004.

Yu, Jiang and Robin W. Shacket. "Alcohol Use in High School: Predicting Students' Alcohol Use and Alcohol Problems in Four-Year Colleges," *American Journal of Drug and Alcohol Abuse* 27, no. 4 (November 2001): 775–793.

Zacny, James, et al. "College on Problems of Drug Dependence Taskforce on Prescription Opioid Non-Medical Use and Abuse: Position Statement," *Drug and Alcohol Dependence* 69, no. 3 (2003): 215–232.

Zhu, Shu-Hong, et al. "Evidence of Real-World Effectiveness of a Telephone Quitline for Smokers," *New England Journal of Medicine* 347, no. 14 (October 3, 2002): 1,087–1,093.

INDEX